Mosby's Textbook of Dental Nursing

Mary Miller MA(Ed)

Principal, Education and Training (Accredited) Assessment Centre for Dental Nurses,
Eastman Dental Institute and Hospital, London, UK

Crispian Scully CBE

MD PhD MDS MRCS BSc FDSRCS FDSRCPS FFDRCSI FDSRCSE FRCPath
FMedSci FHEA FUCL DSc DChD DMed(HC) Dr HC

Consultant and Professor, United Bristol Hospitals NHS Foundation Trust and
University of Bristol, Bristol, UK

Emeritus Professor, University College London, London, UK

Visiting Professor at Universities of Athens, Edinburgh, Granada and Helsinki

Foreword by
Dame Margaret Seward DBE CBE

Former Chief Dental Officer (England)

Former President of the General Dental Council

ELSEVIER
MOSBY

ELSEVIER
MOSBY

ISBN 9780723435068

British Library Cataloguing in Publication Data
A catalogue record for this book is available from the British Library

Library of Congress Cataloging in Publication Data
A catalog record for this book is available from the Library of Congress

Notices
Knowledge and best practice in this field are constantly changing. As new research and experience broaden our understanding, changes in research methods, professional practices, or medical treatment may become necessary.

Practitioners and researchers must always rely on their own experience and knowledge in evaluating and using any information, methods, compounds, or experiments described herein. In using such information or methods they should be mindful of their own safety and the safety of others, including parties for whom they have a professional responsibility.

With respect to any drug or pharmaceutical products identified, readers are advised to check the most current information provided (i) on procedures featured or (ii) by the manufacturer of each product to be administered, to verify the recommended dose or formula, the method and duration of administration, and contraindications. It is the responsibility of practitioners, relying on their own experience and knowledge of their patients, to make diagnoses, to determine dosages and the best treatment for each individual patient, and to take all appropriate safety precautions.

To the fullest extent of the law, neither the Publisher nor the authors, contributors, or editors, assume any liability for any injury and/or damage to persons or property as a matter of products liability, negligence or otherwise, or from any use or operation of any methods, products, instructions, or ideas contained in the material herein.

ELSEVIER your source for books, journals and multimedia in the health sciences

www.elsevierhealth.com

Working together to grow libraries in developing countries

www.elsevier.com | www.bookaid.org | www.sabre.org

ELSEVIER   BOOK AID International   Sabre Foundation

The Publisher's policy is to use **paper manufactured from sustainable forests**

Printed in China

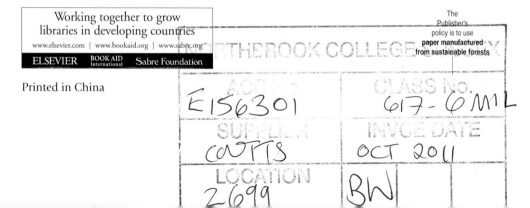

CONTENTS

v

You may be reading this foreword undecided as to whether the contents of this book are of relevance to you. On the other hand, you may already be the proud owner of this book and wondering if it has been a wise purchase. Knowing both authors well, Professor Crispian Scully and Mary Miller, I can assure you that you will not be disappointed because *Mosby's Textbook of Dental Nursing* is an outstandingly readable yet comprehensive text containing all the information you will need to pass your NEBDN examination with flying colours. As an added bonus, the book explores areas such as dental emergencies and general health promotion not covered in the examining board's published syllabus, and the authors have included some very useful features such as Terms to Learn, Key Points and an extensive index.

Delivery of oral healthcare in this twenty-first century is centred on teamwork and each member of the team has responsibility to be well informed and, after qualification, embark on a journey of life-long learning for the benefit of patients and for personal satisfaction. It has taken many decades to achieve this vision, cherished by so many of us, that Dental Care Professionals should be treated as equals and be registered with the General Dental Council. But with the fulfilment of this dream comes the commitment to attain the necessary qualifications and *Mosby's Textbook of Dental Nursing* makes this task achievable and enjoyable.

Finally, it gives me personal pleasure to commend this book written by two authors who possess a wealth of knowledge and experience acquired during a lifetime of teaching in dental hospitals and postgraduate training institutes, and to wish you continuing satisfaction and enjoyment in your chosen career of dental nursing.

Dame Margaret Seward DBE CBE
Former Chief Dental Officer (England)
Former President of the General Dental Council

The final stimulus to produce this book arose from the introduction by the General Dental Council of the UK (GDC) of the requirement for the following dental care professionals (DCPs) to register:

- Dental nurses
- Dental hygienists
- Dental therapists
- Clinical dental technicians
- Orthodontic therapists.

According to the GDC, the purpose or aim of their education is to produce a caring, knowledgeable, competent and skilful DCP who is able, on qualification, to accept professional responsibility for their role in the effective and safe care of patients. In realising this aim, the GDC applies the following principles:

- That those qualifying as DCPs should be required to attain the highest standards in terms of knowledge and understanding, skills (including clinical and laboratory skills), and professional attributes, in particular recognition of their obligation to practise in the best interests of patients at all times.
- That DCP students should be provided with the high-quality learning opportunities and experiences necessary to enable them to achieve those standards, including the opportunity, where appropriate, to undertake clinical and laboratory procedures, and acquire competence across a range of skills.
- That learning opportunities and experiences should be underpinned by adequate and appropriate support, including educational, clinical and laboratory support.
- That learning opportunities and experiences in biomedical sciences, clinical and laboratory subjects should be integrated over the course of the programme.
- That learning opportunities and experiences should be designed to encourage a questioning, scientific and self-critical approach to the practice of dentistry, and to foster the intellectual skills required for future personal and professional development.
- That learning opportunities and experiences should enable students to develop an understanding of audit and clinical governance.
- That learning opportunities and experiences should enable students of the professions complementary to dentistry to work and train as part of the dental team.
- That learning opportunities and experiences should prepare students adequately for the transition to their work role in relation to the practice of dentistry.
- That student progress is effectively monitored to ensure that only those who comply with relevant health and conduct requirements are allowed to complete the programme.

The aims of this book have been to comply with the above. In our task we have been impressed with the scope of the educational needs, have sought advice from a number of sources and have tried to keep abreast of the rapidly changing legislation and guidance facing all dental professionals. Therefore, we are most grateful to our Editorial Advisors who have ably assisted in many ways; however, any errors that might remain are ours.

ix

Mary Miller
Crispian Scully
London 2011

The illustrations and text listed below have been reproduced or adapted with permission from the following publications.

Collins W J, Walsh T, Figures K, 1998, A Handbook for Dental Hygienists, 4th edition, Butterworth-Heinemann (Figures 4.1.1, 4.2.13, AB and 5.1A)

Department of Health (http://www.dh.gov.uk/en/Publicationsandstatistics/Publications/ PublicationsPolicyAndGuidance/DH_109363), Crown Copyright (Figure 1.2.2; Tables 1.2.2 and 1.2.4)

Department of Health (http://www.dh.gov.uk/en/Publicationsandstatistics/Publications/ PublicationsPolicyAndGuidance/DH_109364), Crown Copyright (Figure 1.2.3)

Department of Health (http://www.dh.gov.uk/prod_consum_dh/groups/dh_digitalassets/ @dh/@en/documents/digitalasset/dh_4019034.pdf), Crown Copyright (Figure 3.2.1)

Department of Health, 1997, The Caldicott Committee Report on the review of patient-identifiable information (Box 3.2.5)

Drake R, Vogl A W, Mitchell A, 2009, Gray's Anatomy for Students, 2nd edition, Saunders (Figures 4.1.10, 4.1.11, 4.1.5, 4.1.6, 4.1.7, 4.2.1, 4.2.2, 4.2.5, 4.2.6B, 4.2.8, 4.2.9, 4.2.10, 4.2.11, 4.1.4 and 4.2.15B)

General Dental Council, Speciality definitions (http://www.gdc-uk.org/Search+our+registers/ home/Home.htm). GDC information is correct at time of going to press. Please visit the GDC website to check for any changes since publication (Text in Chapter 3, Box 15.2).

Jevon P, 2006, Emergency Care and First Aid for Nurses, Churchill Livingstone (Figures 2.1AB, 2.1D, 2.1EF and 2.2ABC)

Millet D, Welbury R, 2005, Clinical Problem Solving in Orthodontics and Paediatric Dentistry, Churchill Livingstone (Figures 5.3 and 5.4)

Resuscitation Council, 2006, Medical Emergencies and Resuscitation (Table 2.3)

Rhind J, Greig J, 2002, Riddle's Anatomy and Physiology Applied to the Health Professions, 7th edition, Churchill Livingstone (Figure 4.2.12)

Scottish Government, www.scotland.gov.uk/Publications/2008/08/interimdresscode (Box 6.1.1)

Scully C, 2010, Medical Problems in Dentistry, 6th edition, Elsevier (Tables 2.2, 17.2.2, 17.2.3 and 17.2.4; Box 1.1.3)

Scully C, Flint S, Porter S R, Moos K, 2004, Oral and Maxillofacial Diseases, 3rd edition, Taylor and Francis (Figures 17.1.2 and 17.1.5)

Scully C, Flint SF, Bagan JV, Porter SR, Moos K, 2010, Oral and Maxillofacial Diseases, 4th edition, Informa (Figures 5.1A, 5.2, 5.5, 5.8, 5.10, 5.12 and 11.8)

Scully C, Wilson N, 2007, Culturally Sensitive Oral Health Care, Quintessence (Table 6.2.2; Box 15.1)

Shahid M, Nunhuck A, 2008, Crash Course Physiology, Mosby Ltd (Figures 4.1.8, 4.1.9, 4.1.13 and 4.1.14)

Standring S (ed), 2008, Gray's Anatomy, 40th edition, Churchill Livingstone (Figures 4.2.4, 4.2.6A, 4.2.7, 4.2.14, 4.2.15A and 5.1B)

Trevisi H, 2007, SmartClip™ Self-Ligating Appliance System, Mosby Ltd (Figure 11.2)

ACKNOWLEDGEMENTS

Whaites E, 2006, Essentials of Dental Radiography and Radiology, 4th edition, Churchill Livingstone (Figures 5.7AB, 11.1AB, 14.2ABC, 14.3AB, 14.4, 14.5AB)

Figure 7.4 has been reproduced courtesy of Brian Wetherly of Henry Schein.

Brand names and products have been reproduced with permission from:

Agfa (Figure 14.1)

Colgate Palmolive (Figures 8.1 and 8.5)

GlaxoSmithKline (Figure 8.6). **CORSODYL** is a registered trade mark of the GlaxoSmithKline group of companies. Copyright of the Corsodyl Mint Mouthwash image is owned by the GlaxoSmithKline group of companies.

TePe Munhygienprodukter AB (Figures 8.3 and 8.4)

This textbook has been written specifically for pre-registration Dental Nurses and incorporates all aspects of the National Examining Board for Dental Nurses (NEBDN) pre-registration syllabus. The corresponding section of the syllabus is indicated at the start of each chapter. Some additional related information has also been included, which we believe will help the student dental nurse care better for their patients.

The text is accompanied by several features to engage the reader and help them consider the practical aspects of the theoretical learning:

- *Terms to learn*: boxes in the margins providing definitions of terms used in the text that may be unfamiliar to the reader. These terms are given in bold at the first mention in the book.
- *Key points*: key messages that the reader should always remember.
- *Identify and learn*: tasks which aim to encourage the reader to transfer their learning into their workplace by inviting them to look for various items and understand how they work or what they are used for.
- *Find out more*: sections which give hints on where to look for further information or perhaps find out more about certain topics for greater understanding.

Dental nurses have been an integral part of dentistry since the early twentieth century. They are invaluable and skilled members of the dental or oral healthcare team.

A career in dental nursing is rewarding and involves participation in the care of a variety of patients in different settings ranging from, for example, a dental practice to a dental hospital, a dental department in a general hospital, the community dental service, the armed forces, corporate organisations or the prison service.

When training to become a dental nurse, you will be required to attend a training centre that has been accredited by the National Examination Board for Dental Nurses (NEBDN). After qualifying as a dental nurse, you must register with the General Dental Council (GDC) (see p. 68 for more details) and you must re-register annually.

KEY POINT It is illegal to work as a qualified dental nurse without registration.

As professionals, dental nurses are accountable to their patients, the GDC and to themselves, therefore, you will need to demonstrate that you are participating in continued professional development (CPD). This can be done by attending a variety of **verifiable** and non-verifiable courses, including post-registration courses. There will also be opportunities for further post-registration training to extend your duties in specialist areas of dental practice, for example dental radiography and dental sedation nursing.

KEY POINT The terms in bold italics will be explained in the chapters that follow.

Regardless of where you work as a dental nurse, you will perform a variety of roles or duties, which can be divided into two main categories: clinical and clerical.

CLINICAL DUTIES

The clinical role of the dental nurse includes:

- **Decontamination** of instruments and *infection control* before, during and after a dental procedure
- Helping ensure health and safety in the workplace
- Setting out instruments and items needed for each dental procedure (see below)
- Caring for the patient before, during and after all dental procedures
- Handling and care of *local anaesthetics*
- Assisting the clinician at the chairside in all procedures by anticipating, passing and receiving instruments and items
- Manipulating and handling dental materials
- Recording dental, periodontal and other *charting*
- Processing and *mounting* of radiographs
- Providing oral hygiene instruction in accordance with the dental practice or other workplace guidelines (if trained and qualified to do so).

Term to Learn
Verifiable course:
A course should have specific aims that clearly state what you will have learnt and achieved by the end of the course. You must keep documentary evidence of attendance of such a course. For more details, see the Freelance Dental Nurse website (http://www .freelancedentalnurse .co.uk/index.php/ 2010/03/verifiable-cpd/)

xvii

Term to Learn
Decontamination:
partly or fully removing or destroying harmful (pathogenic) micro-organisms that may be living in an area or on another object, so that they cannot produce an infection or other harmful response in people coming into contact with those areas or objects. Decontamination can be of different levels: simple cleaning; cleaning followed by *disinfection*; and cleaning followed by *sterilisation*.

PREPARING A DENTAL SURGERY

At the Beginning of the Session

- Switch on the main electricity switch, and then all the other switches (including the dental chair) and the water supply in the dental surgery.
- Switch on the *air compressor* if required.
- Ensure the dental chair is working correctly.
- Fill the *steam steriliser* with distilled water, test and record.
- Fill the *ultrasonic bath* and turn on the *washer-disinfector*.
- Flush into the sink, the *3-in-1 dental syringe* and water lines for the dental **handpieces** for two minutes to cleanse the tubing.
- Clean the work surfaces, dental unit and bracket table with a detergent wipe, then wipe with an alcohol-base wipe (do not use an alcohol-base wipe to clean the dental chair).
- Clean the spittoon and flush the water.
- Place a clean disposable cup with a mouthwash tablet on the spittoon.
- Connect the **aspirator tip** and **saliva ejector** to the tubing on the spittoon.
- Place 'cling film' or equivalent on the handles of the dental light, unit and headrest of the dental chair, 3-in-1 syringe, handpiece lines and computer keyboard, if there is one.
- Collect the patient case records for the session, ensuring that all appropriate radiographs and any laboratory work or other necessary items are present.
- Lay out the dental instruments and items in a logical order for the first patient and mount any relevant radiograph on the radiograph viewer.
- Lay out any laboratory work and necessary instruments.
- Place the dental handpieces (in sterile bags) and dental *burs* on the bracket table.
- Ensure the dental surgery is free from unnecessary clutter.

End of the Session

- Reverse the procedure and flush aspirator tubing.

Terms to Learn

Saliva ejector: an instrument that removes saliva, blood or other debris during dental procedures from the patient's mouth to keep the working environment clean and dry and the patient comfortable.

Handpiece: a small drill that is used to power dental burs, for example to cut away the decayed parts of a tooth.

Aspirator: a removable high- or low-speed suction device that removes water, saliva and debris from the patient's mouth. The tip if plastic is disposed off after use.

CLERICAL DUTIES

The clerical role of the dental nurse may include:

- Ordering stock
- Liaising with the dental laboratory
- Managing patient records
- Managing financial records
- Arranging referrals
- Managing appointments and recall systems.

THE THREE 'Cs'

Always remember the three 'Cs' that form a key part of the dental nurse's day-to-day role:

1. *Communication* – communication skills are essential to dental nursing. The role involves working with a range of people, and thus interacting with families, colleagues, patients and others. Therefore, you need to be 'a people person'. Here are some situations where the communication skills of a dental nurse play a key part:
   - Putting nervous patients at ease, as well as any relatives and friends.
   - Giving explanations to patients who ask the dental nurse to explain again what they have been told by the clinician.
   - Reassuring and giving explanations to a dissatisfied patient.
2. *Chaperone* – the dental nurse acts as chaperone at all times for the clinician, as he or she may be required to give an account of a conversation or incident.
3. *Confidentiality* – patients are required to give personal, social and medical details before undergoing a dental procedure. These details must remain within the confines of the dental surgery and out of earshot of the waiting area or other people.

The duties of the dental nurse and the three Cs are covered in greater detail in the rest of the book.

CHAPTER 1

Health and Safety, Occupational Hazards and Infection Control in the Dental Workplace

CHAPTER POINTS

- This chapter covers the requirements of the NEBDN syllabus Section 1: Health and safety and infection control in the workplace.
- The chapter is divided into two subchapters:
  1.1: Health and Safety and Occupational Hazards
  1.2: Infection Control

1.1 HEALTH AND SAFETY AND OCCUPATIONAL HAZARDS

HEALTH AND SAFETY: GENERAL CONSIDERATIONS

- A *hazard* is anything that can cause harm. All workplaces, including the dental surgery and especially the laboratory, contain some hazards.
- A *risk* is the chance of someone actually being harmed by the hazard.

It is essential that dental nurses are aware of the hazards in the dental workplace and the health and safety actions that you can take to avoid harm. Human error is responsible for most risks in a workplace.

In the UK:

- The Health and Safety Executive (HSE) is the government body currently responsible for regulating health and safety in the workplace. All dental surgeries are required to be registered with the HSE.
- The **General Dental Council** (GDC) also lays down particular regulations for dental staff, which include health and safety with regard to dental workplaces.

> **KEY POINT** All dental practices must have in place policies and procedures that guide staff how to respond appropriately when a hazard is anticipated and to reduce risks. Local policies and procedures are based on national health and safety regulations.

> **Term to Learn**
> **General Dental Council:** the body that regulates all dental professionals training and working in the UK.

> **KEY POINT** If an employer or employee does not comply with health and safety regulations, they could be prosecuted.

Health and Safety Legislation

Several government Acts and Regulations deal with health and safety in the workplace; these laws and regulations are enforced by the HSE. Of particular importance to the UK dental environment are:

- Control of Substances Hazardous to Health Regulations (COSHH; 1994)
- Environmental Protection Act (1990)
- Fire Precaution (Workplace) Regulations (amended 1999)
- Health and Safety at Work etc. Act (HSW; 1974)
- Health & Safety (First Aid) Regulations (1981)
- Ionising Radiations Regulations and Ionising Radiation (Medical Exposure) Regulations (IRME; 2000; see Chapter 14)
- Reporting of Injuries, Diseases, and Dangerous Occurrences Regulations (RIDDOR; 1995)
- Special Waste & Hazardous Waste Regulations (England and Wales 2005; see Subchapter 1.2).

As a dental nurse, you need to be aware of these regulations, as they will underpin your day-to-day actions regarding your own and others' health and safety in the dental environment. The most important Act, which was a major advance in health and safety, is the Health and Safety at Work etc. Act 1974.

Health and Safety at Work etc. Act 1974

The Health and Safety at Work etc. Act 1974 applies to all workplace premises, including dental surgeries. It makes it clear that all employers are responsible not only for the health and safety of their staff but also of anyone who might be on their premises, such as patients or suppliers. All staff and visitors to a workplace should also act in a responsible manner and prevent any hazards occurring that may cause injury to themselves or others.

In addition to the Health and Safety at Work etc. Act 1974, the Dentists Act 1984 makes the employing dentist accountable for all faults or omissions made by their staff (including dental nurses).

FIND OUT MORE

If there are five or more employees in the workplace, the employer must have a written health and safety policy statement. Does your workplace require this? If it does, find out where it is located and who is responsible for it.

THE EMPLOYER'S RESPONSIBILITIES

Every employer should:

- Provide a health and safety policy
- Provide a safe working environment with no health risks
- Maintain the workplace (see Box 1.1.1), equipment and all work appliances in a safe condition
- Display the HSE's health and safety law poster in a location where all staff can easily refer to it
- Ensure staff are aware of, and comply with, the provided health and safety policies and procedures

---

BOX 1.1.1 HEALTH AND SAFETY CONSIDERATIONS IN THE WORKPLACE

The workplace room temperature should reach at least 16 °C after one hour and all rooms should have thermometers to check this. Interestingly, there is no legislation covering temperatures that are high!

Enclosed workplaces such as a dental surgery should be ventilated with sufficient fresh or purified air to minimise exposure to dust, mercury, chemicals, nitrous oxide and **disinfectant** vapours. An open window will usually provide adequate ventilation, but mechanical ventilation or air-conditioning units could be considered. These should provide at least 5–8 litres per second of fresh (not recycled) air per occupant. The relative humidity should be between 40% and 70%.

All dental practices should have a first aid kit as well as the required emergency kit (see Chapter 2). All dental surgeries must also keep a stock of emergency drugs on the premises. Surgeries in which **inhalational sedation** is performed have further requirements to fulfil, to ensure nitrous oxide and any other gas levels are minimised.

- Ensure staff are trained in the safe handling and storage of any hazardous substances and equipment
- Ensure risk assessments (see next section) are carried out and recorded
- Review health and safety performance at least annually and be aware of and investigate any failures or concerns.

Usually the employer will have **liability insurance** to cover any injury that occurs on the premises to either staff or visitors (e.g. patients and their accompanying people, contractors etc.).

EMPLOYEES' RESPONSIBILITIES

All employees, including dental nurses, have a duty to take reasonable care of their own health and safety. Therefore you are required to:

- Work to agreed procedures in accordance with the instruction and training given
- Report any suspected health problem related to your work
- Not enter certain designated areas unless you are authorised to do so
- Be trained in the use of the specified materials or equipment
- Not interfere with or misuse any equipment or item that is meant for the purpose of controlling or eliminating risk
- Report to your immediate supervisor or line manager, as a matter of urgency, any apparent faults in procedures or equipment.

RISK ASSESSMENT

A *risk assessment* is simply a careful examination of what, in the workplace, could cause harm to people. Doing a risk assessment helps employers decide whether they have taken enough precautions, or should do more, to prevent harm from occurring to themselves, their staff or others.

A risk assessment should:

- Identify a hazard
- Consider whether anyone (e.g. especially certain staff handling specialised equipment, older people, pregnant women, children, etc.) may be harmed by that hazard
- Evaluate the existing precautions

Terms to Learn
Disinfection: a process by which the number of viable harmful micro-organisms is reduced in an area, e.g. a worktop in a dental practice. Disinfection does not get rid of certain micro-organisms, such as some viruses, or destroy certain forms of harmful micro-organisms, such as spores. Therefore it is only used for cleaning those areas of a dental clinic that only need to be acceptably safe. Disinfection can by carried out using special chemicals called disinfectants or by using heat.

Inhalational sedation: reducing or relieving anxiety using nitrous oxide and oxygen inhalation (in the dental workplace) (see Chapter 13).

Term to Learn
Liability insurance: a type of insurance that protects against claims of negligence or inappropriate action that were alleged to result in bodily injury (or property damage) to another person.

3

- Take action to improve precautions and minimise the risk of the hazard occurring
- Record the findings
- Review regularly the arrangements – at least once a year.

Terms to Learn
Sterilisation: a process by which an object is rendered free from all viable harmful micro-organisms, including viruses and bacterial spores. Therefore this method is used to decontaminate instruments that will be used inside a patient's mouth.
Dental bur: a type of drill bit that is fitted into the dental handpiece and used for cutting or grinding the hard tooth material or bone. Also used in laboratory work.

POSSIBLE RISKS IN DENTISTRY: SOME EXAMPLES

Handling dangerous substances:

- Certain dental materials used in the dental surgery and laboratory (e.g. acids) that could cause bodily harm if not used correctly
- Substances used for developing radiographs (X-ray films) (see p. 327).

Handling dangerous instruments (these may also be dangerous if hot):

- Extraction forceps and other surgical instruments
- Handpieces and **dental burs**
- Orthodontic pliers
- Sharps – instruments, scalpels, needles (see p. 14).

Handling dangerous machinery/equipment:

- Dental handpieces
- Electrosurgery equipment
- Heating equipment
- Laboratory equipment
- Lasers (see p. 16)
- Steam **sterilisers** (autoclaves).

4

IDENTIFY AND LEARN

Identify a pair of extraction forceps, a handpiece, a dental bur and a pair of orthodontic pliers in your workplace.

OCCUPATIONAL HAZARDS RELATED TO DENTISTRY

KEY POINT Dental nursing is one of the safest occupations.

Generally the risk of hazards occurring in the surgery are very low nowadays because of regulation and enforcement of good work practices by government authorities such as the HSE.

Most dental staff are in good general health. The more important concerns in the dental workplace are:

- Accidents
- Allergies
- Assaults
- Burns
- Chemicals
- Electrical
- Eye damage
- Fires and explosions

- Infections and inoculation injuries
- Lasers
- Noise
- Posture
- Pregnancy
- Pressure systems
- Radiation
- Stress.

Government regulations are in place concerning most of the above. The following sections explain how, as a dental nurse, you can reduce the risks by following the regulations.

Accidents

Legislation applying:

- Notification of Accidents and Dangerous Occurrences Regulations (1980)
- Reporting of Injuries, Diseases, and Dangerous Occurrences Regulations (RIDDOR) (1995)

Accidents occur in most workplaces, and dental premises are no exception. Accidents are more likely to happen when staff are not concentrating on their activities or are distracted. Obvious physical dangers to patients, staff and others include:

- Hitting the head or face on the dental light
- Trapping fingers or limbs when opening doors or moving the dental chair
- Being hit by a door opening without warning
- Damage from the dental handpiece or hot or sharp instruments
- Slipping or tripping over objects such as carpet edges and wires.

The hands and eyes are especially vulnerable when caustic fluids, needles, scalpels, wires or lasers, hot or rotating instruments are used. Risks related to the use of needles are explained in more detail in the section on 'Infections and inoculation injuries' (p. 14).

IDENTIFY AND LEARN

Identify a rotary instrument in your workplace.

> **KEY POINT** Staff and patients should always wear glasses or other eye protection during procedures involving the use of dental handpieces/burs, grinding or polishing, cutting wires, use of caustics or instrument cleansing.

THE PREMISES

Careful design and furnishing of clinical premises, especially flooring, and thoughtful behaviour, such as not running, can prevent many accidents (see Box 1.1.1 and 'Accident notification', p. 6).

- Floor coverings in clinics:
  - Should be impervious and non-slip; carpeting must be avoided
  - Should be seam-free; where seams are present, they should be sealed
  - The junctions between the floor and wall and the floor and cabinetry should be covered or sealed to prevent inaccessible areas where cleaning might be difficult.
- Work surfaces:
  - Should be impervious and easy to clean and disinfect (e.g. Corian); check the manufacturer's instructions for suitable products to clean.
  - Joins should be sealed to prevent the accumulation of contaminated matter and aid cleaning.
  - Junctions should be rounded or coved to aid cleaning.

DENTAL EQUIPMENT

Much of the equipment used in dentistry constitutes some hazard to staff and sometimes to the patient or others. All equipment must therefore be carefully and regularly maintained by an appropriately trained person. This is covered in more detail below.

RECORDING AND NOTIFYING ACCIDENTS

All accidents and injuries to staff or patients or visitors while on the premises, however apparently trivial, should be recorded in an accident book. Her Majesty's Stationery Office (HMSO) publishes an 'Accident Book', which is suitable for use in the dental environment.

FIND OUT MORE

Where is the accident book kept in your workplace? Who supplies it?

Employers must notify the HSE of accidents causing death or 'major injury' to any person or 'dangerous occurrences', even if there has been no death or injury. They also have to keep records of the event.

Under the regulation called RIDDOR, any injury occurring in a workplace should be reported if the person:

- Requires 24-hour hospitalisation for treatment

or

- Requires sick leave for three or more days

or if the injury involves any of the following:

- Fracture of skull, spine, pelvis or limbs
- Loss of sight
- Unconsciousness from **hypoxia** or chemical exposure
- Explosions or fires
- Major mercury spillage
- Acute ill health from exposure to a **pathogen**.

Thus, for example, in the dental practice, a compressor or **steam steriliser (autoclave)** explosion could be notifiable, as could a mercury spillage. In case of doubt of whether an injury should be reported, the advice of the local HSE office should be sought.

Reports related to RIDDOR should be immediately given by telephone to HSE, and a completed accident report form (2508) sent to the HSE within 10 days. Incident reporting forms can be downloaded from the HSE website (https://www.hse.gov.uk/forms/incident/f2508.pdf) or obtained from The Stationery Office Bookshop (www.tso.co.uk/contact). A copy of the completed 2508 form should also be kept by the employer.

If the incident does not result in a reportable injury but clearly could have done so, it is classed as a dangerous occurrence and must also be reported immediately by completing form 2508. A full list of what are 'dangerous occurrences' and the employer's responsibilities are given in the RIDDOR 97 leaflet. (A needlestick injury (p. 14), involving an infected patient may also fall in this category.)

> **Terms to Learn**
> **Hypoxia:** the condition in which the cells in the body (especially the brain) receive an inadequate amount of oxygen to carry out their tasks.
> **Pathogen:** an agent that can cause disease, e.g. bacteria.

> **Term to Learn**
> **Steam steriliser (autoclave):** a pressure vessel in which steam at high pressure is produced. When instruments are placed in the steam steriliser for a certain amount of time, the high temperatures in the steam help to kill the harmful micro-organisms or their spores that may be attached to the instruments.

6

FIND OUT MORE

Visit the HSE website (www.hse.gov.uk/riddor) for more information about RIDDOR.

> **KEY POINT** Although RIDDOR applies to all places of work including dental premises it excludes accidents to 'patients when undergoing treatment in a hospital or surgery of a doctor or dentist'. That exclusion only applies to patients when undergoing treatment – the RIDDOR rules do still have to be followed if, for example, a patient breaks a leg on the surgery doorstep.

REPORTING DISEASES UNDER RIDDOR

If the employer is notified by a doctor that an employee has a reportable work-related disease or infection (e.g. occupational dermatitis, occupational asthma, tuberculosis, hepatitis B, legionnaires' disease), the HSE must be sent a completed disease report form (2508A; available at: https://www.hse.gov.uk/forms/incident/f2508a.pdf).

FIND OUT MORE

Of the responsibilities listed in Box 1.1.2 which would be the dental nurse's responsibilities? Make a list and get your supervisor to comment on it.

BOX 1.1.2 MINIMISING ACCIDENTS IN THE DENTAL SURGERY AND LABORATORY

- Avoid unnecessary rushing about and horseplay.
- Paths and doors should not be obstructed by trailing wires or any other hazards.
- Passageways and staircases should be well lit, secure and not obstructed, and cleaned daily.
- Floor surfaces should be clean, non-slip, and have a minimum of joints.
- Furniture should be strong, safe and secured where necessary.
- Staff should use appropriate steps or stepladders when reaching for objects in high places.
- Fires, heaters, Bunsen burners, etc. should be guarded.
- Flammables, explosives and toxic materials including domestic bleach should be safely stored and labelled correctly.
- There should be procedures for regular maintenance of all equipment, especially steam sterilisers and compressors because of the risk of explosion.
- Heat treatment and **casting equipment** should be housed adequately, and tongs used for handling heated casting rings.
- **Acid baths** should be properly housed and protected.
- All electrical equipment should be installed, earthed, fused and connected, and maintained properly.
- Cables and tubing from electrical and other equipment should not trail on the floor.
- All gas appliances should be installed, connected and maintained properly.
- Electrical, radiography, pressure and gas appliances should be turned off outside working hours.
- Staff and others should avoid injuries from sharps by using appropriate waste disposal.
- Staff should wear protective attire as appropriate.
- Staff should adhere to the practice safety policy.
- Staff should not smoke, eat or drink on the premises except in designated areas.
- Staff should know the hazards of, and preferably stop, smoking.
- Safety training and refresher courses should be taken by all appropriate staff.
- Staff should not use radio headsets and iPods and listen to overloud music, all of which isolate the wearer from the surrounding environment, and have resulted in many accidents.

Terms to Learn
Casting equipment: the equipment used in a dental laboratory to make fixed restorations such as crowns (see Chapter 9).
Acid bath: a solution containing acid that is used to stop the developing process for X-rays.

Allergies

Allergic reactions are common and usually minor but some are potentially lethal. People with asthma, eczema and some other conditions often have underlying allergies. Sometimes allergic reactions can be very severe (called anaphylaxis; see Chapter 2).

Many allergies have a hereditary component but the prevalence of allergies appears to be increasing. Table 1.1.1 lists some common allergens.

KEY POINT Some dental materials may produce allergic reactions.

LATEX ALLERGY

Latex allergy has become a significant clinical problem, along with allergies to iodine, plasters (e.g. Elastoplast and Band-aid) and drugs (remember this with the acronym LIED – **L**atex **I**odine **E**lastoplast **D**rugs). Latex products are common in the home and workplace

TABLE 1.1.1 Common Allergens

Source of Allergen	Examples
Food products	Milk, nuts, egg, shellfish
Drugs	Aspirin, penicillins,
Environmental	Animal hair, dust mite, pollen
Latex	Condoms, elastic bands, gloves
Dental materials	Amalgam alloy, gold, mercury, resin-based materials

Term to Learn
Sensitisation: a change in response by the body to a foreign substance, usually an allergen, so that on subsequent exposures to that substance the body shows a heightened immune response (see Subchapter 4.1).
HIV: human immunodeficiency virus, the virus that causes AIDS.
AIDS: acquired immune deficiency syndrome, a fatal disease. People with AIDS have problems with their immune system and so catch infections more easily.

including clinics, wards and operating theatres. Therefore allergy is an important occupational problem, especially with handwashing using abrasive materials, which increases the risk of **sensitisation**. Allergic reactions to latex have become increasingly common since the use of protective medical/dental gloves became mandatory following the advent of **HIV/AIDS**. Latex exposure may occur via the skin, mucous membranes, or respiratory tract (see Subchapter 4.1) with inhalation of latex glove powder (natural rubber latex (NRL) allergens may attach to lubricating powder, and become aerosolised, causing sensitisation; or, in those who are allergic, they can cause respiratory, ocular or nasal symptoms).

'Low-allergen' latex gloves are available but there is little certainty that these offer any real benefit. People who have allergies to one type of substance are more likely to have allergies to others; patients with latex allergy, for example, may react to foods with allergen cross-reactivity such as avocado, banana, chestnut and kiwi.

Many items used in dental practice can sometimes contain latex (Box 1.1.3) and even equipment and laboratory work previously handled with latex gloves may elicit an allergic response.

IDENTIFY AND LEARN

Identify all the dental materials and instruments marked with ** in Box 1.1.3 in your workplace.

Diagnosis of an allergy is based on:

- Clinical history and presentation
- Family history of allergy
- Skin-prick or patch testing
- Elimination diet to identify food allergens.

KEY POINT For latex allergy, anything containing, or contaminated by, latex should be avoided: a latex-free clinic is ideal.

To avoid future allergic reactions, known allergens should be avoided, which is easier said than done. This is because sensitive individuals may react to minute traces of an allergen, and because allergens can be present in the most unexpected places.

BOX 1.1.3 LATEX IN DENTAL ITEMS*

- Equipment and laboratory work previously handled with latex gloves
- Adhesive dressings and their packaging
- Amalgam carrier tips**
- Bandages and tapes
- Chip syringes**
- Dappen pots**
- Endodontic stops**
- Gloves
- Gutta-percha and gutta-balata**
- Headgear and head positioners**
- Induction masks**
- Latex ties on face masks
- Local anaesthetic cartridges**
- Mixing bowls**

- Needle guards
- Orthodontic elastics**
- Prophylaxis cups and polishing wheels and points**
- Protective eyewear
- Rubber dam**
- Rubber gloves
- Rubber sleeves on props, and bite blocks**
- Spatulas**
- Suction tips**
- Surgical face masks and other protective items of clothing e.g. gowns, overshoes
- Tourniquets and blood pressure cuffs
- Wedges

*Latex is present in some rubber dental local anaesthetic cartridges, stoppers or plungers, where either the harpoon penetrates or where the flat piston end of a self-aspirating syringe rests. At the other end of the cartridge is the diaphragm, which the needle penetrates. Any of these components may contain latex. Although there are no documented reports of allergy due to the latex component of cartridges of dental LA, the UK preparation of prilocaine (Citanest) contains no latex. **See 'Identify and Learn' above.

Patients who have had serious allergic reactions such as anaphylaxis (see Chapter 2) are also usually advised to always carry with them adrenaline for **subcutaneous** self-injection in the event of a reaction (e.g. Epipen). Affected individuals are usually advised to wear a warning emblem such as Medic-Alert.

Treatments for allergies include use of various drugs such as antihistamines.

Term to Learn
Subcutaneous: the tissues of the body just under the skin.

Assaults

Occasionally dental staff are victims of assault by patients who may be drunk, stressed, have mental problems or may be drug abusers. Potentially dangerous incidents should be defused where possible. If you are assaulted, the most effective response will be to:

- Stay calm
- Avoid confrontation – verbally, by body language or physically
- Listen to the person
- Empathise with the person
- Seek help if the situation does not resolve.

Guidelines governing the prosecution of violent offenders who target NHS staff have been issued by the Crown Prosecution Service (CPS) and the NHS Security Management Service (NHS SMS).

FIND OUT MORE

To read more about security in the workplace, see the NHS website: www.nhsbsa.nhs.uk/413.aspx.

Burns

Burns can result from chemical (acids) or physical agents (heat, cold, radiation such as X-rays or lasers).

CHEMICAL BURNS

Several acids (e.g. phosphoric acid, chromic acid and trichloroacetic acid) and corrosive agents (e.g. sodium hypochlorite) are used in the dental surgery and can cause burns if they are not used carefully. Many other stronger acids and corrosives are used in the dental laboratory (e.g. hydrofluoric, sulphuric and nitric acids, and caustic soda or sodium bicarbonate). All acids and caustic solutions should be stored safely in appropriate and clearly labelled containers, and proper safety precautions should be taken when handling these materials.

THERMAL BURNS

Thermal burns can happen when taking out hot instruments or materials from steam sterilisers or microwaves. Several dental instruments, such as extraction forceps, elevators and metal mouth gags, in particular, retain heat for several minutes after being sterilised and so can cause burns to staff and to patients if used immediately after sterilisation. Handling dental handpieces that have overheated during use can also cause heat burns. This often happens because of the difficulty in gauging their temperature through the gloves that all staff are required to wear in the clinic.

Hot wax knives and Bunsen burners are also common causes of burns; long hair and gloves or clothing can catch light in a Bunsen flame. Hot air blowers can reduce this danger, although they take somewhat longer to heat objects.

Other possible causes of thermal burns in the dental environment include handling hot gutta-percha, dental composition, wax and boiling water, lasers, diathermy and even heated operating lights. Diathermy accidents have resulted from metallic parts of the dental chair becoming part of the path of the current – the localised increase in current density can then cause superficial burns of the skin.

IDENTIFY AND LEARN

Identify gutta-percha, dental composition, a wax knife, diathermy unit and an elevator in your workplace and find out what they are used for.

COLD BURNS

Cold burns may occur from spillage of liquid nitrogen, which is used, for example, for **cryotherapy** or to freeze some biopsy specimens.

Term to Learn
Cryotherapy: a method of destroying abnormal cells in the skin or mucosa usually by freezing them with an extremely cold liquid or instrument.

Chemicals (Hazardous Substances)

Legislation applying:

- Control of Substances Hazardous to Health Regulations (COSHH) 2002

All dental surgeries and laboratories must undertake risk assessments of all chemical and potentially hazardous substances used in the premises. The results of the assessments must be recorded in a COSHH report. The report must include:

- The hazards a material poses
- How the hazards can be avoided
- How to deal with a hazard should it occur.

Hazardous materials in general include:

- Substances used directly in work activities (e.g. adhesives, cleaning agents)
- Substances generated during work activities (e.g. fumes from soldering)
- Naturally occurring substances (e.g. dust)
- Biological agents, such as bacteria and other micro-organisms.

Hazardous materials in dentistry include:

- Sodium hypochlorite
- Acid etchants
- Mercury
- X-ray fixers
- Flammable materials.

FIND OUT MORE

Read the COSSH reports of five hazardous materials that are used in your dental practice. See also the COSSH publication 'Working with substances hazardous to health' (www.hse.gov.uk/pubns/indg136.pdf).

IDENTIFY AND LEARN

Identify an acid etchant and the X-ray fixer used in your workplace.

Employers are required to:

- Assess the risks to health from chemicals and decide what controls are needed
- Use those controls and make sure staff use them

10

- Make sure the controls are working properly
- Inform staff about the risks to their health
- Train staff.

GASES AND VOLATILE LIQUIDS

A dental nurse may be exposed to anaesthetic gases (nitrous oxide) and vapours for a significant part of their career if the equipment used to administer the gases is faulty, poorly maintained or used without an effective scavenging system, or if the agents are misused. These gases, which are also called inhalational agents, are used in conscious sedation (nitrous oxide) and general anaesthesia (nitrous oxide, isoflurane, enflurane, sevoflurane and desflurane; halothane is no longer commonly used – see below). Anaesthesia is covered in detail in Chapter 13.

Under normal working conditions, our mental and nervous responses, that is, how alert we are and how quickly and appropriately we react to situations, are not much impaired by exposure to inhalational agents. However, if a clinician is exposed to excessive amounts of these gases or over a long period of time, not surprisingly, their responses can be impaired. They may also develop numbness, difficulty in concentrating, paraesthesias ('pins and needles') and dizziness. Nitrous oxide exposure for prolonged periods can also have adverse effects on other organs of the body, for example the heart, liver and bone marrow, and the reproductive organs.

Halothane and some other halogenated inhalational agents (sevoflurane and desflurane) can cause severe liver dysfunction (called hepatotoxicity) and problems with the beating of the heart (called **arrhythmias**). Therefore halothane is no longer recommended for use in adults. Only occasional hepatotoxicity has been reported with enflurane and isoflurane.

Term to Learn
Arrhythmia: when the heart beats too slowly or too rapidly or irregularly or too early.

Clearly, all dental practices should take steps to control and minimise the exposure to inhalational agents (see Box 1.1.4).

A Note about Ventilation

- A dental surgery should be adequately ventilated; often an open window will suffice but, in some cases, especially where gases are used, it might be appropriate to install an extractor fan, or a scavenger system. Recycling air conditioning systems are not recommended.
- Systems should exhaust to the outside of the building without risk to the public or recirculation into any public building.
- Fresh air supply rate should not fall below 5–8 litres per second per occupant and should not create uncomfortable draughts.
- Mechanical systems must be regularly cleaned, tested and maintained according to the manufacturer's recommendations to ensure they are free from anything that may contaminate the air.

IDENTIFY AND LEARN

Identify a vacuum ejector in your workplace.

BOX 1.1.4 PRECAUTIONS TO TAKE WHILE USING NITROUS OXIDE

- Careful use of well-maintained equipment
- Adequate room ventilation
- High-volume vacuum ejectors
- Effective scavenging systems.

11

Electrical Hazards

Regulations applying:

- Electricity at Work Regulations 1989
- Electrical Equipment (Safety) Regulations 1994

QUALITY CONTROL

The Electrical Equipment (Safety) Regulations 1994 state that all electrical equipment should be constructed and designed for safe use when connected. This should be achieved by providing protection against electric shock through a combination of insulation and a protective earthing conductor. The main hazards from electrical equipment are:

- Contact with live parts causing shock and burns (normal mains voltage, 230 volts AC, can kill).
- Faults which could cause fires – where electricity could be the source of ignition in a potentially flammable or explosive atmosphere.
- The risk of injury from electricity is strongly linked to where and how it is used, being greatest:
  - In wet surroundings
  - In cramped spaces.

INSPECTION ROUTINES

Electricity plugs, cables, etc. should be inspected every six months. All electrical equipment should be regularly tested by an appropriately qualified person at least every two to three years, with records kept of the test results.

MEASURES TO REDUCE ELECTRICAL ACCIDENTS

- Instruction of personnel in the correct use of equipment.
- Frequent periodic maintenance of apparatus and wiring.
- Earthing of all apparatus.
- Separation of mains circuits.
- Use of earth leakage circuit breakers.

Eye Hazards

Eyes need protection from foreign bodies, infected material, chemicals and the various forms of radiation used in dentistry – lasers, light sources for **curing** (ultra-violet/visible blue or white halogen light) and X-rays. These are covered in more detail on page 16.

Patients

Patients must always be provided with adequate eye protection – particularly if they are being treated in the supine position (lying on the back) and for procedures being carried out under conscious sedation or general anaesthesia.

Staff

All clinical staff should always wear protective eyewear at work. Objects such as bits of fillings can behave like projectiles and fly out of the mouth at speeds of over 10 m/s when using drills at 250 000 revolutions per minute (rpm). The ends of orthodontic and other wires should be held in mosquito forceps, and when cutting, the wire should always be held between two forceps so that the cut end does not fly off and cause eye damage.

Special eyewear is needed for work with lasers and with curing lights. Remember that ordinary dark glasses do *not* filter the hazardous wavelengths of lasers and curing lights. Rather, because they absorb visible light, they can dilate the pupils (open them wider) and therefore worsen the problem because more of the hazardous light rays can now enter the eyes. Contact lens wearers should be careful not to get powders or other materials behind their lenses.

Term to Learn

Curing: the process of hardening of tooth-coloured materials that are used mainly to fill teeth with cavities. The materials come in paste form and harden either by a chemical reaction or on application of a special light (see Chapter 9).

12

IDENTIFY AND LEARN
Identify a pair of mosquito artery forceps in your workplace.

Fires and Explosions
Legislation applying:

- Fire Precaution (Workplace) Regulations
- Regulatory Reform Fire Safety Order 2006

Human error is responsible for most fires and explosions. The main causes of fire in a dental practice or similar place usually are: electrical faults (see p. 12); careless use of matches; incorrect use of flammable gases (e.g. oxygen) and fluids; and non-electrical heating.

A commonsense approach, particularly avoiding the use of naked flames and taking care in the use and storage of flammable materials, will prevent many problems. For example:

- Gas cylinders should be securely stored so that they cannot fall, in a room separate from flammable materials.
- Steam sterilisers (autoclaves) and surgery air compressors should be used and maintained properly. All pressure vessels must be regularly maintained.

EMPLOYER AND EMPLOYEE RESPONSIBILITIES
Employers must comply with fire safety regulations. This means carrying out a fire risk assessment to determine what precautions are needed and putting in place fire precaution measures. If there are five or more employees, the fire risk assessment must be written down.

- Fire precaution measures could include fire alarm systems and extinguishers as well as clearly signed escape routes (see also Box 1.1.5).
- All flammable materials (e.g. oxygen, gas cylinders, alcohol, monomer, methylated spirits) must be stored in a metal cabinet and never used near flames, or a fire or explosion could result.
- Fire-fighting equipment such as extinguishers and blankets must be kept on the premises, regularly inspected and serviced by an authorised body. Staff should be aware of the location of fire-fighting equipment, as well as the colour coding for use on different types of fire.
- Fire exits must be marked with the appropriate green signs, kept free of any obstruction, and kept unlocked/unbolted during normal working hours, for emergency exit and for access if required by a fire and rescue service (fire brigade).
- The fire regulations should be clearly displayed in the reception area – they must be clearly seen by all staff, patients and visitors. They should also appear in the practice manual and patient leaflets.
- Emergency lighting may be necessary.
- An assembly point must be noted outside the premises.
- The fire drill should be practised regularly.

KEY POINT The safety of employees and visitors in the event of a fire rests with the responsible person of the organisation. If an employer is negligent, they could be prosecuted.

> **BOX 1.1.5 STEPS TO TAKE IN THE EVENT OF A FIRE**
>
> 1. Activate the fire alarm or call out 'fire'.
> 2. Call the Fire and Rescue Service.
> 3. Locate the fire source and extinguish if safe to do so.
> 4. Evacuate all patients and staff from danger.
> 5. Close the doors and windows.
> 6. Assemble all people at the designated assembly point.

13

Infections and Inoculation Injuries

Dental staff are commonly exposed to respiratory infections, mainly 'colds', and other viral throat and chest (respiratory) infections. Other more serious respiratory hazards are 'flu' (influenza), tuberculosis (TB) and, to a much lesser extent, *Legionella* infection (also called legionnaires' disease). All these infections could also be transmitted to patients or others (see Subchapter 1.2).

The main infectious hazard in the dental practice is contact with infected body fluids (blood, saliva, etc.). Infections can be transmitted via sharps injuries (needlestick injury; inoculation, particularly those caused by viruses such as hepatitis B, hepatitis C and human immunodeficiency virus (HIV). **Prions**, which cause Creutzfeldt–Jakob disease (CJD), are virtually impossible to destroy. MRSA (meticillin-resistant *Staphylococcus aureus*) infection is mainly a healthcare-associated infection **(HCAI)**.

INOCULATION (SHARPS OR NEEDLESTICK) INJURIES

Inoculation injuries include all incidents where a contaminated object or substance enters the body through a breach in the skin or a mucous membrane (see Subchapter 4.1) or comes into contact with the eyes. Typical examples of inoculation injuries are:

- Sticking or stabbing with a used needle or other instrument – particularly when re-sheathing a needle
- Splashes with a contaminated substance to the eye or other open lesion
- Cuts with contaminated equipment
- Bites or scratches inflicted by patients.

Inoculation injuries must be dealt with promptly and correctly:

1. The wound should be allowed to bleed, but do not scrub it.
2. Wash the wound thoroughly with running water and cover with a waterproof plaster.
3. Assess hepatitis B antibody status of the injured person and establish **viral carriage status** of the source patient.

If a dental nurse receives a sharps injury during a treatment session and there is reason for concern, the injured nurse should be referred to an infectious disease consultant (consultant in communicable disease control) or consultant microbiologist. It is necessary to follow the local procedures for seeking urgent advice, and follow-up action, including **serological surveillance**. Ideally, all dental practices should have formal links with an occupational health service, so that management of sharps injuries is undertaken promptly and according to accepted national protocols. Every primary care trust (PCT, see Chapter 3) will have at least one designated specialist who can be contacted for advice on post-exposure prophylaxis (PEP; see p. 15). Every practice should have details of the local contact displayed prominently.

Make a full record of the incident in the accident book. Include details of:

- Who was injured
- How the incident occurred
- What action was taken
- Which clinicians were informed and when
- If known, the name of the patient being treated.

Both the injured person and the clinician in charge should countersign the record.

Terms to Learn
Prion: a microscopic protein particle that can cause disease.
HCAI: infection that is caught by a patient from another patient, staff or visitor during stay in a hospital or visit to another healthcare facility.

KEY POINT Sharps injuries are one of the main hazards for dental nurses. The clinician or you must dispose of needles into a special sharps container (see p. 40) to avoid the risk of injury.

Term to Learn
Viral carriage status: a check to see whether the source patient has or may have an infection such as hepatitis or HIV.

KEY POINT Standard (universal) **infection control** procedures must be used with all patients undergoing dental treatment to avoid the risk of transfer of infection. See Subchapter 1.2 and the British Dental Association website (www.bda.org) for more details.

Terms to Learn
Serological surveillance: the procedure of keeping a close check on whether a person develops a disease by testing the blood at regular intervals.

14

CONTACT INFORMATION FOR ADVICE ON INOCULATION INJURIES

England: the duty doctor at the Health Protection Agency, 61 Colindale Avenue, London NW9 5EQ (tel: 020 8200 6868).

Scotland: Scottish Centre for Infection and Environmental Health (SCIEH), Clifton House, Clifton Place, Glasgow G3 7LN (tel: 0141 300 1100).

Wales: Public Health Laboratory (PHL) Cardiff, University Hospital of Wales, Heath Park, Cardiff CF14 4XW (tel: 02920 742718).

Northern Ireland: Director of Public Health at your local Health and Social Services Board.

POST-EXPOSURE PROPHYLAXIS

The risk of acquiring a viral infection such as hepatitis B or HIV following an inoculation injury is usually small but on occasion it can be greater. If the source patient is infected, and if the assessment of the injury suggests that there is a significant risk for transmission (e.g. Box 1.1.6), post-exposure prophylaxis (PEP) is recommended. In terms of hepatitis this means immunoglobulins usually, or in terms of HIV it means taking a short course of **anti-retroviral drugs** (four weeks), starting as soon as possible after exposure (ideally within one hour). The aim is to reduce the risk of infection with HIV following exposure. During this time, the injured person should practise **safer sex**, and may need to avoid exposure-prone procedures (see below), After 12 weeks after the injury, the person should have a serological test to check whether HIV transmission has occurred.

FIND OUT MORE

- What are your local arrangements for urgent access to PEP?
- Where is your occupational health department located?
- Who is your local consultant in communicable diseases?

INOCULATION INJURIES: KEY MESSAGES

- A needlestick injury from a used needle can present a risk of infection.
- The clinician should remove the needle from the device and dispose of the needle into a rigid sharps container.
- A needlestick injury from a used needle should be washed under running water and the needle safely discarded into a sharps container.
- A senior clinical staff member (the designated doctor) should be informed.
- The local occupational health person or accident and emergency department should be contacted immediately about PEP.
- If there has been significant exposure, the HIV status of the source patient should be established with 8–24 hours. Hepatitis B and C virus status may also need to be determined.
- PEP should be started within the first 72 hours (the recommended follow-up period after occupational exposure to HIV has been shortened and is now a minimum of 12 weeks after the HIV exposure or, if PEP has been taken, a minimum of 12 weeks from when PEP was stopped).
- Injured staff may need to change their clinical work practice (but see p. 16 regarding EPPs).
- The accident should be recorded in the accident book (see p. 5).

IF THE DENTAL HEALTHCARE WORKER HAS AN INFECTION

The risk of infection transmission is considered greater if an infected healthcare worker undertakes **exposure-prone procedures** or EPPs. These are **invasive procedures** where there

---

Terms to Learn—cont'd
Infection control: the activities carried out by healthcare professionals to prevent the spread of pathogens (harmful micro-organisms) between patients or from the healthcare workers to the patients and vice versa, e.g. proper hand washing, wearing personal protective equipment (PPE). Dental nurses play a key role in infection control in the dental surgery.

Terms to Learn
Anti-retroviral drugs: drugs that act against a particular class of viruses called retroviruses, which includes HIV.
Safer sex: practising sex with due regard to the use of more effective methods to prevent the spread of infection, e.g. always using condoms.

Term to Learn
Exposure-prone or invasive procedures: procedures in which a clinician's gloved hands may be in contact with sharp instruments, needle tips and sharp tissues (spicules of bone or teeth) inside a patient's open body cavity, wound or a confined space within the body, where the clinician's hands or fingertips may not be completely visible at all times.

15

> **BOX 1.1.6 FACTORS ASSOCIATED WITH HIV TRANSMISSION BY NEEDLESTICK INJURY**
>
> - Deep injury to the healthcare worker.
> - Visible blood on the device causing injury.
> - Device previously placed in a blood vessel in the source patient.
> - Source patient is within last 60 days of life (i.e. has late-stage AIDS).

is a risk that injury to the healthcare worker may result in exposure of the patient's open tissues to the blood or body fluids of the healthcare worker.

THE GDC's VIEW ON INFECTED DENTAL STAFF AND EPP

'All healthcare workers have an overriding ethical and legal duty to protect the health and safety of their patients and those who carry out exposure-prone procedures (EPP) should be immune to or non-infectious for hepatitis B. A dental clinician who believes he or she may be infected with a blood borne virus or other infection has an ethical responsibility to obtain medical advice, including any necessary testing. If a clinician is found to be infected, further medical advice and counselling must be sought. Changes to clinical practice may be required and may include ceasing or restricting practice, the exclusion of exposure-prone procedures or other modifications. An infected clinician must not rely on his/her own assessment of the possible risks to their patients. Failure to obtain appropriate advice or act upon the advice given would almost certainly lead to a charge of serious professional misconduct.'

(General Dental Council (1997) Maintaining Standards)

If a dental nurse is found to be infected with a blood-borne virus following a needlestick injury, his or her employer has to undertake a risk assessment. This is done to determine whether there is a risk to patients and whether the dental nurse should be permitted to work within the practice. The risk assessment must take into account the duties performed by the dental nurse and the likelihood that the infection could be transmitted to a patient or another member of staff.

An infected dental nurse must not undertake EPP, so as to remove, as far as is possible, the risk of transmitting infection. There may be employment issues that need to be considered and the dental nurse should seek advice from an occupational health doctor.

Lasers

Legislation applying:

- Care Standards Act 2000
- Nursing Homes (Laser) Regulations (1984)

Laser is the acronym for **L**ight **A**mplification by **S**timulated **E**mission of **R**adiation. In dentistry lasers are used in a variety of ways as a sharp cutting tool to remove decayed tooth material or take a biopsy specimen, or to enhance the effect of a tooth-whitening material. All lasers are potentially hazardous, mostly because of the risk of eye damage, burns and fire or electric shock, but some lasers are less damaging than others.

Types of Laser

Lasers used in medicine and dentistry are categorised into four classes according to the amount of damage they are likely to cause (see Table 1.1.2). Class 3B and 4 are more commonly used in dental practice. Some examples of these lasers are:

- CO_2 (short for carbon dioxide) lasers – these are used to 'cut' the soft tissues (e.g. overgrown gingivae) and are potentially dangerous as they burn. In dentistry, they are

TABLE 1.1.2 Safety Concerns with Lasers	
Laser Classes	**Safety Concerns**
1	Safe under all conditions of normal use
2	Safe because the blink reflex will limit the exposure
3	Hazardous if the eye is exposed directly
4	Can burn the skin, in addition to potentially devastating and permanent eye damage as a result of direct or diffuse beam viewing. Can also be a fire risk

Terms to Learn
Oral surgery: the branch of dentistry involved with tooth extractions and other surgical procedures carried out within the oral cavity (mouth).
Dentine: one of the tissues of the teeth (see Chapter 4).
Retina: the lining of the back of the eye that senses the light coming into the eye, which then forms the image we see.

mostly used in **oral surgery** and rarely for other kinds of dental treatment. They burn any tissues exposed to them, including the eyes!

- Nd:Yag (short for **ne**odymium, **y**ttrium-, **a**luminium-**g**arnet) lasers and krypton lasers – these are used for cutting **dentine** and soft tissues. They have wavelengths in the spectrum of visible light and are absorbed preferentially by the **retina** of the eye, which can then be damaged if this kind of laser is shone into the eye.
- Argon lasers – these are mainly used for curing some tooth-coloured filling materials called composite resins (see p. 223). They also have wavelengths in the spectrum of visible light and are absorbed preferentially by the retina, which can be damaged if a laser of this type is shone into the eye.

Lasers and the Law

- Current legislation – the Care Standards Act 2000 – requires that all premises operating a class 3B or class 4 laser or an intense pulse light (IPL) source for the purposes of treating humans must register with the Care Quality Commission (www.healthcarecommission.org.uk). This includes all hospitals, dental surgeries, cosmetic clinics and health centres.
- A nominated user who is skilled in the safe use of the laser should always be present whenever a class 3B or 4 laser is used medically and should also be registered with the Care Quality Commission.
- Any dental practice using lasers should have a policy about laser use and a designated laser controlled area.
- Laser warning signs must be provided at every entrance to the laser controlled area. Figure 1.1.1 shows a typical laser safety hazard symbol. This symbol is usually accompanied by some text depending on the kind of laser in use, for example, the sign will say that class 3B laser radiation is being used and to 'Avoid exposure to the beam' or that class 4 laser radiation is being used and to 'Avoid eye or skin exposure to direct or scattered radiation'.
- All laser products must also carry clearly visible labels indicating the laser class, precautions required, maximum laser output and wavelength.
- Class 3B and 4 lasers must have a red emergency shut-off switch in a prominent, accessible position. Class 3A, 3B and 4 lasers must have a **master control** that will only function when the key is inserted and operated, and must give an audible or visible warning when the laser is switched on and operating or not discharged.
- Laser foot switches must be shrouded to prevent accidental operation.

KEY POINT Lasers must always be used with great care and *never* shone into the eyes, in unintended directions, or onto brightly plated instruments that reflect the laser.

17

FIGURE 1.1.1
A typical laser warning sign.

KEY POINT Before a laser is operated, the operator should orally warn staff in the vicinity that the laser is about to be fired. All staff and patients should be wearing protective eyewear *suitable for the laser wavelength being used.*

Light

Light is used for curing, and as far as possible, staff should avoid directly viewing ultra-violet (UV) or blue halogen lights. Protective glasses should be used to filter out all light of wavelength under 500 nm. Therefore glasses with red, orange or yellow coloured lenses of sufficient **optical density** are recommended when using blue or other coloured lights in dental treatment.

Ultra-Violet Light

UV-A light (wavelength between 320 nm and 400 nm) is possibly the most dangerous light. It can cause long-term damage to the retina and also result in the formation of cataracts – especially if there has been a low-dose exposure over a long period of time. Although nowadays UV-A light sources have largely been replaced by the safer blue halogen light sources, these lights may still be used for some procedures such as curing some tooth-filling materials and fissure sealants.

IDENTIFY AND LEARN

Identify a curing light and a fissure sealant in your workplace.

Blue Halogen Light

Visible blue halogen light (wavelength 400–500 nm) was developed to replace UV-A light, but even this light is not entirely safe. It may also damage the retina.

White (Visible) Light

Visible white light (wavelength 400–700 nm) is much safer than UV or blue light but it also contains some blue and green lights and minute amounts of UV-A. So, although the risks to the eyes are very small, protective eyewear that absorbs these wavelengths should still be worn when curing dental materials with a visible light source.

Noise

Noise-induced hearing loss is irreversible and thus prevention is crucial. Dental staff are, however, much more likely to have leisure-related hearing loss (e.g. from loud music) than they are from work-related problems.

In the past there was concern over possible hearing damage from dental handpieces and turbines and other rotary and ultrasonic instruments. However, research has not found clear evidence for damage from noise produced by air turbines, especially with the use of the quieter, modern handpieces. Nevertheless, clinicians are recommended to consider their quietness when choosing high-speed dental handpieces, and dental nurses should ensure they are well maintained. Noise associated with the use of ultrasonic scalers is not considered to affect the hearing of dental staff. All other unnecessary noise arising in a dental surgery should be eliminated.

IDENTIFY AND LEARN

Identify an air turbine and an ultrasonic scaler in your workplace.

Posture and Manual Handling

Dentistry is a sedentary occupation, and many staff work in a somewhat hunched position. Dentists have more neck, shoulder and lower back pain than do other healthcare practitioners; moreover, a higher percentage of women than men develop neck/shoulder pain.

Four-handed dentistry in theory can help reduce stresses and strains. However, you should take as many short breaks as reasonable in the day, stretching and moving around as much as you can. In general, exercise is important to health (see Chapter 17).

Repetitive movements are common in dental work, for example, while **scaling** and **root planing**. Chronic musculo-skeletal pain associated with repetitive movements has been reported by clinicians and also dental nurses. Carpal tunnel syndrome, which is associated with a feeling of tingling (dysaesthesia) in the upper extremities, has also been reported, especially after a prolonged scaling session.

> **GUIDELINES FOR GOOD POSTURE IN THE DENTAL CLINIC**
> - The feet should be flat on the floor.
> - The angle between the calf and thigh should be more than 90°, usually 90°–115°.
> - The torso should be vertical.
> - Staff should move about, and arch and straighten their back, from time to time.
> - Awkward movements such as twisting should be avoided.
> - Heavy equipment or material should be lifted correctly.

For information regarding safe manual handling please see http://www.hse.gov.uk/pubns/indg143.pdf

Pregnancy Hazards

A pregnant dental nurse may be concerned about potential hazards to her unborn baby. However, current evidence suggests that there is little if any specific occupational risk in dentistry to the outcome of pregnancy. In the past the possible hazards of exposure to anaesthetic gases, mercury, ionising radiation and infections had raised concern.

Pressure Systems

Regulation applying:

- Pressure Systems Safety Regulations 2000

These regulations apply to benchtop sterilisers and compressor(s). All medical devices marketed in the European Union (EU) carry a 'CE' mark, which indicates that the device satisfies the requirements of the EU directive (regulation) and is 'fit for the intended purpose'.

Dental practices must have a written scheme of inspection and pressure vessel insurance cover against the explosion of such vessels, i.e. third-party liability insurance to cover the particular risks associated with pressurised equipment and steam (e.g. steam steriliser).

A new steriliser has to be installed, commissioned and **validated** by an accredited engineer before use. Employers should retain all records (for 11 years) of these activities in the steriliser logbook for future reference. An **a**uthorised **p**erson (AP sterilisers) can provide advice about the validation of a new steriliser, and a qualified competent person (pressure vessels) should carry out the validation tests for a vacuum steam steriliser.

> **Term to Learn**
> **Validation:** the process that demonstrates that the right conditions for sterilisation are being achieved; validation is usually undertaken by an appropriately trained engineer.

19

APPROPRIATE USE OF PRESSURE SYSTEMS

Manufacturers must, by law, provide instructions for re-processing instruments (decontamination) using pressure systems. This includes methods for cleaning and packaging the instruments before placing them in the steriliser. The instructions must also state whether there is any limit to the number of times an item can be sterilised. Failure to comply with the manufacturer's decontamination instructions may put patients and staff at risk. It may also mean that the warranty is no longer valid and the person re-processing the item or the person who authorised the re-processing is now responsible for the risk.

Employers must ensure that there is a set of operating instructions for the steriliser, safety devices and pipe work, including instructions for emergencies. They must ensure that staff are fully trained in the operation and use of the equipment and the management of steam-related injuries (scalds/burns) and also ensure regular maintenance.

An operator or owner who does not comply with the safety regulations regarding pressure systems might be held responsible for injury or damage to people or property. They could even be committing a criminal offence.

Radiation

Legislation applying:

- Ionising Radiations Regulations (IRR) 1999 and 2000
- Ionising Radiation (Medical Exposure) Regulations (IMER 2000)

Radiation hazards mainly involve **ionising radiation**, such as X-rays. However, provided the rules of radiation protection are carefully followed, even radiographers or radiologists – who are more exposed to X-rays than dental nurses – appear to be at no significant risk. See Chapter 14 for a full discussion of this topic. Here we have summarised the key points.

JUSTIFICATION FOR TAKING X-RAYS

A patient should only be exposed to radiation if the benefit of having the test will outweigh the risks of exposure to radiation for that patient. This is one of the key principles of radiological protection as laid down by the International Commission on Radiological Protection (ICRP). These principles also form the basis of the radiological protection framework in the UK.

IRR regulations relate to protection of the public, through legislation for the safe use of X-ray equipment. Specific guidance notes for dental practitioners on the safe use of X-ray equipment have been published (see www.hpa.org.uk).

RESPONSIBILITIES OF THE EMPLOYER

- The dental practice must notify the HSE of the routine use of X-ray equipment on the premises and of any changes such as change in ownership.
- A risk assessment must be performed regularly and equipment must be checked by a qualified engineer.
- All rooms containing X-ray machines must be so labelled (using the correct yellow and black warning labels).
- The 'legal person' must provide written procedures to be followed by all staff for the safe use of X-rays.
- A **r**adiation **p**rotection **s**upervisor (RPS) must be appointed (usually the senior dentist).
- All staff who are involved with X-ray procedures must have written proof of their adequate training for these roles and should wear monitoring badges.
- The principles of ALARA ('**A**s **L**ow **A**s **R**easonably **A**chievable') should be applied at all times when taking X-rays
- A **r**adiation **p**rotection **a**dvisor (RPA; the 'legal person') must be appointed if there is a **cephalostat** in the practice.
- Staff must be appointed to roles as follows, dependent on their training and qualifications:
  - Practitioner: clinician
  - Referrer: clinician referring patient for X-ray exposure
  - Operator: clinician.

Dental nurses who have passed the Dental Radiography Examination for Dental Nurses are legally permitted to take X-rays.

Term to Learn
Ionising radiation: certain kinds of radiation, such as X-rays, that have high-energy photons, which on striking an object, cause the atoms in that object to release electrons and thus become ions.

Term to Learn
Cephalostat: an X-ray machine that takes special radiographs called cephalograms for orthodontic purposes (see Chapter 11).

KEY POINT All members of the dental team have a responsibility to keep up to date and implement the appropriate regulations to ensure health and safety in the dental practice.

Stress

A little stress is necessary for everyone, otherwise there is a risk of boredom and de-motivation. Excess stress, however, can damage health.

1.2 INFECTION CONTROL

Infection control can be defined as: the formal policies and procedures that are required to be followed in all healthcare facilities, including dental workplaces, to reduce the risk of spread of infection. As discussed in Subchapter 1.1, healthcare associated infections (HCAI; see p. 14) can be a problem both for patients and staff.

For the dental nurse, infection control includes:

- Following personal and hand hygiene measures
- Using personal protective equipment (PPE)
- Following surface and equipment decontamination procedures:
  - For decontamination of equipment
  - For decontamination and storage of instruments
- Following water hygiene measures
- Following measures to deal with blood spillages
- Appropriate waste management.

RELEVANT GUIDANCE

The GDC publication *Maintaining Standards* states that 'Failure to employ adequate methods of cross-infection control would almost certainly render a clinician liable to a charge of serious professional misconduct'. In other words, infection control is an important duty for both you as the dental nurse and your employer to help avoid the spread of infection.

In the past the British Dental Association (BDA) Advice Sheet *A12 Infection Control in Dentistry* was often used for guidance, but in 2008, this was superseded by the Department of Health document often referred to as 'HTM 01-05': *Health Technical Memorandum 01-05: Decontamination in Primary Care Dental Practices*. A new edition of this HTM was published in April 2009.

FIND OUT MORE

HTM 01-05 forms the cornerstone of the infection control practices that a dental nurse needs to know about and apply in day-to-day practice. You can access this memorandum at the Department of Health website (http://www.dh.gov.uk/en/Publicationsandstatistics/Publications/PublicationsPolicyAndGuidance/DH_109363).

THE HCAI PROBLEM

HCAI at any one time affected up to 8% of in-patients in the UK. During 2001–2006, meticillin-resistant *Staphylococcus aureus* (MRSA) was implicated in 5109 deaths and *Clostridium difficile* in 13 189 deaths. However, with increasing awareness and prevention, between 2007 and 2008 male deaths because of MRSA infection decreased by 31%.

Healthcare staff have the greatest potential to spread the micro-organisms that cause infection because their hands can:

- Transfer the patient's own micro-organisms into sterile areas of the patient's body during care or treatment
- Transfer micro-organisms from one patient to other patients
- Transfer micro-organisms from the environment and equipment to a patient
- Acquire micro-organisms as a result of their contact with patients, which places healthcare staff themselves at risk of infection.

HAND HYGIENE
Handwashing or Handrub
HANDWASHING

Hands should always be cleaned with liquid (never solid) soap and water when:

> **KEY POINT** Good hand hygiene contributes significantly to the reduction of HCAI.

- They are visibly soiled
- The patient has been vomiting and/or has diarrhoea
- There is direct hand contact with bodily fluids if gloves were not worn
- There is an outbreak of norovirus, *Clostridium difficile* or other diarrhoeal illnesses.

Liquid soap and water is the most reliable way of decontaminating hands, but alcohol handrubs are more frequently used for 'non-soiled' hands.

ALCOHOL HANDRUBS

Alcohol handrubs are the most acceptable method for decontamination of non-soiled hands because they are:

- Better tolerated by the hands, that is they are gentler on the hands and reduce the risk of drying and cracking, which could lead to infection.
- Quicker to use
- Easy to provide at the **point of care** in which healthcare staff to patient contact or treatment is taking place.

Risks associated with the use of alcohol handrub in clinical areas are particularly related to the management of patients who **misuse alcohol** and patients at risk of **deliberate self-harm**. Alcohol rub-related risks and their management are shown in Table 1.2.1.

The Point of Care as the Crucial Moment for Hand Hygiene

The point of care represents the moment in time and the place at which there is the highest likelihood of transmission of infection of HCAI via healthcare staff. The World Health Organization (WHO) 'five moments for hand hygiene', which are endorsed by NPSA, are shown in Box 1.2.1.

22

Terms to Learn
Point of care: the patient's immediate environment.
Alcohol misuse: drinking harmful amounts of alcohol regularly.
Deliberate self-harm: having a mental disorder that predisposes patients to attempt suicide.

TABLE 1.2.1 Management of Risks Associated with Alcohol Rubs

Risk	Management
Ingestion	National Poisons Information Service provides advice via TOXBASE (www.toxbase.org) or its 24-hour telephone service (0844 892 0111)
Eye exposure	Should be managed by irrigation. Contact TOXBASE for further advice
Skin irritation	The NHS Employers Healthy Workplaces website provides advice on this (http://www.nhsemployers.org/HealthyWorkplaces)
Storage	The National Patient Safety Agency (NPSA) and the Department of Health (England) state that only minimum quantities of alcohol-based handrub should be stored

---

BOX 1.2.1 THE FIVE MOMENTS FOR HAND HYGIENE

1. Before patient contact
   When?
     - Clean your hands before touching a patient when approaching him/her.
   Why?
     - To protect the patient against harmful germs carried on your hands.
2. Before an aseptic task
   When?
     - Clean your hands immediately before any aseptic task.
   Why?
     - To protect the patient against harmful germs, including the patient's own, from entering his/her body.
3. After body fluid exposure risk
   When?
     - Clean your hands immediately after an exposure risk to body fluids (and after glove removal).
   Why?
     - To protect yourself and the healthcare environment from harmful patient germs.
4. After patient contact
   When?
     - Clean your hands after touching a patient and his/her immediate surroundings when leaving the patient's side.
   Why?
     - To protect yourself and the healthcare environment from harmful patient germs.
5. After contact with patient surroundings
   When?
     - Clean your hands after touching any object or furniture in the patient's immediate surroundings when leaving – even if the patient has not been touched.
   Why?
     - To protect yourself and the healthcare environment from harmful patient germs.

A hand hygiene policy must be available within the dental surgery and should contain, at least, the following practices (see also Table 1.2.2):

- Hands should be decontaminated between each patient treatment, and before donning and after removal of gloves.
- Bar (solid) soap must no longer be used, or made available, in the dental workplace.
- Antibacterial-based handrubs/gels formulated for use without water can be used on visibly clean hands, in conjunction with a good hand wash technique, for invasive dental procedures (Figure 1.2.1).
- Antibacterial-based handrubs/gels can also be used between patients during surgery sessions: 20–30 seconds are required for this (Figure 1.2.1A). For hand wash, 40–60 seconds are required (Figure 1.2.1B). Guidance is required on the maximum number of applications of antibacterial-based handrubs/gels that can be used on physically clean hands before handwashing. If hands become 'sticky' because of a build-up of the product, they must be washed as normal using a proper hand hygiene technique.
- Alcohol-impregnated wipes used for cleaning surfaces are not effective in hand decontamination and therefore should not be used in place of handrubs/gels.
- Do not use scrub or use nail brushes because these can abrade the skin where micro-organisms can reside.
- Nails should be kept short and clean, using a blunt 'orange' stick, and kept free of nail art, permanent or temporary enhancements (false nails) or varnish.

TABLE 1.2.2 Levels of Hand Hygiene

	Level 1: Social	Level 2: Hygienic	Level 3: Surgical Scrub
Why?	To render the hands physically clean and to remove transient micro-organisms, picked up during social activities	In addition to level 1, to destroy micro-organisms and to provide residual effect during times when hygiene is particularly important in protecting yourself and others	In addition to level 2, to substantially reduce the numbers of resident micro-organisms that normally live on the skin during times when surgical procedures are being carried out
When?	Before: • Commencing/leaving work • Using computer keyboards • Eating or handling food or drinks • Preparing or giving medications • Direct patient contact where no exposure to blood or other bodily fluids or non-intact skin has occurred After: • Becoming visibly soiled • Visiting the toilet • Patient contact even where no exposure to blood or other bodily fluids, or non-intact skin has occurred • Using computer keyboard • Handling laundry, equipment or waste • Blowing, wiping or touching nose	Before: • Aseptic procedures • Contact with immunocompromised patients • Wearing gloves and carrying out minor surgical or routine dental procedures After: • Contact with blood, other bodily fluids, excretions, secretions, mucous membranes, non-intact skin, wound dressings, spore-forming organisms	Before: Surgical or invasive procedures, oral surgery, perio or implant surgery (specific policies and procedures on surgical preparation should be available at local level)
What hand hygiene to use?	Mild liquid soap – does not need to be antibacterial or antiseptic Antibacterial-based handrubs/gels can be used when hands have not been soiled Bar soap should not be used	An approved antibacterial hand cleanser (e.g. 2–4% chlorhexidine, 5–7.5% povidone iodine, 1% triclosan or plain soap from a dispenser) Antibacterial-based handrubs/gels can be used following handwashing (e.g. when performing aseptic techniques) to provide further cleansing and residual effect, and may be used with plain (liquid) soap where necessary	An approved antibacterial hand cleanser (e.g. chlorhexidine gluconate 4%, povidone iodine 7.5%) People who are sensitive to antiseptic cleaners can wash with an approved plain liquid soap followed by two applications of an antibacterial-based hand-rub/gel. Skin problems should be reported and discussed with a general practitioner or occupational health, and a local procedure followed
How long for?	10–15 seconds	15–30 seconds	2–3 minutes, ensuring all areas of hands and forearms are covered

Wash hands only when visibly soiled! Otherwise use handrub!

Wet hands with water

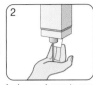
Apply enough soap to cover all hand surfaces

Rub hands palm to palm

Dispense a little of the handrub product (about 3ml) into cupped hand

Rub hands palm to palm

Right palm over left dorsum with interlaced fingers and vice versa

Palm to palm with fingers interlaced

Backs of fingers to opposing palms with fingers interlaced

Right palm over left dorsum with interlaced fingers and vice versa

Palm to palm with fingers interlaced

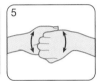
Backs of fingers to opposing palms with fingers interlaced

Rotational rubbing of left thumb clasped in right palm and vice versa

Rotational rubbing, backwards and forwards with clasped fingers of right hand in left palm and vice versa

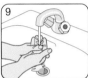
Rinse hands with water

Rotational rubbing of left thumb clasped in right palm and vice versa

Rotational rubbing, backwards and forwards with clasped fingers of right hand in left palm and vice versa

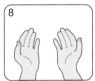
Hands are dry now and safe to use

Dry thoroughly with a single-use towel

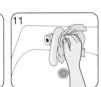
Use towel to turn off tap

...and your hands are safe

(A) Duration of the entire procedure: 20–30 seconds

(B) 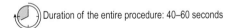 Duration of the entire procedure: 40–60 seconds

FIGURE 1.2.1
Techniques for (A) using handrub without water and (B) handwashing.

- Good-quality (soft) paper hand towels should be used after handwashing to avoid skin damage.
- Hand cream can be used after handwashing at the end of a session to avoid dryness. Cream should not be used under gloves since it may encourage the growth of micro-organisms.
- Foot- or sensor-operated waste bins should be used.

PERSONAL PROTECTIVE EQUIPMENT

As a dental nurse, you are required to wear personal protective equipment (PPE), as are other clinicians, when carrying out duties that may involve possible exposure to blood or other body fluids, or splashing from cleaning processes. PPE includes face and eye protection

25

(masks, protective eyewear), gloves and aprons. Clinical and decontamination clothing should not be worn outside the practice. Footwear should also be appropriate for a clinical environment and should protect against material or instruments that may accidentally fall on the feet, and should be stable and without heels.

- Face and eye protection – the face and eyes should be protected by a visor or face shield which are single use; they should be disposed of as clinical waste.
- Gloves
  - Clinical disposable gloves – to protect the hands from becoming contaminated, and prevent contact with chemicals. All clinical gloves are single use and should be discarded as clinical waste (see p. 39). Gloves must fit properly; powder-free latex gloves are used frequently although some users report allergies (see Subchapter 1.1, p. 8), when vinyl or nitrile gloves may be used instead.
  - Heavy-duty household gloves – these are used during cleaning instruments and equipment, and can be washed with detergent and hot water for re-use.
- Aprons – a disposable plastic apron should be worn during all decontamination procedures. Treat it as a single-use item and change it at the end of each procedure and dispose of as clinical waste (see p. 39).
- Clothing and footwear – you should wear a freshly laundered uniform each day. Machine washing the uniform with a suitable detergent at a minimum temperature of 65 °C will reduce microbial contamination. Short sleeves are recommended but nurses can protect their forearms and also comply with their religious guidance where relevant, by wearing long-cuffed gloves or disposable sleeves or disposable long-sleeved gowns.

PPE should be removed in the following order:

1. Gloves (ensuring they end up inside out)
2. Aprons – the neck straps can be broken and gathered together, touching the inside surfaces only
3. Face mask – the straps can be broken or lifted over the ears to avoid touching the outer surface
4. Eye protection – the outer surfaces should not be touched.

After removing PPE, wash your hands thoroughly.

SURFACE AND EQUIPMENT DECONTAMINATION

All dental practices should have a policy outlining cleaning schedules and maintenance of simple records on decontamination. Cleaning staff should also be briefed specifically on cleaning patient care areas and decontamination rooms.

ROLE OF THE DENTAL NURSE IN DECONTAMINATION

- *Between patients,* clean the work surfaces, the dental chair, dental light, dental unit, UV light, spittoons and aspirator (the treatment area). Surfaces can be effectively cleaned using commercial alcohol-based cleaning agents and wipes, or water with suitable detergents provided that the surface is then dried. Following initial deep cleaning of a surface, subsequent use of a wet or dry microfibre cloth can achieve satisfactory removal of infectious agents. Computer keyboards should be either washable or provided with covers that can be easily decontaminated.
- *At the end of each session,* clean the treatment area and adjacent areas (the taps, drainage points, splashbacks, cupboard doors and sinks) using disposable cloths or microfibre materials. Aspirators, drains and spittoons should be cleaned with a surfactant/detergent and a non-foaming disinfectant.

Wipe down the decontamination area after each decontamination cycle or after each patient.

INSTRUMENT DECONTAMINATION

Clinicians need to use sterile instruments, and they have three options:

- Use sterile single-use devices
- Use re-usable devices sterilised by a certified sterile services unit such as a hospital Central Sterile Supply Department (CSSD)
- Decontaminate and sterilise the devices themselves.

HTM 01-05 gives detailed guidance on infection control in the dental workplace following the essential principles for the effective prevention and control of HCAI defined in the 'Health and Social Care Act 2008: Code of Practice for the NHS on the prevention and control of healthcare associated infections and related guidance' (the HCAI Code of Practice).

HCAI CODE OF PRACTICE

- Requires that effective prevention and control of HCAI should be embedded in everyday practice.
- Establishes a duty to provide and maintain a clean and appropriate environment for healthcare.
- Notes that use of disposable equipment and instruments is one helpful and effective way to reduce the risk of infection.

FIND OUT MORE

Look out for a circular symbol showing a crossed out '2' – if an instrument or its packaging has this sign it means the material or instrument is for single use only. How many of these can you find in your practice?

HTM 01-05 provides guidance for decontamination of re-usable instruments in primary care dental services (general dental practices, salaried dental services and where primary care is delivered in **acute settings**). It outlines 'locally conducted decontamination procedures' – this means that both the instrument user and the person carrying out the decontamination are employees of the same organisation and work in the same or related premises. It is therefore intended to raise the quality of decontamination. The guidance principally covers two areas:

- Essential quality requirements
  - All primary care dentistry is required to be carried out at or above the 'essential quality requirements'
- Best practice
  - All dental practices need to demonstrate that they have assessed and, where possible, planned for the improvements necessary to implement best practice.

At present, not all practices will be (immediately) able to fully adopt best practice requirements but it should be implemented as far as possible.

Essential Quality Requirements

To achieve the essential requirements, a dental practice should have in place:

- A lead member of staff for infection control and decontamination
- An infection control policy, which includes requirements for instrument decontamination
- Procedures for managing single-use and re-usable instruments (segregation, disposal and re-processing)

Term to Learn
Acute settings: hospitals where patients are treated and cared for after surgery or a severe illness or injury; usually the care is provided by highly specialised healthcare professionals, including doctors and specialist nurses, using sophisticated medical equipment.

- Dedicated equipment for re-processing re-usable instruments
- A dedicated sink for handwashing and two dedicated sinks for decontamination (not used for handwashing)
- An **ultrasonic bath** (covered during use to restrict aerosols) or clear procedures for manual cleaning of instruments. (A **washer-disinfector** (see p. 31) enhances cleaning but is not an essential requirement)
- Schedule for instrument inspection to ensure they are free from contamination, salt deposits or marked discoloration
- Systems to ensure sterilised instruments are used within specified times:
  - Non-vacuum autoclaves/steam sterilisers (instruments sterilised in these are either stored in covered trays and used within that treatment session, or dried and packaged and used within 21 days)
  - Vacuum autoclaves (the instruments are packaged before being sterilised and should be used within 30 days)
- Decontamination procedures separated from clinical procedures by using either a designated room or a designated area within the surgery with a dirty to clean workflow (Figures 1.2.2 and 1.2.3). In other words, decontamination areas must be separate from clinical areas. (See below for more details)
- Decontamination equipment fit for purpose and validated, commissioned, maintained and periodically tested by a competent person
- Procedures for safe storage, preparation and use of decontamination materials and chemicals in line with COSHH (see Subchapter 1.1) requirements
- Storage area for instruments as far from the dental chair as reasonably practicable
- Arrangements for waste segregation and appropriate disposal

28

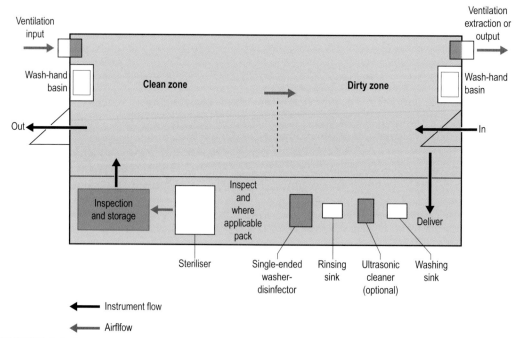

FIGURE 1.2.2

Example layout for single decontamination room. The single-ended washer-disinfector is the only item not part of the HTM 01–05 essential requirements. Where decontamination is done within the surgery, the decontamination area should be as far from the dental chair as possible. Procedures that could generate aerosols or splashing (manual washing, ultrasonic cleaners, decontamination) should never be carried out with the patient present. A dirty to clean workflow should be maintained so that the risk of used instruments coming into contact with decontaminated instruments is minimised and to enhance distinction between clean and dirty workflows. If there is no ultrasonic cleaner, the washing sink should be located near the rinsing sink to avoid handling problems. Alternatively, a double-bowl sink assembly can be installed that incorporates both sinks. (The number of washer-disinfectors and sterilisers could be increased if the practice requires this, depending on the number of patients, etc.).

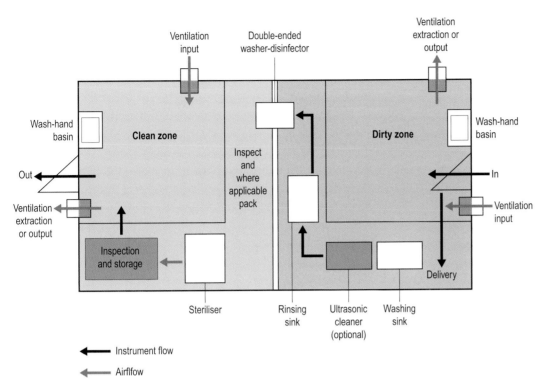

Instrument flow

Airflow

FIGURE 1.2.3

Example layout for two decontamination rooms. Contaminated instruments are received into the dirty zone. The washing and rinsing sinks or bowls should be installed adjacent to the receiving area. The cleaner should be adjacent to the rinsing sink/ bowl well away from the receiving area. For instruments to be inspected after cleaning and disinfection, a dedicated clean area of work surface with task lighting is needed. The steam steriliser should be situated well away from other activities, with a clean area furthest away for unloading, inspection and wrapping (where appropriate). A transfer hatch between the two rooms or the use of double-ended washer-disinfectors helps reduce the risks associated with manual handling. However, a single-ended washer-disinfector that has been validated will also satisfy the requirements of HTM 01-05. As for the single decontamination room, an ultrasonic cleaner is optional and if not installed the same alternatives may be followed.

- Training and immunisation facilities (against **hepatitis B** virus infection and tetanus if required) for staff involved with decontamination
- Audit procedures (annual) for infection control.

Box 1.2.2 summarises the *essential requirements* for dental practices with regard to infection control.

BOX 1.2.2 ESSENTIAL REQUIREMENTS FOR INFECTION CONTROL

Policies:

- For minimising the risk of transmission of blood-borne viruses (e.g. HIV, hepatitis viruses), including needlestick injuries
- For hand hygiene
- For decontamination and storage of dental instruments
- For clinical waste disposal
- For decontamination of new and re-usable instruments.

Procedures:

- For personal protective equipment use
- For cleaning, disinfection and sterilisation of dental instruments
- For use, storage and disposal of disinfectants within the practice
- For dealing with spillage
- For transfer of contaminated items from the treatment to decontamination area
- A documented training scheme with individual training records for all staff engaged in decontamination.

Best Practice Requirements

HTM 01-05 requirements for best practice include:

- A modern, validated washer-disinfector (p. 31) to remove the need for manual washing.
- Improved separation of decontamination processes by, for example, a separate decontamination room.
- Suitable instrument storage away from the surgery to reduce exposure to air and possible contamination (see p. 33).
- Robust systems to ensure sterilised instruments are used within the specified timescales outlined in essential requirements.
- A protocol for the safe transfer of contaminated items from the treatment room to the decontamination area, ensuring separation of contaminated and clean/sterile instruments. Containers for transporting instruments should be leak-proof, easy to clean, rigid and capable of being closed. They should be cleaned and dried after each use, or discarded.

Best practice suggests that decontamination/re-processing should take place in a separate room or rooms (Figure 1.2.2).

Hand Hygiene during Decontamination

Social hand hygiene (Table 1.2.2) is sufficient for decontamination processes, and will render hands physically clean, and should be practised:

- After washing instruments
- Before contact with sterilised instruments (wrapped and unwrapped)
- After cleaning decontamination equipment
- At completion of decontamination work.

The dedicated wash-hand basin should not have a plug or overflow and should not have the U-bend directly under the waste. The water mixer tap should be sensor- or lever-operated and should not discharge directly into the drain opening. Wall-mounted liquid handwash dispensers with disposable cartridges should be used.

A poster depicting a six- or eight-step method should be displayed above every clinical hand-wash basin in the practice.

FIND OUT MORE

Draw a diagram of the decontamination layout in your workplace. Is it similar to Figure 1.2.2 or 1.2.3?

Cleaning Instruments

Cleaning instruments before they are sterilised reduces the risk of transmission of infection. Wherever possible, this should be done using an automated and validated washer-disinfector rather than manually. The disinfection stage of a washer-disinfector renders instruments safe for handling and inspection. Manual cleaning should only be considered when the instrument manufacturer's instructions specify that it should not be cleaned in an automated device or when the washer-disinfector is unavailable and if it is carried out following an appropriate protocol.

KEY POINT Instruments should be cleaned as soon as possible after use and, where this is impossible, they should be immersed in water to prevent drying.

Where recommended by the manufacturer, instruments and equipment consisting of more than one component should be dismantled to allow each part to be cleaned. See also Chapter 12.

CLEANING USING A WASHER-DISINFECTOR

A washer-disinfector is a device that both cleans and disinfects instruments by application of heat rather than chemicals. To ensure effective cleaning, washer-disinfectors must be loaded correctly:

- Do not overload instrument carriers or overlap instruments
- Open instrument hinges and joints fully
- Attach instruments requiring irrigation (e.g. handpieces) to the irrigation system correctly.

A typical washer-disinfector cycle includes five stages:

1. Flush – gross decontamination using water at less than 45 °C
2. Wash – removes soil remnants using detergents
3. Rinse(s) – removes detergents using water
4. Thermal disinfection – temperature raised for required time: for example 80 °C for 10 minutes or 90 °C for one minute
5. Drying – heated air removes residual moisture.

Dental nurses should be trained in and follow the manufacturer's instructions when using the washer-disinfector, including understanding the recommendations for water quality/ type, detergents and/or disinfectants and instrument loading. You must also know how to perform daily tests to check that the machine is working properly. Records of training must be maintained. Washer-disinfector logbooks and records should include cycle parameters (temperature, time etc.) and details of routine testing and maintenance, and the records should be kept for at least two years.

CLEANING USING ULTRASONIC CLEANERS

Ultrasonic cleaners use energy from sound waves to loosen and shake off debris stuck to instruments, e.g. dried blood on a dental instrument. They can be effective, but they must be maintained according to the manufacturer's recommendations, with testing every three months to ensure they are fully functional.

After instruments have been used, you should immerse them in cold tap water (with detergent) to remove visible soiling, ensuring the joints and hinges are fully open and instruments disassembled as appropriate. Place the rinsed instruments in a suspended basket (avoid overloading and overlapping) and fully immerse in the cleaning solution of the ultrasonic cleaner. Then set the timer, close the lid and wait until the cycle is completed. Drain the basket of instruments and rinse the instruments using clean, fresh reverse osmosis (RO) or distilled water to remove residual soil and detergent. Instruments that will be wrapped and sterilised in a vacuum autoclave must be dried. You should change the ultrasonic cleaner water/fluid at the end of the clinical session or more frequently if it becomes heavily contaminated.

MANUAL CLEANING

Manual cleaning is difficult to validate as it is not possible to ensure that it is carried out effectively each time. It also carries a greater risk of inoculation injury. However, you can do manual cleaning when other methods are not appropriate or available.

Instrument Inspection

Always inspect instruments after cleaning and before sterilisation, for cleanliness and to check for wear or damage.

- Working parts should move freely. A non-oil-based lubricant may be needed.
- Edges of clamping instruments should not be rough or meet with overlap.
- Edges of scissors should meet to the tip and move freely across each other with no rough edges or overlap.
- All screws on jointed instruments should be tight.

If you find instruments to be faulty or damaged, take them out of use or report them to your supervisor. If they are to be sent for repair, you should decontaminate them and label as decontaminated before sending for repair.

Instrument Sterilisation

The essential requirements state that instruments should be re-processed using a validated decontamination process and a validated steam steriliser (autoclave) and, at the end of the re-processing cycle, the instruments should be sterile. Steam sterilisers are pressure vessels in which steam at high pressure is produced. This 'steam under pressure' will kill the harmful micro-organisms or their spores that may be attached to the instruments after clinical use. For moist heat sterilisation using steam as the sterilant, it is crucial that all the surfaces of the items requiring sterilisation are subjected to saturated steam:

- At a pre-determined temperature and pressure
- For a pre-determined period of time.

The steam steriliser if working properly will kill virtually all bacteria, viruses and fungi, but not prions.

There are three types of steam steriliser but two bench-top sterilisers are commonly used (Table 1.2.3). Bench-top steam sterilisers are used to sterilise re-usable invasive medical devices (RIMDs) and are considered medical devices in this capacity. They are regulated as class IIa medical devices in accordance with the Medical Devices Directive 93/42/EEC and must bear a CE mark.

- *Before use each day*: You should clean the rubber door seal of the steam steriliser with a clean, damp, non-linting cloth; check the chamber and shelves for cleanliness and debris; and fill the reservoir with fresh distilled or RO water.

32

TABLE 1.2.3 Steam Sterilisers

Class	Type	Use	Designed for Decontaminating	Comments
N	Non-vacuum steam sterilisers	Passive displacement of air with steam	Unwrapped, non-hollow and non-air retentive instruments such as probes, mirrors or elevators. They are *not* capable of sterilising porous devices, devices that are hollow, have lumen or are pre-wrapped	Unwrapped sterilised instruments are intended for immediate use or for non-sterile storage, transportation or application. Instruments risk becoming contaminated once the steriliser is opened. You can wrap dried instruments only after sterilisation using sealed view packs. If you need to store trays of instruments, the entire tray should be placed in a sealed pack. Instruments can be stored for up to 21 days. Alternatively, instruments can be covered and used within the current session
B	Vacuum steam sterilisers	A vacuum created before steam is introduced into the chamber allows fast and more positive heat to penetrate the entire steriliser load	Hollow, air retentive and packaged loads such as aspirators	Requires a vacuum or 'leak rate test', in addition to an air removal and steam penetration test (Bowie-Dick test) each day. Dried instruments can be pre-wrapped. Once sterilised, you may store the instruments for up to 30 days.

- *After final use of the day*: Drain the chamber, clean and dry and leave the door open. Carry out the daily tests and housekeeping tasks and record the results in the logbook. Daily tests include an automatic control test (all small sterilisers) and a steam penetration test e.g. Helix or Bowie-Dick test (vacuum sterilisers only).

> **KEY POINT** A steriliser that fails to meet any of the test requirements should be withdrawn from service and advice sought from the manufacturer and/or maintenance contractor.

FIND OUT MORE

Which kind of daily tests are carried out on the steam sterilisers in your workplace?

Causes of Failure of Attempted Sterilisation Using a Steam Steriliser

- Use of the wrong type of steriliser.
- Use of the wrong type of steriliser cycle.
- Failure to follow manufacturer's instructions.
- Failure to properly install, calibrate and validate steriliser.
- Ineffective cleaning of devices to be sterilised.
- Inappropriate wrapping or packaging of devices.
- Inappropriate loading of steriliser.
- Supply of poor quality water or facilities.
- Inadequate management of training, validation, calibration, use, maintenance, servicing or audit.

You should never use the following appliances for sterilising instruments:

- Microwave ovens
- Pressure cookers
- Incubators
- Ultraviolet cabinets
- Boiling water units
- Ultrasonic cleaners and similar appliances.

Remember: These appliances will not effectively sterilise instruments and consequently may spread infectious diseases.

Instrument Storage

Instruments must be protected against recontamination by wrapping or storing in a covered container. The steam steriliser used, however, affects the wrapping and storing options (Table 1.2.3).

Disposable non-linting cloths should be used to dry instruments and then disposed of after each sterilisation load. Storage systems must ensure easy identification of instruments and monitoring of storage times to ensure recommended intervals are not exceeded. The area where sterilised instruments are packaged for storage should be wiped clean with detergent and alcohol wipes at the start of each session.

Instruments should be stored in a dedicated secure, dry and cool area away from direct sunlight. Best practice requires instruments to be stored in a separate environment.

Wherever possible, air flow should be from clean to dirty areas. Where the storage area is in the surgery, it is an essential requirement that it should be as far from the dental chair as reasonably practicable.

33

> ## BOX 1.2.3 STAGES IN DECONTAMINATION OF INSTRUMENTS (SOURCE HTM 01-05)
>
> Collect the instruments.
> ↓
> Clean the instruments:
> - With a washer-disinfector (WD)
> - With or without an ultrasonic cleaner
> - Manually.
> ↓
> Disinfect if used a WD.
> ↓
> Inspect the instruments. Repeat cleaning if required.
> ↓
> Steam sterilisation and storage:
> - Package the instruments and steam sterilise in a vacuum steriliser (type B or S). Store for maximum 30 days
> - Steam sterilise unwrapped instruments in type N steriliser. Package the instruments and store for maximum 21 days.
> ↓
> Use the instrument.
> ↓
> Start again by collecting the instruments.

Before use, check the instrument packaging is intact; the sterilisation indicator confirms the pack has been sterilised (if a type B steam steriliser has been used) and visible contamination is absent.

Box 1.2.3 gives an overview of the various stages in the process of decontamination following HTM best practice recommendations.

DECONTAMINATING DENTAL IMPRESSIONS AND APPLIANCES

Immediately after removal from the mouth, rinse the impression or appliance under cool running tap water until it is visibly clean.

Prostheses and devices for oral use should be disinfected according to the manufacturer's instructions. You will need to use specific cleaning materials noted in the CE marking instructions. After disinfection, the device should again be thoroughly washed in clean cool running tap water. This process should occur before any device is placed in a patient's mouth.

If the device is to be returned to a supplier/laboratory or to be sent out of the practice for some other reason, affix a label to the package to indicate that a decontamination process has been used.

DENTAL WATER SUPPLY

Legislation applying to the dental water supply includes:

- Water Supply (Water Fittings) Regulations 1999
- Water Supply (Water Quality) Regulations 2000

Drinking water (potable water) must meet a certain standard with respect to concentrations of contaminants and chemicals.

Dental Unit Water Lines

Without regular maintenance, the quality of water delivered by dental units would not meet the standard

> **KEY POINT** During surgical procedures that require irrigation, sterile water or sterile isotonic saline from a separate single-use source must be used.

for drinking water. This water is unsuitable for **irrigating** surgical wounds – in such instances, sterile water or sterile isotonic saline from a separate single-use source must be used.

Although there is no evidence that water from dental unit water lines is otherwise harmful to patients, the United States Centers for Disease Control and Prevention (CDC) has stated that 'Exposing patients or dental health care staff to water of uncertain microbiological quality, despite the lack of documented adverse health effects, is inconsistent with generally accepted infection control principles.'

Risks Associated with Dental Unit Water Lines

The small diameter of dental unit water lines, combined with their design and flow rate, enables bacteria and other micro-organisms to form a biofilm, which coats the inside of the tubing. As water then travels through the waterlines micro-organisms may slough off, contaminating the water. Various micro-organisms can thus be found in some dental water lines.

The bacterium *Legionella pneumophila* and related bacteria are not only found naturally in rivers, lakes and reservoirs, usually in low numbers, but may also be found in purpose-built water systems, including dental unit water lines. Under favourable conditions *Legionella* may grow and, occasionally and chiefly in people susceptible because of older age, illness, immunosuppression (see Chapter 5), smoking, it can cause a potentially fatal lung infection (Legionnaires' disease).

Legionnaires' disease has been reported from hotels, spas, etc. but despite evidence of infection in some dental hospitals' water lines, disease has not been reported to arise from dental sources. Nevertheless, dental practices, through their registered manager, should seek advice for guidance on dental unit water lines. Primary care trusts and representatives from professional organisations (such as the Legionella Control Association) may recommend a suitable contractor.

No currently available single method or device will completely eliminate such bio-contamination of dental unit water lines, or exclude the risk of cross-infection. Thus to reduce the risk of contamination, a combination of methods should be used.

> **Term to Learn**
> **Irrigation:** the process of 'washing' a surgical wound or even a tooth cavity or root canal. This may be done while the clinician is drilling to ensure a clear field of work or in between to wash out the debris.

> ## BEST PRACTICE GUIDELINES ON THE CONTROL OF *LEGIONELLA*
>
> The Health and Safety Commission's Approved Code of Practice L8 'Legionnaires' disease – the control of Legionella bacteria in water systems. Approved Code of Practice & Guidance' gives practical advice on how to comply with UK health and safety law with respect to the control of *Legionella* bacteria. Guidance is also available from the Department of Health's Technical Memorandum 04-01, 'The control of *Legionella*, hygiene, 'safe' hot water, cold water and drinking water systems'.
>
> If a healthcare organisation, such as a dental practice, were to be prosecuted for a breach of health and safety law, and it is held that it did not follow the relevant provisions of the code L8, the organisation would need to demonstrate that it had complied with the law in some other way, or a court would find it at fault. Guidance from L8 includes:
>
> 'Water systems at risk of harbouring *Legionella*, particularly those used with the patient, should be drained down at least at the end of each working day. Where manufacturers provide protocols for daily cleaning, these should be applied.
>
> Remove any self-contained water bottles (bottled water system), flush with distilled or RO water and leave them open to the air for drying overnight. The bottles should be stored inverted. Where visual contamination is present, flushing with a suitable disinfectant followed by thorough washing is necessary. The manufacturer's instructions will specify the disinfectant to be used and may also require the continuous presence of antimicrobial agents to prevent the build-up of biofilms. Self-contained water supplies used for dental care systems should use freshly distilled or RO water. (If self-contained water bottles are not used, a type A air gap should separate the dental unit water lines from the mains water supply.)'

Dental unit water lines should be flushed for at least two minutes at the beginning and end of the day and after any significant period when they have not been used (e.g. after lunch breaks), and for at least 20–30 seconds between patients. Care should be taken to minimise the occurrence of splashing and aerosol formation.

Dental unit water lines should be periodically disinfected. Sodium hypochlorite and isopropanol are effective in biofilm removal and reduction of microbacterial contamination, but should only be used where recommended by the manufacturer. Following this the dental unit water lines should be carefully flushed before being returned to clinical use. In all cases, the manufacturer's instructions should be consulted.

Dental equipment requiring protection against backflow should have anti-retraction valves incorporated on all handpieces or waterlines. Responsible persons should ensure these are fitted where required. They must be regularly monitored and maintained.

Dental equipment requiring backflow protection includes:

- Dental spittoons
- **3-in-1 syringes**
- Ultrasonic scalers
- Wet-line suction apparatus
- Self-filling automatic X-ray processors (where still used).

> **Term to Learn**
> **3-in-1 syringe:** an attachment on the dental unit that is used to spray water, air or a combination of air and water in the mouth.

IDENTIFY AND LEARN

Identify a 3-in-1 syringe and wet-line suction apparatus in your workplace.

Where in-line filters are used, these will require treatment using an appropriate cleansing solution at intervals recommended by the manufacturer – but always at the end of each session. This step should be performed after first flushing the dental unit water line. If the line has disposable filters, they should be replaced daily.

Water Supply Hygiene

After any installation work, all piping, fittings and associated services used for the conveyance of water for domestic purposes must be disinfected before being brought into use. The method generally used for disinfection is chlorination carried out in accordance with **British Standard** (BS) EN 806-2:2005, BS EN 806-3:2006 and BS 6700:2006 (see also HTM 04-01 Part A Chapter 17; www.wales.nhs.uk/sites3/docmetadata .cfm?orgid=254&id=66958) and under the direct supervision of a nominated person.

To reduce the risk of outbreaks of disease related to treated water supplies, the design should eliminate:

- Direct contact with the internal parts of water pipes and structures by people, animals or birds (e.g. ensure covers are in place on storage tanks/cisterns)
- Backflow (back-siphonage) of contaminated water into systems conveying potable water (mains and storage structures).

> **Term to Learn**
> **British Standards:** the standards set by the British Standards Institute. The BSI maintains standards for almost any thing that is used or manufactured in the UK.

Water Treatment

In a properly installed and commissioned hot water system, it should be possible to maintain a temperature of at least 55 °C at the furthest draw-off point in the circulating system, and 50 °C in the circulating system's return connection to the calorifier. Where

36

automatic equipment is used for disinfection, it should indicate any change in the amount or concentration of material injected into the water so that immediate action can be taken. A regular flushing programme for all outlets should also be implemented. The continuous chlorination of hot and cold water service systems to control the growth of *Legionella* is not generally recommended. Treatment using chlorine dioxide or copper/silver ionisation can be used. Advice should be sought from the primary care trust's responsible person (water).

Drinking water

If separate drinking water supplies are provided, reference should be made to HTM 04-01.

The registered manager should ensure that arrangements are in place such that a dental practice is consistently compliant with these regulations. Registration with the Legionella Control Association or other recognised body is recommended.

Blood and Body Fluid Spillages

If blood or a body fluid is spilled – either from a container or as a result of an operative procedure – the spillage should be dealt with as soon as possible. The spilled liquid should be completely covered with disposable towels (which are then treated with 10 000 ppm sodium hypochlorite solution or with sodium dichloroisocyanurate granules). At least five minutes must elapse before the towels, etc. are cleared and disposed of as clinical waste.

The dental nurse who deals with the spillage must wear appropriate PPE, including household gloves, protective eyewear and a disposable apron. In the case of an extensive floor spillage, waterproof protective footwear must be worn.

Good ventilation in the area is essential.

BIOPSY SPECIMENS SENT THROUGH THE POST

A dental practice may use Royal Mail to send **non-fixed specimens** to pathology laboratories for diagnostic opinion or tests. If this is the case, it must comply with the UN 602 packaging requirements. The 602 packaging requirements ensure that strict performance tests (including drop and puncture tests) have been met. In practice this means:

- The outer shipping package must bear the UN packaging specification marking. Only first class letter post, special delivery or data post services must be used. Parcel Post must not be used
- Every pathological specimen must be enclosed in a primary container that is watertight and leak-proof
- The primary container must be wrapped in sufficient absorbent material to absorb all fluid in case of breakage
- The primary container should then be protected by placing it in a second durable watertight, leak-proof container
- Several wrapped primary containers may be placed in one secondary container provided sufficient additional absorbent material is used to cushion the primary containers
- Finally, the secondary container should be placed in an outer shipping package which protects it and its contents from physical damage and water while in transit
- The shipping package must be conspicuously labelled 'PACKED IN COMPLIANCE WITH THE POST OFFICE INLAND LETTER POST SCHEME'
- The sender must also sign and date the package in the space provided
- Information concerning the sample, such as data forms, letters and descriptive information should be taped to the outside of the secondary container
- A clinician sending a pathological specimen through the post without complying with the above requirements may be liable to prosecution.

Fixed specimens should be enclosed in a primary container and sealed securely. Following this:

Term to Learn
Biopsy: the procedure involving removal of a small sample of tissue from a living person for the purpose of making a diagnosis. The sample is also called a specimen and it is examined by a specialist doctor (pathologist or histopathologist).

Terms to Learn
Non-fixed specimens: specimens that are simply prepared for examining under a microscope as opposed to fixed specimens.
Fixed specimens: specimens that have been immersed in a solution called a fixative to denature the proteins. This is part of an elaborate process to produce high-quality specimens for examination by the pathologist.

37

- The container must be wrapped in sufficient absorbent material to absorb all leakage if it is damaged, and then sealed in a leak-proof plastic bag
- The specimen should be placed in a padded bag and labelled 'PATHOLOGICAL SPECIMEN – FRAGILE WITH CARE'
- The bag must show the name and address of the sender to be contacted in case of damage or leakage.

WASTE MANAGEMENT

Legislation applying:

- Hazardous Waste (England and Wales) Regulations 2005
- List of Wastes Regulations 2005

Laws in Other Parts of the UK

Dental practices have a duty of care to ensure all healthcare waste is managed and disposed of in accordance with current waste regulations (Box 1.2.4). Dental healthcare waste can consist of:

- Hazardous waste (see next section)
- Non-hazardous waste (waste which is not classified as hazardous)
- Trade waste (any waste other than domestic waste).

The current colour coding system for waste disposal is shown in Table 1.2.4.

PPE for Waste Handling

Protective clothing (heavy-duty gloves, aprons) should be worn for the handling and movement of clinical and hazardous waste when deemed necessary by the dental practice's COSHH assessment, and if spillages occur.

Hazardous Waste

Hazardous waste is any waste listed as hazardous in the List of Wastes (England) Regulations 2005 or equivalent legislation in Northern Ireland, Scotland or Wales. Clinical waste should all be disposed of as hazardous waste. Clinical waste is defined as:

Any waste which consists wholly or partly of human or animal tissue, blood or other bodily fluids, excretions, drugs or other pharmaceutical products, swabs or dressings, syringes, needles or other sharp instruments, being waste which unless rendered safe may prove hazardous to any person coming into contact with it.

38

BOX 1.2.4 HEALTHCARE WASTE POLICY

- A policy is required that identifies who is responsible for healthcare waste and how it should be managed.
- The policy should also identify each waste stream as hazardous, non-hazardous or offensive.
- How the waste is segregated, stored and handled should be documented along with the practice arrangements for collection and record keeping.

TABLE 1.2.4 Waste Segregation and Classification

Container Type	Example Waste Description	Contents	Classification and EWC Codes	Disposal
Sharps box (yellow lid) (Note: orange lids must not be used)	Clinical waste: mixed sharps and pharmaceutical waste for incineration only	Hypodermic needles, syringes and syringe barrels including those contaminated with medicines (not cytotoxic and cytostatic) Used medicine vials Other sharp instruments or items including teeth without amalgam fillings	18 01 03* & 18 01 09 Hazardous	Incineration only
Soft clinical wastes (orange bag)	Clinical waste: infectious, suitable for alternative treatment	Body-fluid-contaminated dressings, PPE and swabs, and other waste that may present a risk of infection **NO** medicinally, chemically or amalgam contaminated wastes	18 01 03* Hazardous	Alternative treatment or incineration
Medicines (rigid leak proof container)	Non-cytotoxic and cytostatic medicines, clinical waste, for incineration only	Non-cytotoxic and cytostatic medicines including used and out-of-date stock	18 01 09 Non-hazardous	Incineration only
Offensive or hygiene wastes	Offensive/hygiene waste from dental care suitable for landfill	Gowns, gloves, tissues, X-ray film and other items from dental care which are not contaminated with bodily fluids, medicines, chemicals or amalgam	Non-hazardous 18 01 04	Landfill
	Municipal offensive/ hygiene waste suitable for landfill	Hygiene waste from toilets only	Non-hazardous 20 01 99	
Amalgam waste	Dental amalgam: infectious, clinical waste, for recovery	Teeth with amalgam fillings	Hazardous 18 01 10*	Metal recovery
	Dental amalgam and mercury: non-infectious, for recovery	Dental amalgam and mercury including spent and out-of-date capsules, excess mixed amalgam, and contents of amalgam separators		
X-ray fixer (container type not specified)	Photographic fixer	Waste photographic fixer from X-ray (must be kept separate from developer)	Hazardous 09 01 01*	Recovery (various)
X-ray developer (container type not specified)	Photographic developer	Waste photographic developer from X-ray (must be kept separate from fixer)	Hazardous 09 01 04*	
Lead foils (container type not specified)	X-ray lead foils from dentistry	Lead foils from X-ray film packaging	Hazardous 15 01 04	
Municipal waste	Mixed municipal waste	Domestic type refuse: food packaging, paper/magazines that cannot be recycled, paper towels (no hazardous wastes)	Non-hazardous 20 03 01	Landfill or municipal waste incinerator

Term to Learn
Incineration: the process by which substances are burned completely to reduce them to ash.

SHARPS WASTE

Sharps waste (items that could cause cuts or puncture/inoculation/needlestick wounds) should be collected in yellow-lidded receptacles (Table 1.2.4), which require disposal by **incineration**. Sharps include needles, syringes with needles attached, broken glass ampoules, scalpels and other blades and some teeth (provided no amalgam is present, see below).

LOCAL ANAESTHETIC CARTRIDGES

Local anaesthetic cartridges are hazardous waste and always disposed of via the sharps container.

Term to Learn
Local anaesthetic: a substance that is used to block the sensation of pain in a small area of the body, e.g. a patch of skin or just one quadrant of the mouth. It may be a gel that is just rubbed gently into the area to be anaesthetised or it may be given as an injection.

DENTAL AMALGAM

Dental amalgam is a tooth-filling material that contains an alloy of silver and mercury. Waste dental amalgam is classified as hazardous/special waste. It must be stored, transported and disposed of as hazardous/special waste to make sure there is no risk to human health or the environment. Waste dental amalgam in any form and materials contaminated with amalgam include:

- Unwanted amalgam
- Old amalgam fillings
- Teeth with amalgam fillings
- Grindings
- Surplus amalgam that cannot be re-used
- Residues containing amalgam, e.g. from separators (see below)
- Packaging such as capsules containing residues.

40

KEY POINT Extracted teeth *without* amalgam should be disposed of in the dental sharps box. Never put amalgam-filled extracted teeth in the sharps container. This is because amalgam must not be incinerated. But you can dispose of these teeth with waste amalgam, provided care is taken (as the teeth will be contaminated with blood, they must first be decontaminated).

Waste collection agencies often provide special containers for the disposal of amalgam-filled teeth (Table 1.2.4). It is also possible to send decontaminated amalgam-filled teeth (and non-filled teeth) through the post to dental schools for teaching and research purposes but the patient's consent must be obtained first (and recorded in the clinical records). It is important to ensure that extracted teeth sent through the post are packaged securely to avoid the package being split open during transit. Some dental schools provide a container and disinfectant suitable for decontamination, storage and transport.

Waste amalgam must be stored in an air-tight container (often in old X-ray fixer) until collected. The waste is collected by a suitably licensed or permitted waste management collector with facilities where the waste undergoes a mercury recovery process prior to final disposal.

Particles of amalgam produced during the cleaning, drilling and filling of teeth must be prevented from exiting with the waste water. An amalgam separator is needed to remove particles of amalgam from waste water, so they can be disposed of as hazardous waste. Separators must be positioned to protect all routes by which amalgam may enter the drains and must meet the requirements of British Standard dental equipment – amalgam separators (BS EN ISO 11143:2000). Simple filters and gauze material do not comply with the current legislation.

KEY POINT Dental amalgam must be treated using a mercury recovery process before final disposal.

LEAD FOILS

The lead foil present in X-ray films (see Chapter 14) is also hazardous waste. (Any packaging containing residues of, or contaminated by, dangerous substances is classified as hazardous waste.)

X-RAY FIXER AND DEVELOPER SOLUTIONS

Waste X-ray fixer and developer solutions (see Chapter 14) are also classified as hazardous. They should be collected by a suitably licensed company or waste facility for material recovery. If recovery is not appropriate, the fixer and developer solution is incinerated at suitably licensed or permitted facilities.

DENTAL MATERIALS, CHEMICALS AND DRUGS

Dental materials, chemicals and drugs should never be disposed of down the sink or drains. Expired emergency drugs are best taken to a pharmacy for disposal.

Waste Storage and Collection

Healthcare waste should be collected at regular intervals to reduce build-up on the premises. If to be stored, the storage must be secure and not accessible to interference. If patients are treated in their home, any waste produced is considered to be healthcare waste of the dental professional. If hazardous, the waste should be taken back to the practice for appropriate disposal. Healthcare waste should not however, be moved between dental practices.

For radiographic developer and fixer solutions, dental amalgam and waste containing drugs, the practice should have collection containers supplied by the licensed waste collection companies (Table 1.2.4). Waste radiographic developer and fixer solutions should be stored in leak-proof containers. White rigid containers with a mercury suppressant are preferred for dental amalgam waste storage.

Waste Disposal Documentation

A key element of the dental nurse's duty of care is keeping track of waste. The holder of waste is responsible for:

- Taking adequate steps to ensure that waste is managed safely and kept secure
- Transferring it only to an authorised or exempt person.

HAZARDOUS WASTE CONSIGNMENT NOTE

Before the waste is removed from premises on the collection route, the dental practice (as producers of the waste) is responsible for filling in the notification details and the description of the waste in the 'waste consignment note' and signing the note. The carrier may obtain these details from the dental nurse and complete them on the nurse's behalf, enabling the carrier to take appropriate measures to ensure wastes are packaged, labelled and handled correctly, and that the consignee (the person who receives the waste for final disposal) is able to take it. In each case however, the dental practice must ensure that the carrier has completed the note correctly (notification and waste details) and that the carrier is registered to collect such waste. The dental practice responsibility also includes declaring that the waste is packaged and labelled correctly.

An 'annual transfer note' may be used to cover all the movements of regular consignments of the same waste, between the same parties.

A consignment note must state:

- The quantity of waste transferred, by weight where possible
- How it is packed
- The type of container
- A description of the waste.

> ### BOX 1.2.5 EUROPEAN WASTE CATALOGUE (EWC) CODES
>
> Code description (*denotes a hazardous waste):
> - 09 01 03* Solvent-based developer solutions
> - 09 01 04* Fixer solutions
> - 15 01 10* Packaging containing residues of or contaminated by dangerous substances (e.g. lead foil)
> - 18 01 01 Sharps (except 18 01 03)
> - 18 01 02 Body parts and organs including blood bags and blood preserves (except 18 01 03)
> - 18 01 03* Clinical waste
> - 18 01 04 Offensive waste
> - 18 01 08* Cytotoxic and cytostatic medicines
> - 18 01 09 Medicines other than those mentioned in 18 01 08
> - 18 01 10* Dental amalgam waste

- The description of the waste must provide enough information to enable subsequent holders to avoid mismanaging the waste and should include:
  - The European Waste Catalogue (EWC) code (Box 1.2.5)
  - The type of premises or business from which the waste comes
  - The name of the substance or substances
  - The process that produced the waste
  - A chemical and physical analysis.

Any special problems:

- Any special containment requirements
- Type of container required, and material the container is made of
- Can it be safely mixed with other wastes or are there wastes with which it should not be mixed
- Can it be safely crushed and transferred from one vehicle to another
- Can it be safely incinerated or does it require specific minimum temperatures or combustion times
- Can it be disposed of safely to landfill with other waste
- Is it likely to change physical state during storage or transport
- Any information, advice or instructions about the handling, recovery or disposal of the waste by the waste regulators or suppliers etc.
- Details of problems previously encountered with the waste
- Changes to the description since the previous load
- Anything unusual about the waste that may pose a problem.

GOOD PRACTICE POINTS: WASTE MANAGEMENT

- Label drums and containers with the description of the waste.
- Copies of waste consignment notes should be retained by all parties for a minimum of two years.
- If you are aware of any particular handling issues with the waste you should inform either your supervisor or the carrier about them.

Usually the carrier will be collecting more than one consignment of waste from different premises. If this is the case then a multiple collection consignment note will be used. After the carrier has signed the annex, they need to give the practice a copy of the annex and a copy of the multiple collection consignment note for them to keep for three years. See HTA 01-05 for examples of consignment notes (producer's copy).

Hazardous waste collection companies are entitled to pass on a consignment note fee each time hazardous waste is collected.

HAZARDOUS WASTE RETURNS

The waste collection company is also required to send the dental practice each quarter year a return which is a record of what has happened to the waste, and the return should be kept with other waste records.

The return may be provided as:

- A form

or

- A copy of the consignee's copy of each consignment note, together with a description (or confirmation) of the method of disposal or recovery applied to the waste.

The return contains the information on the quantity, nature, origin, destination, frequency of collection, mode of transport, waste carrier and the disposal or recovery operation applied, of the waste received, as required by the regulations.

If the dental practice does not have these returns the records will be incomplete. Where the waste contractor has not provided returns, request them in writing from the waste contractor (see below). If this is unsuccessful consider making alternative arrangements for waste until the waste contractor complies with the law, and pass their details to the Environment Agency.

WASTE REGISTRATION WITH THE ENVIRONMENT AGENCY

Practices can register via the Environment Agency website (www.environment-agency.gov.uk). However, not all dental practices need to do this: they are exempt from notifying the Environment Agency as long as the total amount of hazardous waste produced in any 12-month period is less than 200 kg. There is no limit on the number of consignments that can be made from the premises under the registration exemption.

In cases where a practice owner has first considered that less than 200 kg of hazardous waste (such as developer and fixer solution, dental amalgam, etc.) would be produced from the practice, but later anticipates this limit will be exceeded, they must notify the agency before the limit is exceeded.

COSHH regulations (see Subchapter 1.1) are also applicable to dental healthcare waste. To comply with the regulations, clinicians must, among other things:

- Assess the risks to employees and others from healthcare waste
- Make arrangements for renewing the assessment as and when necessary
- Aim to eliminate or prevent these risks; if this is not possible, adequately control the risks
- Provide suitable and sufficient information, instruction and training for employees about the identified risk and controls
- Offer immunisation where appropriate.

Training in Waste Management

All staff who work with dental waste need to be adequately trained. Training needs vary depending on the job and on the individual. All dental staff involved in handling healthcare waste need training, information and instruction in:

- The risks associated with healthcare waste, its segregation, handling, storage and collection
- Personal hygiene
- Any procedures which apply to their particular type of work
- Procedures for dealing with spillages and accidents
- Emergency procedures
- The appropriate use of personal protective equipment (PPE).

43

> ## BOX 1.2.6 DEALING WITH MERCURY SPILLAGES
>
> Use a *mercury spillage kit*. This should include:
>
> - Disposable plastic gloves
> - Paper towels
> - Bulb aspirator for the collection of large drops of mercury
> - Vapour mask
> - Suitable container fitted with a seal
> - Mercury absorbent paste (equal parts of calcium hydroxide, flowers of sulphur and water).
>
> Steps to clear a mercury spillage:
>
> 1. Combine the droplets of mercury if possible.
> 2. Pick up as much mercury as you can using the syringe (never use a vacuum cleaner).
> 3. Apply the absorbant to the affected area.
> 4. Contain the waste mercury in the clearly labelled plastic container with a lid.
> 5. Ventilate the room well.
> 6. Send the waste mercury for reclaiming or disposal as toxic waste.
>
> In the case of larger spillages, a paste of calcium hydroxide or flowers of sulphur should be painted around and over the spillage, and then collected in disposable paper towels (wearing gloves).

Information should be provided by the employer to reflect the outcomes of the COSHH assessment and should:

- Be written in a way which can be understood by those who need to follow them, including those who may not have a good command of English
- Take account of different levels of training, knowledge and experience
- Be up to date
- Be available to all staff including part time, shift, temporary, agency and contract staff.

KEY POINT Never use a vacuum cleaner or aspiration unit to clean a mercury spillage, as this will vent mercury vapour into the atmosphere.

Mercury Spillages

Clinicians who use mercury should carry out a risk assessment for dealing with mercury spillages and produce written procedures.

If there is mercury spillage, you must report the incident to a clinician and follow the steps outlined in Box 1.2.6

Term to Learn
Sero-convert: when a person becomes infected by a blood-borne pathogen so that the blood is now positive for the disease on testing.

IMMUNISATION

Employees handling clinical waste who are not vaccinated against hepatitis B should be offered immunisation without charge. Staff must be informed of the benefits (e.g. protection against serious illness, protection against spreading illness) and drawbacks (e.g. reactions to the vaccine) of vaccination. Employers need to establish arrangements for dealing with staff who decline to accept the immunisation offered and those who do not **sero-convert**.

CHAPTER 2

Medical Emergencies and First Aid in the Dental Surgery

CHAPTER POINTS
- This chapter covers the requirements of the NEBDN syllabus Section 2: Emergencies in the dental surgery.

INTRODUCTION

A medical emergency is an injury or illness that poses an immediate threat to a person's life or long-term health. Box 2.1 lists the warning signs of a medical emergency that you may encounter as a dental nurse.

Emergencies are best prevented where possible. Since emergencies are more likely to occur in people with existing medical problems, the clinician will take a medical history so that they are as forewarned as possible.

RISK ASSESSMENT

Healthcare aims to improve the health of patients but can itself carry risks, so the first principle must be to do no harm ('primum non nocere' – from the Latin). Dentists and dental nurses can be involved in using local anaesthesia (LA) and conscious sedation, procedures that are safer than general anaesthesia (GA), which is now only carried out in hospitals with critical care facilities. Most dental procedures are safe, although surgical procedures may be less safe. Patients with medical problems are generally more likely to have complications, including emergencies, than are healthy individuals. Thus a **non-invasive procedure** such as applying a fissure sealant on a healthy child, is likely to be far safer than, for example, a surgical operation in an older person with a heart by-pass who is being treated with anticoagulants (Box 2.2).

The taking of a medical history aims to elicit such risks, following which steps are then taken to reduce the risks (Table 2.1).

MEDICAL HISTORY

The relevant medical history (RMH) taken by the clinician includes any past medical and surgical problems. Patients are also asked if they carry a medical warning card or device.

Term to Learn
Non-invasive procedure: a procedure, usually an investigation that aids in the diagnosis of a disease, in which no instrument enters the body tissues.

BOX 2.1 WARNING SIGNS OF A MEDICAL EMERGENCY

- Change in mental status (e.g. unusual behaviour, confusion, difficulty arousing, aggression, collapse).
- Chest pain.
- Continuous bleeding.
- Coughing up or vomiting blood.
- Difficulty breathing, shortness of breath or choking.
- Fainting or loss of consciousness.
- Severe or persistent vomiting.
- Sudden dizziness, weakness or change in vision.
- Sudden, severe pain anywhere in the body.

BOX 2.2 FACTORS INFLUENCING THE EFFECT OF HEALTHCARE PROCEDURES ON A PATIENT (THE OUTCOME)

- Health of patient.
- Type of procedure.
- Duration of procedure.
- Degree of trauma and stress.
- Degree of urgency of procedure.
- Skill and experience of operator.
- Skill and experience of anaesthetist/sedationist.

TABLE 2.1 Operative Risk Assessment and Management

Risks Increased by	Risks Reduced by
Increasing age	Planning treatment properly
Medical treatments	Non-invasive procedures
Surgical treatments	Monitoring
Lengthy dental procedures	Reassurance
Drug use – medication or recreational	

Term to Learn
Warfarin: a drug used for blood thinning (an anti-coagulant).

Careful note should be taken of it, particularly in respect of corticosteroid or **warfarin** use, a bleeding disorder or diabetes. It is far more helpful to be aware of a medical condition before undertaking dental treatment for a patient than trying to find out that history during an emergency. For example, managing a fit in a known epileptic person is far easier and less stressful for staff than managing a fit in a person not known to be epileptic. In the latter situation, there can be considerable uncertainty about what could be causing the problem and what is happening.

The relevance of many common medical conditions is discussed in Chapter 17. An easy to recall alphabetical list for the RMH is shown in Table 2.2.

FIND OUT MORE

What are the oral complications of Crohn's disease and coeliac disease (mentioned in Table 2.2)?

TABLE 2.2 Relevance of Medical History to Dentistry

Condition	Relevance in Dentistry
Allergies	These range in severity from a localised rash to collapse from anaphylaxis. Common allergies are to LIED (see p. 7). Anaesthetics, analgesics (e.g. aspirin or codeine) and antibiotics (e.g. penicillin) and latex are the main offending agents
Bleeding disorders	Bleeding and/or bruising are a significant hazard to any surgery
Cardio-respiratory disorders	Wheezing, cough, shortness of breath (dyspnoea), chest pain, swelling of ankles, palpitations, hypertension may be a contraindication to GA or conscious sedation
Drug treatment	Drug use may be the only indication of serious underlying disease. Treatment will need to be deferred until the drugs are identified. Most serious interactions with drugs or herbal medicines are with GA or conscious sedation agents. Aspirin and other similar drugs may be a hazard in anticoagulated, asthmatic, diabetic or pregnant patients, those with peptic ulcers, or children under 16 years. Recreational drugs may cause behavioural problems.
Endocrine disorders	Diabetes mellitus may lead to collapse. Hypoglycaemia (low blood sugar) is the main problem
Fits or faints	Fainting and epilepsy may result in injury to the patient
Gastro-intestinal disorders	Crohn's disease or coeliac disease may have oral complications such as ulceration, and gastric disorders may increase the risk of vomiting during GA or conscious sedation
Hospital admissions and attendances	Hospital admissions may indicate presence of a disease A history of operations may provide knowledge of possible reactions to GA, sedation and surgery Operations on the retina (part of the eye) may use intraocular gases and such history would be a contraindication to GA or conscious sedation, which may cause rapid expansion of the ocular gas, leading to blindness
Infections	The transmissibility of infections must be considered. People who have attended a clinic for sexually transmitted infections (STI), or been admitted to hospital for an infection, or who have been refused for blood donation may be at risk. Carriers of meticillin-resistant *Staphylococcus aureus* (MRSA), tuberculosis, or of *Neisseria meningitidis* may be a particular hazard to others
Jaundice and liver disorders	A history of jaundice or other liver disease may mean the patient is prone to prolonged bleeding or impaired drug metabolism, and may imply carriage of hepatitis viruses
Kidney and genitourinary disorders	Excretion of some drugs may be impaired. Tetracyclines should be avoided or given in lower doses
Likelihood of pregnancy	Any essential procedures involving drugs (even aspirin), elective operative dentistry (restorative or surgical), radiography or GA should be arranged during the middle trimester
Mental state	Anxiety is common before dental treatment. Anxious patients may sometimes react aggressively, and anxiety may limit extent of dental treatment that can be provided under LA
Neurological	Movement disorders can significantly disrupt operative procedures

47

MANAGING A MEDICAL EMERGENCY

- All clinical staff must be trained in the management of emergencies.
- All dental practices are required to have an emergency kit readily available.
  - o All practices should have a designated **first responder**. Depending on the severity of the emergency, a trained first aider, a dental nurse or a clinician may be the most appropriate person to act as first responder.
  - o The first responder should designate a specific person to call the emergency services. Another person should be sent to wait for the arrival of the emergency services and direct them to the location of the emergency.
- Note that trained first aiders should only act within the boundaries of their knowledge while awaiting help from the appropriately qualified staff.
- Dental nurses can also be helpful in ensuring that onlookers are separated from the ill patient, allowing the responder adequate space to work.

Term to Learn
First responder: the person who is the first to take action in the event of a medical emergency.

ROLE OF THE DENTAL NURSE IN A MEDICAL EMERGENCY

According to the General Dental Council (p. 71), dental nurses should be:

- Able to *identify* a medical emergency
- Able to *provide support* for the individuals involved in a medical emergency and those managing the emergency
- Able to *carry out resuscitation* (see below)
- Familiar with the principles of *first aid*.

KEY POINT Ensure you keep the emergency kit and yourself up to date (e.g. attend resuscitation training at least once a year and make sure the drugs are not out of date).

The most important tool that you, as a dental nurse, will have in any emergency is the ability to remain calm and focused. By keeping your knowledge up to date and practising procedures, you can ensure that you will act effectively and confidently during any emergency. Crucial to this is:

- *Advanced preparation* – it is essential that you are aware of the location of the emergency kit and the telephone number for calling an ambulance or a doctor at all times. You should also know the location and quickest route to the nearest emergency department. Emergency phone numbers should be posted by the phone (police, fire and rescue department, poison control centre, and ambulance services as well as the doctor's surgery). Indeed, all staff should know when and how to call these numbers.
- *Contact* – the patient may have contact numbers for their workplace, partner, or neighbour or nearby friend or relative. Some may have this on their mobile phone under 'ICE' (**In Case of Emergency**).
- *Planning* – the dental practice must have an agreed plan of action in the event of an emergency.
- *Regular practice* – to stop emergencies from becoming disasters.

FIND OUT MORE

What is the plan of action in an emergency at your workplace? How often are emergency procedures practised?

THE EMERGENCY KIT

The emergency kit should consist of the equipment and drugs listed in Table 2.3. Where possible all emergency equipment should be meant for single use only and latex-free to avoid allergies. Note that the recommended kit includes only drugs meant for injecting into the *muscles* (intramuscular, short form: IM) and not into *veins* (intravenous, short form: IV).

ACTIONS A DENTAL NURSE SHOULD TAKE IN A MEDICAL EMERGENCY

- Keep calm.
- Shout for help.
- Clear the area of unnecessary people.
- Keep clear and accurate records, including records of the time of events and procedures (not least because **medico-legal cases** are increasingly common).

Term to Learn
Medico-legal case: when a patient is not happy with advice or treatment provided by a clinician and takes them to court for compensation.

TABLE 2.3 Suggested Minimal Equipment and Drugs for Emergency Use in Dentistry

Equipment	Comments
Portable apparatus for administering oxygen	Portable oxygen cylinder (D size) with pressure reduction valve and flow meter. The cylinder should be of sufficient size to be easily portable and also to allow for adequate flow rates, e.g. 10 litres per minute, until the arrival of an ambulance or the patient fully recovers. A full D size cylinder contains 340 litres of oxygen and should allow a flow rate of 10 litres per minute for up to 30 minutes. Two such cylinders may be necessary to ensure oxygen supply does not fail Oxygen face mask with tube Basic set of oropharyngeal airways (sizes 1, 2, 3 and 4) Pocket mask with oxygen port Self-inflating bag valve mask (1 litre size bag) for use by staff who have been appropriately trained Variety of well-fitting adult and child face masks for attaching to self-inflating bag
Portable suction	Portable suction with appropriate suction catheters and tubing, e.g. the Yankauer sucker
Spacer device for inhalation of bronchodilators	
Automated external defibrillator (AED)	
Automated blood glucose measuring device	
Equipment for administering drugs intramuscularly	Single-use sterile syringes (2 ml and 10 ml sizes) and needles (19 and 21 gauge)
Drugs as below	

Emergency	Drugs Required (Dosage Given is for Adults)
Anaphylaxis	Intramuscular adrenaline (0.5 ml of 1 in 1000 solution; repeat at five minutes if needed)
Hypoglycaemia	Oral glucose solution/tablets/gel/powder (proprietary non-diet drink or 5 g glucose powder dissolved in water) – for example, GlucoGel, formerly known as Hypostop gel (40% dextrose) Glucagon injection (intramuscular 1 mg) – for example, GlucoGel, GlucaGen, HypoKit
Acute exacerbation of asthma	Beta 2 agonist – for example salbutamol aerosol inhaler (100 micrograms/activation, activations directly or up to six into a spacer)
Status epilepticus	Midazolam (10 mg) (buccal or intranasal use)
Angina	Glyceryl trinitrate (GTN)* (two sprays of 400 micrograms/metered activation)
Myocardial infarction	Dispersible aspirin (300 mg chewed)

No corticosteroid is included.
Other agents (e.g. flumazenil) and equipment (e.g. pulse oximeter) are needed if conscious sedation is administered in the surgery.
*Do not use nitrates to relieve an angina attack if the patient has recently taken sildenafil (e.g. Viagra or Cialis) as there may be an abrupt fall in blood pressure; analgesics should be used.

This is because IM injections are generally easier and safer to give. IM injections are best given into the side of the thigh.

BASIC LIFE SUPPORT

Regardless of the nature of an emergency, the first aim of managing it is to ensure basic life support (BLS), that is, adequate oxygenation and maintenance of adequate airways and blood pressure. The standard, well-tested approach to BLS (called the primary survey) includes:

1. Rapidly assessing any **D**angers, and the patient's **R**esponsiveness and **A**irways, **B**reathing and **C**irculation (DRABC)

   and

2. Carrying out *cardiopulmonary resuscitation* (CPR), to help the person start to breathe again and to help the person's heart pump blood around the body.

> **KEY POINT** As a dental nurse you should be aware of the most up-to-date guidelines issued by the Resuscitation Council. You can find these at the council's website (http://www.resus.org.uk).

In the UK, the Resuscitation Council is responsible for providing guidelines for how to carry out CPR. The BLS sequence described below is based on the UK Resuscitation Council Resuscitation Guidelines (2005). Box 2.3 provides an aide mémoire for adult BLS.

Adult BLS Sequence (Figure 2.1)

1. Make sure the person having the problem, any other people around, and you are safe.
2. Check if the person is responsive. Gently shake them by their shoulders and ask loudly, 'Are you all right?'
3. (A) If the person responds:
   - Leave them in the position in which they already are, provided there is no further danger.
   - Try to find out what is wrong with them and get help if needed.
   - Reassess them regularly.
   (B) If the patient does not respond:
   - First of all shout for help.
   - Then lay the person on their back and open the airway by tilting their head backwards and lifting their chin (Figure 2.1A,B).
4. Keeping the airway open, look for chest movement and check if the person is breathing normally by listening near their mouth for breath sounds and feeling for air on your cheek (Figure 2.1C). Do this only for about 10 seconds – if you have any doubt, act as if the breathing is not normal. Remember that in the first few minutes after a cardiac arrest

---

BOX 2.3 SUMMARY OF BASIC LIFE SUPPORT

1. Check whether the patient is conscious or unresponsive
   - If *conscious*: monitor
   - If *unresponsive*: shout for help.
2. Check breathing
   - If breathing (conscious or unresponsive): monitor
   - If not breathing:
     ○ Call the emergency services, e.g. 999
     ○ Give 30 chest compressions
     ○ Give two rescue breaths using a mouthpiece
     ○ Give 30 chest compressions
     ○ Continue the above until help arrives.

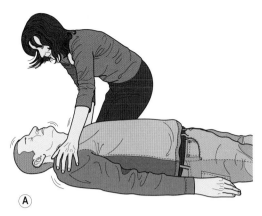

(A)

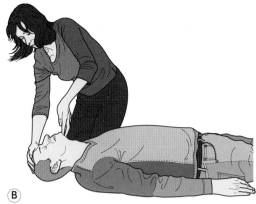

(B)

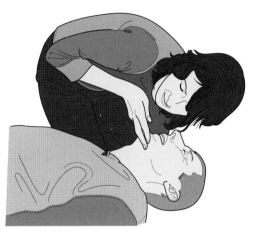

(C)

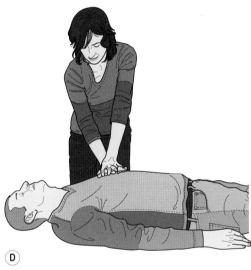

(D)

FIGURE 2.1
Cardiopulmonary resuscitation (CPR) on a child of 8 years or older or an adult. (A) Lay the person down on a hard, flat surface. Put on disposable gloves and check their mouth and throat to ensure that no object is present. If there is, try to sweep it out with your fingers. If the person vomits, turn them on their side and sweep the vomit out of the mouth with two fingers. If the person is rigid or having a seizure, do not try the above. (B) Place one hand on the forehead to tilt the head backwards and place your fingertips under the point of their chin to tilt it to open the airway. (C) Look, listen and feel. If the person is at all responsive (if he or she is moaning, breathing, blinking, or moving any part of the body), his or her heart is beating, do not perform steps 6 or 7. (D) Position yourself vertically above the person's chest to perform chest compression (see text for details). (E, F) Performing mouth-to-mouth resuscitation. (G) A mouthpiece.

51

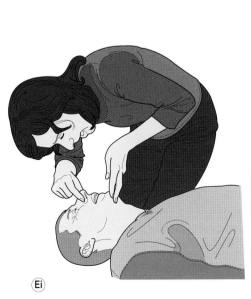

(Ei)

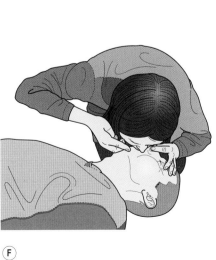

(F)

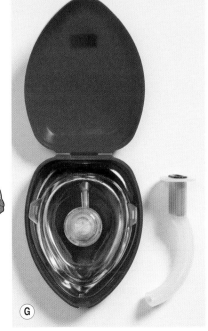

(G)

(when the heart stops beating; see p. 50), a person may be barely breathing, or may be taking infrequent, noisy, gasps (do not confuse this with normal breathing).

5. Ask someone to call for an ambulance or, if you are on your own, do this yourself. You may need to leave the person to do this.

6. (A) If the person is breathing normally now, turn them into the recovery position (Figure 2.2) and check again that they are breathing.
   (B) If the person is not breathing normally go to step 7.

7. Start chest compression:
   - Kneel by the side of the person
   - Place the heel of one hand in the centre of the person's chest.
   - Place the heel of your other hand on top of the first hand.
   - Interlock the fingers of your hands and ensure that you are not applying pressure on the person's ribs, the upper abdomen or the bottom end of their sternum (breastbone) (Figure 2.1D).
   - With your arms straight, press down 4–5 cm on the sternum.
   - Then release all the pressure on the chest but do not lift your hands from the sternum. Repeat the action at a rate of about 100 times a minute (which means almost but not quite two full compressions in one second) 30 times. Release for the same amount of time as compressing the chest.
   - After 30 compressions open the airway again by tilting the head and chin and move to step 8.

8. (A) Start combined compression and mouth-to-mouth breathing:
   - Close the person's nose by pinching the soft part with the index finger and thumb of your hand which should rest on their forehead (Figure 2.1E).
   - Let the person's mouth open, but make sure the chin is still lifted (Figure 2.1F).
   - *Place a mouthpiece (Figure 2.1G) around the mouth,* ensuring the seal is good.
   - Take a normal breath and blow steadily into the person's mouth. At the same time watch for their chest to rise; an effective rescue breath will take about one second to make the chest rise as in normal breathing.
   - Still maintaining the head and chin lift, take your mouth away and check whether the chest falls as air comes out.

52

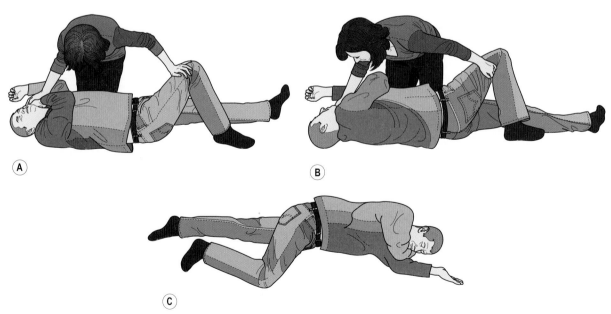

(A)

(B)

(C)

FIGURE 2.2 A–C

Recovery position: extend one arm of the person above their head as shown in the figure and place the other arm on their chest. Bend one knee and then roll the person onto their side.

- Repeat the process by taking a normal breath to give another effective rescue breath, and without any delay perform another 30 chest compressions, with your hands on the correct position on the sternum.
- Continue with chest compressions and rescue breaths in a ratio of 30:2.
- Do not stop unless the person starts breathing normally. However, you should not try to attempt more than two breaths before returning to chest compressions. If there is more than one rescuer present, switch between rescuers every two minutes to prevent fatigue and for minimum delay during the changeover.

    *If the person's chest does not rise when you give the rescue breath, before trying again, check:
- The person's mouth again for any obstruction.
- There is adequate head tilt and chin lift.

8. (B) Continuing chest only CPR. If you are not able to give rescue breaths, continue with the chest compressions at the rate mentioned in step 7, stopping only if the person starts to breathe normally.
9. CPR should be continued until:
    - Qualified personnel arrive and take over
    - The person starts to breathe normally
    - You are too tired to continue.

CPR on Children

The UK Resuscitation Council considers BLS for infants and children (until puberty) separately. It recommends that in children:

- Lay rescuers should use a ratio of 30 compressions to two breaths.
- Two or more rescuers with a duty to respond should use a ratio of 15 compressions to two breaths.

53

FIND OUT MORE

To read more about BLS in children and infants, visit the UK Resuscitation Council website (http://www.resus.org.uk).

MANAGING SPECIFIC EMERGENCY SITUATIONS
Collapse

The commonest cause of collapse in a dental practice is fainting (see next section). Therefore where possible, patients should be treated in a flat (supine) position, especially when giving injections or performing surgery, because it prevents fainting.

If a patient collapses, lay them flat, and reassure the patient and any accompanying person(s).

RESUSCITATING THE COLLAPSED PATIENT (ABC)
Airway

- ○ Check the airways are patent (clear)
- ○ Put the patient in the recovery position (see p. 52) on their side with face down so that any fluids etc. will run out of the mouth
- ○ Suck the airway clear and extend the neck
- ○ Give oxygen.
- If the airway is obstructed:
    - ○ Try to get the patient to cough

Terms to Learn
Expired air respiration: mouth-to-mouth resuscitation.
Carotid artery: the main artery (see Chapter 4) that carries the blood to the face and brain, passes through the side of the neck, where it can be palpated to check the pulse.
IV infusion: also called IV drip, it involves giving of fluids (drugs or blood or other fluids) directly into a person's veins (see Chapter 4).

○ Give an abdominal thrust (stand behind the patient, put your arms around them, clench your hands together and pull upwards on the upper abdomen)

Breathing

- Listen and feel for breathing, while looking for chest expansion. Give oxygen: if the patient is not breathing, give them 100% oxygen *or* use **expired air respiration** (but this only supplies less than 20% oxygen).
- Give rescue breaths.

Circulation

- Check the pulse at the **carotid artery** in the neck (Figure 2.3) and blood pressure with a sphygmomanometer.
- If there is no pulse, resuscitate as given above.
- A doctor needs to treat the patient if they are in shock (e.g. with an **IV infusion**).

FIND OUT MORE

What device is used for expired air respiration in your workplace?

Fainting (Syncope)

Fainting is caused by a reduction of blood flow to the brain. It can be brought on by various stimuli (anxiety, pain, fatigue, fasting, high room temperature or even the sight of a needle – a common cause in dental practice). It particularly occurs in patients undergoing tooth extraction and may occur before or after the treatment.

Fainting may be prevented by:

- Ensuring the patient has eaten something before undergoing treatment under local anaesthesia
- Adopting a reassuring manner and not causing undue anxiety
- Laying the patient supine before giving any injections
- Keeping instruments (particularly any sharps) out of the patient's view
- Not causing the patient pain or anxiety.

CLINICAL FEATURES OF A FAINT

The patient may feel:

- Dizzy
- Weak
- Light-headed
- Sick (nauseous)
- Warm but the skin will be cool and sweaty (moist or clammy).

They may appear very pale, with a slow and thin pulse initially, which becomes faster later and they eventually lose consciousness.

MANAGEMENT

- Immediately lay the patient flat on the back with the legs raised above the level of the head to increase the flow of blood to the heart and brain. If the fainting patient is not laid flat, they may have a vaso-vagal attack. This involves slowing of the heart rate so that the blood flow to the brain reduces (called cerebral hypoxia), which leads to fainting; the patient can also have a convulsion.
- Loosen the patient's collar.

FIGURE 2.3
Feeling the carotid pulse.

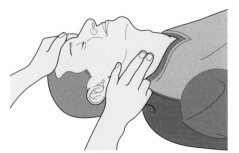

54

- Wait to see if they spontaneously recover (this should only take a few seconds).
- If the patient does not immediately recover, check the carotid pulse (see Figure 2.3):
  - ○ If the pulse is slow, the patient may have had a vaso-vagal attack. This may require an IV injection of a drug called atropine.
  - ○ If the pulse is absent, the patient is in cardiac arrest.
- If loss of consciousness occurs in the supine position or if the patient does not quickly resume consciousness when placed in the supine position, there could be other possible causes for the collapse that require urgent medical attention. Therefore, call an ambulance.

Postural Hypotension

Rapidly bringing a patient upright from lying down may cause a sudden fall in their blood pressure and therefore a temporary reduction in the flow of blood to the brain. This is called postural hypotension. It particularly occurs after a person gets up suddenly after lying down for a long time. Older patients and those taking certain medications such as **anti-hypertensive drugs**, **tricyclic antidepressants** or **atropinics** are particularly prone to this.

Hypoglycaemia

Hypoglycaemia is the term used for low blood sugar (glucose). Hypoglycaemia is common in people with diabetes who have missed a meal or taken an overdose of insulin. It can also occur in anyone if too much alcohol is consumed.

After fainting, hypoglycaemia is the next most common cause of collapse in dental practice. If a patient is suspected to be hypoglycaemic, their blood sugar level can be quickly tested by using a BM stick.

> **Terms to Learn**
> **Anti-hypertensive drugs:** drugs taken to reduce blood pressure.
> **Atropinics:** drugs for certain heart diseases
> **Tricyclic antidepressants:** one of the kinds of drugs used for the treatment of depression.

> **KEY POINT** Remember that in late pregnancy, pressure from the uterus inhibits blood flow back to the heart. This happens because the main vessel that takes blood back to the heart (the inferior vena cava) is compressed when the patient lies down (this is called *supine hypotensive syndrome*). Therefore, women in late pregnancy should be positioned slightly sideways in the dental chair.

55

FIND OUT MORE

Look for a BM stick in your workplace and explain how it is used.

FEATURES OF HYPOGLYCAEMIA

A hypoglycaemic patient may collapse but beforehand may:

- Show aggression and irritability
- Have sweaty, warm skin
- Have a rapid, bounding pulse
- Be anxious and have tremors
- Have tingling sensation around the mouth
- Be confused and disoriented.

MANAGEMENT

- Pre-empt the situation in patients with diabetes (give them sugar or glucose).
- If the patient does become hypoglycaemic, give glucose, preferably orally if the patient is not unconscious but otherwise intravenously. A sugar lump placed inside the mouth between the cheek and teeth (in the buccal sulcus), or a sugar solution or GlucoGel (formerly called Hypostop) can also be used. An IM injection of glucagon (a hormone) is another alternative.
- If the patient does not immediately recover, an ambulance/hospital transfer may be needed.

Anaphylaxis

CAUSES

Anaphylaxis is a severe allergic reaction. It involves rapid release of a specific **antibody** called IgE into the blood that sets off a series of reactions in the body which can be fatal (see below for details). The blood pressure plummets and there may be wheezing and rashes. A variety of allergens can cause anaphylaxis, most commonly the drug penicillin and others such as codeine, aspirin, some general anaesthetics, latex, or certain foods (e.g. peanuts) and insect bites.

Anaphylaxis can occur between one and 30 minutes after drug administration. It is more liable to occur in patients known:

- To be allergic to the particular, or a related, drug (for example if a patient known to be allergic to penicillin is given a related drug such as amoxicillin)
- To have allergies (for example asthma, eczema or hay fever).

> **KEY POINT** When using a local anaesthetic or any injection (particularly IM injection) the patient should be in the supine position so they are less likely to faint. If the injection is given to a standing patient, there may be a delay in distinguishing anaphylaxis from a simple faint (although the latter has a more rapid onset). Collapsing patients can also injure themselves as they fall.

However, anaphylaxis can occur even in the absence of a prior history of allergy to the drug, or even, occasionally, in the absence of any known previous exposure to the drug.

PREVENTION

Taking a good medical history, including history of drugs and allergies, and avoiding the use of potential allergens will help prevent anaphylaxis.

RECOGNISING ANAPHYLAXIS

Anaphylaxis has the following signs and symptoms:

- Feeling of itchiness, paraesthesiae ('pins and needles'), nausea or abdominal pain
- Weak and rapid pulse
- Low blood pressure – that is, acute (sudden) hypotension
- Wheezing – this is because of laryngeal oedema (swelling inside the throat, which causes difficulty breathing) or bronchoconstriction (narrowing of the airways, also causing difficulty breathing)
- Angio-oedema – swelling of lips, tongue and eyelids
- Cold and clammy skin
- Urticarial rash – 'hives' (red itchy swelling)
- Collapse
- Circulatory and respiratory failure – coma and death may result.

MANAGEMENT

Remember: ABC (see pp. 53–54) plus drugs.

- Lay patient flat with legs raised.
- Maintain the airway.
- Give 100% oxygen.
- Summon expert help.
- Give immediately: 0.5 mg (0.5 ml) of 1 in 1000 adrenaline IM.

Patient may need further expert management, possibly in hospital.

Epilepsy

Epilepsy is the term used when a person has a seizure (a 'fit'). There are several types of seizure or epilepsy. A major epileptic attack has several phases: it starts with the person getting a strange feeling (called an aura), followed by loss of consciousness, and then severe muscle spasm (tonic phase). The patient may stop breathing temporarily and become incontinent (that is, they may urinate or defecate spontaneously) followed by repeated twitching and convulsions (clonic phase).

MANAGEMENT

- Remove any objects in the mouth that could obstruct the airway.
- Protect the patient from injury; move equipment away.
- Administer oxygen.
- Wait for the seizure to stop spontaneously.

If the fit *does not* terminate within 5 minutes:

- Call for help and ambulance
- Start BLS (see p. 50).
- During a second fit:
  - ○ Continue giving oxygen
  - ○ Prepare midazolam (a kind of *benzodiazepine* drug) for administration in the buccal sulcus/vestibule of the mouth.
- On third fit:
  - ○ Give midazolam.
- When the fit stops, transfer to hospital.

Myocardial Infarction

Myocardial infarction (also called an 'MI', 'heart attack' or 'coronary' or 'coronary thrombosis') is the condition in which the blood supply to the heart muscle gets blocked, causing part of the heart to die. It is life-threatening condition, and one of the main causes of death. People with a disease called arteriosclerosis and *ischaemic* or *coronary heart disease* are more prone to myocardial infarction.

RECOGNISING MYOCARDIAL INFARCTION

- Patient complains of central 'crushing' chest pain that radiates to the arm, back, jaw.
- They remain conscious but feel they are 'about to die'.
- They are pale, sweaty, nauseated.
- There is a rapid weak pulse and fast respiration.

MANAGEMENT

- Ensure the airway is clear; remove any object that may cause obstruction.
- Sit the patient upright.
- Summon expert help.
- Give glyceryl trinitrate spray (or tablet) **sublingually** – wait for 10 minutes only.
- If patient does not improve, give oxygen, and aspirin (one 300 mg tablet of dispersible aspirin, to be crushed in the mouth).
- Remain with patient, who must be admitted to hospital.

Term to Learn
Sublingual: a drug given sublingually is placed under the tongue, where it dissolves to enter the blood stream.

Cardiac Arrest

Cardiac arrest is when the heart stops beating. The main sign of cardiac arrest is the absence of breathing in a non-responsive patient. The commonest cause of cardiac arrest, especially outside hospital, is **ventricular fibrillation**. This usually happens after a myocardial infarction and it can be life-threatening. Therefore urgent defibrillation is required (see management below)

RECOGNISING CARDIAC ARREST

Cardiac arrest has the following features:

- Sudden loss of consciousness
- Absent arterial pulses (carotid or femoral, which is the pulse felt in the groin)

Term to Learn
Ventricular fibrillation: when the heart beat becomes irregular due to rapid but unco-ordinated contractions of the lower chambers of the heart (see Subchapter 4.1).

57

- Gasping or absent respiration (after 15–30 seconds)
- Pupils begin to dilate (after about 90 seconds).

> **KEY POINT** Assessment of cardiac arrest should be done simultaneously with management to avoid losing any time.

MANAGEMENT

The immediate management of cardiac arrest is BLS (see p. 50), which aims to restore the flow of blood to the brain.

1. Approach the patient with care and shake the patient gently and shout: 'Are you all right?'
2. If the arrest is witnessed by the person providing BLS and they are certain it is a cardiac arrest, they should give a praecordial thump (hit the sternum – centre of chest) (Figure 2.4)
3. Call for assistance:
   - In general practice – from another colleague and an ambulance
   - In hospital – call the resuscitation team and for a **defibrillator**.
4. Clear and maintain the airway (p. 53)
5. Look, feel and listen for breathing (up to 10 seconds); give two effective rescue breaths (up to five attempts, looking for rising of chest wall). Use a face mask (that is, deliver air with mouth-to-mask technique, or using an Ambu bag, ideally connected to an oxygen delivery device).

> **Term to Learn**
> **Automated external defibrillator (AED):** a machine that gives a controlled electric shock to the heart to restart or normalise the heart beat.

IDENTIFY AND LEARN

Identify a face mask and Ambu bag in your workplace.

6. Check the carotid pulse in the side of the neck (for up to 10 seconds):
   - If pulse is present, continue with 10–15 breaths per minute
   - If pulse is absent or inadequate, place the patient on a firm surface and start CPR (see pp. 50–3).

FIND OUT MORE

What is the procedure for delivering rescue breaths in BLS in your workplace?
Is there a defibrillator? If yes, who is trained to use it?

FIGURE 2.4
Giving the praecordial thump.

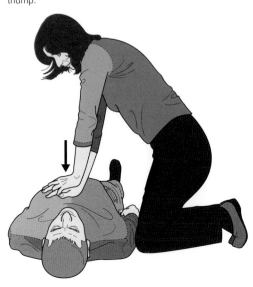

Chest Pain

There are many causes of chest pain, but severe pain may indicate myocardial infarction or angina (partial block of blood supply to the heart muscle but without death of the muscle).

FEATURES OF ANGINA

- Central chest pain that may or may not radiate to the arm.
- Patients with angina remain conscious.
- Usually there is a previous history of angina.
- Pulse may be fast.

MANAGEMENT

1. Reassure and calm the patient.
2. Ensure the airway is clear; remove any object that may cause obstruction.
3. Sit the patient upright.
4. Give GTN spray/tablet sublingually (two puffs of spray or one tablet).

If pain is not relieved rapidly, or if there is sweating, nausea, vomiting, breathlessness, arrhythmia, or loss of consciousness, it may be myocardial infarction. In this situation:

- Summon medical help.
- Give oxygen.
- Give the patient a 300 mg tablet of aspirin to chew.

Respiratory Obstruction

If breathing is obstructed in any way, it can rapidly starve the brain of oxygen (called cerebral hypoxia). If the breathing is obstructed for more than about three minutes, it can cause brain damage or death. Respiratory obstruction in the dental surgery is mainly caused by:

- Mechanical obstruction of the airways by an object (foreign body)
- Pressure on the airways
- Bronchospasm (narrowing of the airways) in a patient with chronic **obstructive airway disease (COAD)**.

CAUSES AND PREVENTION

Unfortunately, despite safety recommendations during dental treatment, inlays (see p. 225), crowns (see p. 226), endodontic instruments (see p. 233) and extracted teeth or roots or other small items continue to be inadvertently dropped into the airway.

A relatively common error is to collect extracted teeth or tooth fragments in a swab and then by mistake use the same swab again in the patient's mouth for **haemostasis**. This can transfer the removed teeth or tooth fragments back into the mouth.

Use of rubber dam in restorative dentistry (see p. 217) can reduce many of the mishaps that can lead to respiratory obstruction.

> **Term to Learn**
> **Obstructive airway disease:** a kind of disease of the respiratory system in which the airways get obstructed, for example by over-production of mucus or constriction of the muscles in the walls of the airways. This causes difficulty breathing. The two forms of COAD are chronic bronchitis and emphysema.

> **Term to Learn**
> **Haemostasis:** the process by which bleeding is stopped, for example by applying pressure on the bleeding site.

59

■ IDENTIFY AND LEARN
Identify the various parts of a rubber dam used in your workplace.

MANAGEMENT OF OBJECTS THAT CANNOT BE ACCOUNTED FOR

> **KEY POINT** Only use clean swabs for post-operative haemostasis.

If a lost item such as a crown, an extracted tooth, or a broken bur cannot be found lying free in the mouth, it could be:

- Within the tissues of the mouth (for example, inside the mass of the cheek)
- Somewhere in the respiratory system (the throat, the airways or the lungs)
- In the digestive tract, or it may have fallen outside the body.

In this situation:

- Check the mouth and throat carefully.
- Check the area around the patient.
- Check in the suction tubing and container.

If the object is within the throat and the patient is conscious, encourage them to cough out the object. Do not perform a blind finger sweep of the throat, as this may push the foreign body further into the throat.

Young children should be held upside down. In other children, back blows or chest thrusts may assist in retrieving the object. Older children and adults may benefit from the abdominal thrust.

If the object cannot be found, X-rays of the neck, chest and abdomen are required. Depending where the object is found it may need to be removed by endoscopy or open operation, unless the doctor predicts it will pass in the faeces.

> **KEY POINT** Do not slap the back of a patient sitting upright, as this might actually cause the object to fall further into the respiratory tract. However, if the obstruction is complete (e.g. the object is lying between vocal cords), slapping the back may partially free the airway.

Asthma

In asthma the airways become hyper-reactive and tend to swell up in response to a variety of stimuli, sometimes allergic. This causes narrowing of the airways and difficulty breathing.

An asthma attack can sometimes be triggered by an inhaled drug or one that is circulating in the blood. It may also be a manifestation of anaphylaxis.

RECOGNISING ASTHMA

The patient may:

- Be breathless
- Have a wheeze
- Have a cough
- Have difficulty speaking
- Feel panic.

MANAGEMENT

Mild Asthma

- Use a salbutamol (Ventolin) inhaler.
- Give oxygen.
- Sit the patient upright.
- Repeat the inhaler as required.
- If the response within 10 minutes is poor – call an ambulance and transfer to hospital.

Severe Asthma

- Call ambulance immediately.
- Use the salbutamol inhaler.
- Give oxygen.
- Sit the patient upright.
- Transfer to hospital.

Stroke

Stroke (also called cerebral vascular accident (CVA)) usually occurs when a blood vessel in the brain bursts or gets blocked and causes brain damage. It is more common in older people. **Atherosclerosis** is the main cause of strokes, but hypertension during a stressful situation (e.g. dental treatment) may also lead to a stroke.

Term to Learn
Atherosclerosis: the accumulation of fats (cholesterol and lipids) in the walls of the arteries.

FEATURES

- Airways, breathing and circulation are usually intact.
- Rapidly altered level of consciousness or cognition (mental status).
- Motor deficits – that is, paralysis of one side of the face (facial palsy), and either one or more limbs, and inability to speak due to tongue muscles being affected.
- Sensory deficits – that is, loss of sensation, e.g. numbness in the fingers.

MANAGEMENT

- Call an ambulance.

- Place the patient in the recovery position.
- Give oxygen.

Bleeding

Life-threatening bleeding (*haemorrhage*) from dental treatment is rare, though implant placement or oral surgery may injure the blood vessels in the face (e.g. lingual or other arteries). Patients who have undergone a treatment called 'radical neck dissection' (e.g. those with oral cancer) may occasionally have sudden, life-threatening haemorrhage. This occurs if the flap of skin covering the surgical wound in the neck gets infected and the infection spreads inwards and erodes the main neck artery (the carotid artery).

> **KEY POINT** FAST – Face, Arm, Speech, Time to call the emergency services – is a simple test to help recognise the signs of stroke and understand the importance of emergency treatment. The faster a stroke patient receives treatment, the better their chances are of survival and of lesser long-term disability.

MANIFESTATIONS OF BLEEDING

- Rising pulse rate
- Falling blood pressure
- Collapse.

MANAGEMENT

- Prevent further blood loss by immediately applying direct pressure over the wound or, if indicated, by suturing and/or packing the wound.
- Set up an IV infusion.

Adverse Drug Reactions

Adverse drug reactions are harmful or unpleasant reactions to medicines that require altering or completely stopping the drug treatment. Unlike side effects, which are usually known reactions that may occur, adverse drug reactions are not always predictable. They also do not always occur on first exposure to a drug. The clinical features of the reaction vary depending on the severity of the reaction. Very severe reactions involving collapse and breathing difficulties can result in anaphylaxis.

Local anaesthetics are the main cause of adverse drug reactions in dentistry. However, lidocaine (formerly called lignocaine), which is the most commonly used local anaesthetic in dentistry, is a very safe drug if administered properly. But if too much is given, or if the drug is injected into a vein instead of the surrounding tissues, it may reach the brain, causing disorientation, agitation, or occasionally, collapse and fits.

PREVENTION

- Stick to recommended doses of local anaesthetic.
- Always use an aspirating syringe to give LA, especially for inferior dental block injections.

MANAGEMENT

- Stop administering the drug immediately if the reaction occurs during that time

or

- Stop the procedure, lay the patient supine and give oxygen, reassuring them all the time.
- Summon medical help.

Conscious sedation agents, such as benzodiazepines (e.g. midazolam), can severely depress the respiratory centre in the brain that controls breathing. Flumazenil is a drug that counteracts this reaction and should be given to patients having a respiratory arrest as a reaction to benzodiazepine administration.

61

General anaesthetics may cause particularly dangerous adverse reactions, particularly in the central nervous system (CNS).

Psychiatric (Mental Health) Emergencies

Many psychiatric emergencies are primarily related to anxiety and use of alcohol or other recreational drugs. Most mentally ill patients can be persuaded to accept help voluntarily. If the patient is highly disturbed and disruptive, the clinician and nurse will need to take some decisive action. If the patient is mute, amnesic (not able to remember things), withdrawn or depressed there is usually less urgency (unless the patient shows signs of suicidal intent).

Suicidal patients need urgent psychiatric assessment. If the patient appears to be at risk, the clinician should contact the psychiatrist urgently and make sure a nurse remains with the patient. Actively suicidal patients almost invariably need admission to hospital and compulsory detention if need be (see next section). Most patients who attempt deliberate self-harm have a mental disorder.

OUT-PATIENTS

Hysteria

Many psychiatric emergencies lead to a crisis out of proportion to the patient's actual problem. The stress of visiting a dentist can lead susceptible individuals to become hysterical. Symptoms such as overbreathing (hyperventilation), crying, etc. make the diagnosis obvious, but patients may still collapse.

Management Be calm and reassuring. Breathing with a paper bag around the mouth and nose may prevent **respiratory alkalosis**, but could also further upset the patient. In unconscious patients, follow the basic principles of ABC (see BLS, p. 50).

Disturbed or Violent Patients Patients with mental health problems such as *schizophrenia* or *mania* may be **delusional** or they may **hallucinate** or behave inappropriately. These patients are often incorrectly treated as if they had no intelligence or awareness of their surroundings. However, they may well understand what is being said to them, even though they may not respond; or they may respond inappropriately.

Management

- Try to make contact with the patient.
- Do not ask too many questions, but offer an explanation of the situation.
- Tell the patient where they are and what is happening.

If the patient is considered a danger to themselves or others and refuses help, compulsory detention in a hospital will usually be required (called *sectioning*). The clinician will need to contact the patient's psychiatrist, who is responsible for carrying out formal sectioning procedures.

This may happen if the patient has a mental problem of such a nature or degree to warrant detention under observation for at least a limited period. To be detained is in the interest of the patient's own health or safety, and/or with a view to the protection of other people.

Alcohol-related problems do not qualify for sectioning under the Mental Health Act.

IN-PATIENTS

In an emergency, the clinician may have to act (detain patient) under **common law**. In the UK, under the Mental Health Act 1983, a patient who is in hospital for other reasons but is suddenly at danger because of a compromised mental state (e.g. post-operative delirium)

KEY POINT As a dental nurse, you should:

- Know where the emergency kit is in your workplace
- Know what drugs/items are in the emergency kit
- Keep the emergency kit up-to-date
- Know what to do in an emergency
  - Keep up to date with resuscitation training.

Term to Learn
Respiratory alkalosis: when a person hyperventilates, that is breathes much more and much harder than the body requires, the alkalinity (pH of their blood) rises as too much carbon dioxide is lost too rapidly.

Terms to Learn
Delusions: firm beliefs that the person hold to be true but actually are fanciful and not true.
Hallucinate: seeing or hearing imaginary things, for example people who are not really there.

Term to Learn
Common law: this refers to law that is derived from decisions taken by judges in courts and other tribunals, rather than through, for example, government legislation. In the UK, this includes judicial decisions made going back to ancient times.

62

can be detained for up to 72 hours against their will, following the recommendation of the doctor in charge of their care (this may be a consultant). Sectioning of an out-patient (or sectioning an in-patient for more than 72 hours) requires the involvement of a psychiatrist.

Disorientated Older Patients

Disorientated older patients are best managed by having a close relative or other accompanying person constantly with them.

FIRST AID

All dental staff and patients should be able to receive immediate first aid attention and, if required, receive treatment from the ambulance service.

> **KEY POINT** Effective first aid can prevent minor injuries and occurrences becoming major ones and save lives.

The Health and Safety (First Aid) Regulations 1981 requires employers to:

- Provide suitably trained personnel to administer first aid for employees who may become ill or injured in the workplace. To cover for temporary and exceptional absences of trained first aiders, the regulations allow for a competent person, known as an 'appointed person', to take charge (see below)
- Provide adequate and appropriate facilities and equipment
- Inform their employees of the arrangements made for first aid 'including the location of equipment, facilities and personnel'.

In addition, employers need to consider:

- The number of people employed – is the number of first aiders and appointed persons as per the recommendations of the HSE (Table 2.4)? The number of suitably trained personnel and appropriate equipment and facilities depends on the size of the practice (or hospital).
- Are all inexperienced staff trained in first aid – trainees, newly qualified clinicians, unqualified dental nurses and students all need special training in first aid.
- Are there any employees and patients with disabilities and special health problems – consider the location of equipment and the use of special equipment.
- Do employees work different hours? There needs to be first aid provision at all times of work.

63

TABLE 2.4 Suggested Numbers of First Aid Personnel

Level of Risk	Examples	Number of Employees	First Aid Personnel Needed
Lower risk	Shops, offices and dental environments	Fewer than 50 50–100 100 or over	At least one appointed person At least one first aider One first aider per 100 employees
Medium risk	Light engineering and warehouses	Fewer than 20 20–100 100 or over	At least one appointed person At least one first aider for every 50 employed One first aider per 100 employees
High risk	Most construction work, and working with dangerous machinery	Fewer than 5 5–50 50 or over	At least one appointed person At least one first aider One additional first aider for every 50 employed

- Is the workplace remote from emergency medical services? Inform and consider special arrangements with the medical services.
- Do employees work at other sites? Arrangements must be made to ensure provision at all sites.
- Do members of the public visit? There is no legal responsibility in regard to first aid to patients, contractors or other members of the public but provision is recommended by the HSE (and is common sense).

The First Aider

A first aider is an employee who has undergone an approved Health and Safety Executive (HSE) training course in first aid at work.

The Appointed Person

An appointed person is an employee who:

- Takes charge when another employee becomes ill or injured
- Calls an ambulance
- Ensures the first aid box is stocked and replenished as required
- Is on site when people are at work and arranges cover as necessary.

An appointed person cannot administer first aid if they are not trained to do so.

There may be a need for more than one appointed person depending on the size and activity of the dental workplace. The numbers of first aid personnel depend on the risk categories of the workplace (Table 2.4). Dentistry falls into the lower and medium risk categories.

> **KEY POINT** The first aid box is *not* the emergency kit, and tablets, pills or medicines should not be kept in it.

The First Aid Box

The HSE has provided guidelines for the contents of a first aid box, as each workplace environment will have differing needs. First aid boxes can be obtained from the HSE.

Where there is no special risk in the workplace the minimum items in a first aid box will include:

- The HSE leaflet giving basic advice on first aid at work
- 20 individually wrapped sterile adhesive dressings of assorted sizes
- Two sterile eye pads
- Four individually wrapped triangular bandages (preferably sterile)
- Six safety pins
- Six medium-sized (12 cm × 12 cm) individually wrapped sterile unmedicated wound dressings
- Two large (18 cm × 18 cm) individually wrapped sterile unmedicated wound dressings
- One pair of disposable gloves.

The contents and location of the first aid box need to be reviewed on a regular basis.

FIND OUT MORE

Consider the location of the first aid box in your workplace: is it easily accessible?

First Aid Courses

BASIC FIRST AID FOR APPOINTED PERSON – ONE-DAY COURSE
Pre-requisites

None, but the person must be physically able to carry out the procedures in the course contents.

Who is the Course for?

This course is for any person:

- Wishing to learn basic first aid
- Acting as the appointed person in the workplace
- Supporting a qualified first aider
- Employed in a low-risk working environment with fewer than 50 employees.

Course Content

- Personal safety, assessing the incident
- Priorities: danger, response: airway, breathing check and obtaining help
- Unconscious person
- Resuscitation (adults)
- Choking
- Dealing with blood loss and shock
- Burns and scalds
- Fractures
- Heart attack
- Diabetes
- Strokes
- Seizures
- Reporting and recording of incidents as required by HSE
- Contents of HSE approved first aid kit

Qualification

Appointed Person Certificate – valid for three years.

FIRST AID AT WORK – FOUR-DAY COURSE

Pre-requisites

- Candidates must be physically able to carry out the procedures in the course contents.
- Candidates must attend all sessions to be eligible for assessment.

Who is the Course for?

- This course is meant for employees who require a First Aid at Work Certificate.

Course Content

- Priorities of first aid
- Managing an incident
- The role and responsibilities of employers/employees at work
- Care of the unconscious person
- CPR
- Disorders of the airway
- Dealing with bleeding and shock
- Causes of unconsciousness
- Burns and scalds
- Injuries to bones, muscles and joints
- Poisoning
- Recognition and management of major illnesses
- Recognition of minor illnesses and appropriate action
- Eye injuries
- Miscellaneous injuries
- Record keeping and accident reporting
- Infection control

- Communication and delegation in an emergency
- Management of transportation of a casualty.

Qualification

- Recognised First Aider in the workplace
- First Aid at Work Certificate – valid for three years.

FIRST AID AT WORK REFRESHER – TWO-DAY COURSE
Who is the Course for?

This course is meant for employees who need to renew a valid First Aid at Work Certificate.

Pre-requisites

Candidates must:

- Be physically able to carry out the procedures in the course
- Hold and produce a First Aid at Work Certificate or First Aid at Work Refresher Certificate. The Certificate can be renewed three months before the expiry date. The unexpired months will be added on to the new certificate.

FIND OUT MORE

Useful links:

- Health and Safety Executive. 2006 Basic advice on first aid at work. Poster. Sudbury: HSE books. Gives practical guidance on complying with first aid at work. Available at: http://books.hse.gov.uk/hse/public/saleproduct.jsf?catalogueCode=9780717661954
- Health and Safety Executive. 2009 First aid at work. Your questions answered. Sudbury: HSE books. Available at: http://books.hse.gov.uk/hse/public/saleproduct.jsf?catalogueCode=INDG214REV13.
- Health and Safety Executive 2006 Basic advice on first aid at work. Leaflet. Sudbury: HSE Books. Available at: http://books.hse.gov.uk/hse/public/saleproduct.jsf?catalogueCode=INDG347REV1
- Health and Safety Executive 2006 Electric shock: first aid procedures Leaflet. Sudbury: HSE Books. Available at: http://books.hse.gov.uk/hse/public/saleproduct.jsf?catalogueCode=9780717662036
- Health and Safety Advisory Committee, British Association of Dental Nurses, PO Box 4, Room 201, Hillhouse International Business Centre, Thornton-Cleveleys FY5 4QD (tel: 01253 338360; http://www.badn.org.uk)

Law and Ethics

3.1 REGULATION OF DENTAL NURSING IN THE UK, SCOPE OF PRACTICE, TRAINING AND QUALIFICATIONS

REGULATION

The Regulatory Bodies

In the UK, all healthcare professionals are accountable to a regulating body. There are in total nine regulating bodies:

- General Dental Council (GDC) – regulates all dental professionals
- General Medical Council (GMC) – regulates doctors
- Nursing and Midwifery Council (NMC) – regulates nurses, midwives and specialist community public health nurses
- Health Professions Council (HPC) – regulates 14 professions (art therapists, biomedical scientists, chiropodists/podiatrists, clinical scientists, dieticians, occupational therapists, operating department practitioners, orthoptists, paramedics, physiotherapists, practitioner psychologists, prosthetists and orthotists, radiographers, speech and language therapists)
- General Optical Council (GOC) – regulates dispensing opticians and optometrists
- General Chiropractic Council (GCC) – regulates chiropractors
- General Osteopathic Council (GOsC) – regulates osteopaths
- Royal Pharmaceutical Society of Great Britain (RPSGB) – regulates pharmacists
- Pharmaceutical Society of Northern Ireland (PSNI) – regulates pharmacists.

Each regulator maintains 'registers', which contain names and other details of healthcare professionals who are considered fit to practise in the UK. The regulators' functions include:

- Setting standards of behaviour, education and ethics
- Dealing with concerns about professionals who are unfit to practise because of poor health, misconduct or poor performance. Regulators can remove people from the register and therefore prevent them from practising.

67

The General Dental Council

The GDC is the organisation that regulates all dental professionals training and working in the UK. Dental professionals include dentists and all dental care professionals. The dental care professionals are:

- Dental nurses
- Dental technicians
- Clinical dental technicians
- Dental hygienists
- Dental therapists
- Orthodontic therapists.

The aims of the GDC are to:

- Protect patients
- Promote the confidence of the patients and public in all dental professionals
- Assure the quality of dental education for all dental professionals in the UK
- Ensure dental professionals keep their knowledge up to date
- Help patients with complaints.

The GDC achieves these aims by setting the standards and principles for ethical dental practice in the UK. These are covered in detail in Subchapter 3.2.

REGISTERS FOR DENTAL PROFESSIONALS IN THE UK

The GDC maintains 'registers' for dentists and dental care professionals:

- Dentists – the Dentists Register
- Dental care professionals – the Dental Care Professionals Register.

The registers include the names of all the dentists and dental care professionals who are registered to practise in the UK, regardless of whether they work in the National Health Service (NHS), private practice or any other form of practice. Thus all dental nurses must be registered with the GDC's Dental Care Professionals Register. Those who are registered are called registrants.

FIND OUT MORE

All dental nurses should have a copy of the Standards for Dental Professionals booklets as well as the additional supporting documents. You can download them from the GDC website (http://www.gdc-uk .org/Current+registrant/Standards+for+Dental+Professionals/).

The GDC itself is regulated by the Council for Healthcare Regulatory Excellence (CHRE).

The Council for Healthcare Regulatory Excellence

The CHRE is a UK-wide organisation that oversees the nine regulators of healthcare professionals in the UK. It is itself accountable to Parliament. The CHRE's mission is to protect the public by:

- Helping regulatory bodies become better regulators
- Setting and driving standards up for professional regulation
- Ensuring greater harmonisation of regulatory practice and outcomes
- Anticipating any problems in the future.

The CHRE fulfils its mission by:

- Reviewing the final stages of cases in which a healthcare professional's fitness to practise has been challenged
- Monitoring how the regulators carry out their functions
- Promoting good practice
- Advising health ministers
- Influencing national and international policy on health regulation
- Promoting data protection and freedom of information (see pp. 86–7).

The Care Quality Commission and the Care Commission

Another, independent, regulatory body that dental nurses need to be aware about is called the Care Quality Commission (CQC) in England and the Care Commission in Scotland. The aim of the CQC is 'to ensure better care for everyone in hospital, in a care home and at home'. Thus the CQC ensures the safety and quality of the care provided to patients through various assessment, monitoring and inspection procedures, and this includes dental professionals.

In April 2010, CQC introduced a registration system for all providers of health and social care which was introduced gradually across the care sector with the aim of incorporating primary care services that provide dentistry (NHS and private sector) by 1 April 2011. Thus, in addition to standards set by GDC, it is mandatory for dental practices to register with CQC and comply with its Essential Standards of Quality and Safety (standards that outline the ideal outcome patients should experience when using a service). Each practice will need to be able to demonstrate compliance with the regulations in the following areas:

- Care and welfare of service users
- Assessing and monitoring the quality of provision
- Safeguarding vulnerable service users
- Management of medicines and medical devices
- Cleanliness and infection control
- Meeting nutritional needs
- Safety and suitability of premises
- Safety, availability and suitability of equipment
- Respecting and involving service users
- Consent to care and treatment
- Complaints
- Records
- Competence and suitability of workers
- Staffing
- Effective management of workers
- Cooperating with other providers.

The Dentists Act 1984 (Amendment) Order 2005

The Dentists Act in the UK was passed in 1984. The title 'dental nurse' is now protected by law through an amendment to the Dentists Act, known as Statutory Instruments 2005 No. 2011, Health Care and Associated Professions: Dentists.

If an individual is not registered with the GDC and uses the title 'dental nurse', or any other title that misleadingly implies that the person is a dental nurse, they can be prosecuted in court. This will also put at risk the registration of the dentist who is employing them.

The Health and Social Care Act (2008)

In recent years, the UK law has undergone several changes to enhance public and professional confidence in the delivery of healthcare. That is, the law now aims to ensure that all health professionals continue to earn the trust that patients place in them by:

- *Improving public and professional confidence in the impartiality of fitness-to-practise decisions by the health regulators.* For example, if a patient files a complaint against a dentist or dental nurse it is the duty of the GDC to conduct a fair inquiry.
- *Harmonising the standard of proof across all the health and social care regulators.* This means that for all healthcare professionals, similar levels of proof should be required to convince the courts that a given allegation made is true. The level of proof differs in civil and criminal cases.
- *Better handling of concerns about doctors* by local employers and authorities. Senior doctors called Responsible Officers monitor the conduct and performance of local doctors to take whatever immediate action is needed to safeguard patients.

The changes have also strengthened clinical governance (see p. 8), and have happened as part of the government's response to a number of official inquiries into doctors who have harmed their patients. One example is the Shipman Inquiry, which investigated the conduct of Dr Harold Shipman from Manchester, who was imprisoned in 2000 for 15 murders, but is alleged to have killed 218 patients.

THE NATIONAL HEALTH SERVICE (NHS)

The NHS is the name commonly used to refer to the UK's publicly funded healthcare system, which was set up in 1948. It is now called by different names in different parts of the UK:

- In England, the 'National Health Service' is responsible to UK Government
- In Ireland, 'Health and Care Northern Ireland' is responsible to the Northern Ireland Executive
- In Scotland, 'NHS Scotland' is responsible to the Scottish Government
- In Wales, 'NHS Wales' is responsible to the Welsh Assembly.

However, a person who lives in one part of the UK can receive treatment under the relevant NHS in another UK country without being discriminated against.

70

STRUCTURE OF THE NHS

The NHS is divided into two sections: primary and secondary care.

- *Primary care* – this is the most common 'front-line' service, that is, it is the first point of contact with the NHS for most people. Primary care is delivered by a wide range of healthcare professionals such as doctors, dentists, pharmacists and optometrists. It also includes NHS Direct and walk-in centres. The government bodies in charge of primary care are the primary care trusts (PCTs). These not only provide some primary and community services but PCTs also commission them from other providers. They are involved in commissioning secondary care (see below). PCTs control 80% of the NHS budget as well as overseeing general medical (GPs) and dental practitioners.
- *Secondary care* (also known as acute healthcare) can be either *elective care* or *emergency care*. Elective care means specialist medical care or surgery that has been planned in advance and it usually follows referral from a primary or community health professional. Emergency care is unplanned care, for example following a car accident. The bodies in charge of providing secondary care in the UK include foundation NHS trusts, acute NHS trusts, mental health NHS trusts and NHS ambulance services trusts. The NHS care trusts provide both health and social care.

The strategic health authorities (SHAs) oversee the work of PCTs and other NHS trusts in a particular region and provide the link between the Department of Health and the NHS at the local level.

Term to Learn
NICE: the UK government agency that is responsible for deciding which treatments or investigations are required most commonly and are the most cost-effective (http://www.nice.org.uk).

Several healthcare-related government agencies (e.g. National Institute for Health and Clinical Excellence (**NICE**) and the National Patient Safety Agency (NPSA)) also come under the umbrella of the NHS.

FIND OUT MORE

What is the mission of the NPSA (http://www.npsa.nhs.uk)?

Allocating National Health Resources

The NHS has to run as cost effectively as possible so as to avoid wasting precious resources, while delivering the best possible care to all patients irrespective of where they live in the UK. (Difference in care in different parts of the UK has been termed 'postcode rationing'.) The organisations that are responsible for ensuring this are:

- In England and Wales: NICE (http://www.nice.org.uk)
- In Scotland:
  ○ NHS Quality Improvement Scotland (http://www.nhshealthquality.org)
  ○ Scottish Intercollegiate Guidelines Network (SIGN) (http://www.sign.ac.uk)
  ○ Scottish Medicines Consortium (SMC) (http://www.scottishmedicines.org.uk).

DENTAL NURSES' SCOPE OF PRACTICE

The material in this section is largely adapted from the GDC's 'Scope of Practice' publication, which states that:

> The scope of your practice is a way of describing what you are trained and competent to do. It describes the areas in which you have the knowledge, skills and experience to practise safely and effectively in the best interests of patients.

> Your scope of practice is likely to change over the course of your career. Some registrants will expand their scope by developing new skills, while some may narrow their scope but deepen their knowledge of a particular area by choosing more specialised practice.

> You should only carry out a task or type of treatment or make decisions about a patient's care if you are sure that you have the necessary skills.

> You should only ask someone else to carry out a task or type of treatment or make decisions about a patient's care if you are confident that they have the necessary skills.

SCOPE OF DENTAL NURSE PRACTICE ON QUALIFICATION

Roles permissible:

- Preparing and maintaining the clinical environment, including the equipment
- Carrying out infection control procedures to prevent physical, chemical and microbiological contamination in the surgery or laboratory
- Recording dental **charting** carried out by other appropriate registrants
- Preparing, mixing and handling dental materials
- Providing chairside support to the operator during treatment
- Keeping full and accurate patient records
- Preparing equipment, materials and patients for dental radiography
- Processing and **mounting** dental radiographs
- Monitoring, supporting and reassuring patients
- Giving appropriate advice to patients
- Supporting the patient and their colleagues if there is a medical emergency
- Making appropriate referrals to other health professionals.

Roles that are *excluded*: dental nurses do not undertake any of the skill areas described in Chapter 15, as these are within the roles of the dental technician, clinical dental technician, dental hygienist, dental therapist, orthodontic therapist or dentist.

Terms to Learn

Charting: filling in the dental record sheet (called a chart) for a patient, e.g. recording which teeth are present, missing or decayed (see Chapter 7).

Mounting: the procedure of correctly displaying dental radiographs for the clinician to see. For example, ensuring the radiograph is the correct side up and the correct side is facing the clinician.

GDC Guidance on the Various Areas of Dental Nurse Roles in 'Scope of Practice'

INFECTION CONTROL

- Applying the principles of infection control when:
  ○ Setting up environment for clinical procedures

71

     ○ Assisting during clinical procedures
     ○ Clearing away after clinical procedures.
- Knowing the different cleaning, disinfecting and sterilisation techniques and their uses
- Understanding how to protect the patient, themselves and other members of the dental team.

CARDIOPULMONARY RESUSCITATION AND MEDICAL EMERGENCIES

- Being able to identify a medical emergency
- Providing support for individuals concerned and those managing the emergency
- Being able to carry out resuscitation techniques
- Being familiar with the principles of first aid.

HEALTH AND SAFETY

- Understanding the basic principles of the Heath and Safety at Work etc. Act as it affects clinical practice.

DENTAL RADIOGRAPHY

- Understanding the principles which underpin dental radiography
- Understanding the hazards of ionising radiation
- Understanding the relevant regulations
- Being able to prepare equipment, materials and patients for dental radiography.

PERSONAL DEVELOPMENT

- Understanding what lifelong learning is and why it is important
- Being able to assess own strengths and weaknesses.

WORKING WITH PATIENTS

- Understanding their role within the team and in a clinical environment
- Being able to communicate with patients, their carers and other members of the team
- Understanding the need for confidentiality
- Being able to cope with difficult or aggressive patients
- Understanding patients' rights and the need to handle complaints sensitively.

Additional Skills that a Dental Nurse Could Develop during Their Career

With additional training, dental nurses may also be involved in expanded duties such as:

- Providing oral health education and oral health promotion
- Assisting in the treatment of patients under conscious sedation
- Assisting in the treatment of patients with special needs
- **Intra-oral** photography
- Shade taking
- Placing rubber dam
- Measuring and recording plaque indices (see Chapter 7)
- Pouring, casting and trimming study models
- Removing sutures after the wound has been checked by a clinician
- Applying fluoride varnish as part of a programme that is overseen by a consultant in dental public health or registered specialist in dental public health
- Constructing occlusal registration rims and special trays
- Repairing the acrylic component of removable appliances
- Tracing cephalograms.

Term to Learn
Intra/extra-oral:
inside/outside the mouth.

IDENTIFY AND LEARN

Identify a shade guide, special tray, occlusal registration rim, cephalogram, topical anaesthetic and vacuum-formed retainers in your workplace.

ADDITIONAL SKILLS WITH ADDITIONAL TRAINING AND ONLY ON PRESCRIPTION (SEE BELOW FOR DETAILS OF TRAINING)

Taking radiographs to the prescription of a clinician (but see Chapter 14; certificate in dental radiography is required)

- Applying **topical** anaesthetic to the prescription of a clinician
- Constructing mouth-guards and bleaching trays to the prescription of a clinician
- Constructing vacuum-formed retainers to the prescription of a clinician
- Taking impressions to the prescription of a clinician (where appropriate).

> **Term to Learn**
> **Topical:** when a drug, for example in a cream formulation, is applied to a local area of the body it is called topical application.

DENTAL NURSE TRAINING AND QUALIFICATIONS

> **KEY POINT** Dental nurses are never permitted to diagnose disease or plan the treatment.

Several different routes lead to a qualification in dental nursing. This is because a route that may be suitable for some may be less suitable for others. Dental nurse training providers in England, Wales and Northern Ireland are listed in Table 3.1.1. For details about the Scottish Vocational Qualification (SVQ) in Oral Healthcare: Dental Nursing Level 3, contact the Scottish Qualifications Authority (see p. 78 for contact details).

Pre-registration Certificates

Appropriate pre-registration certificates are offered by:

- National Examination Board for Dental Nurses (NEBDN)
- City & Guilds of London Institute (City & Guilds).

TABLE 3.1.1 Accessing Dental Nurse Training (England, Wales and Northern Ireland)

Qualification	Awarding Body	Details of Study and Examinations Available from
The National Certificate – Dental Nursing	National Examining Board for Dental Nurses (NEBDN)	NEBDN (http://www.nebdn.org/)
The City & Guilds Level 3 NVQ in Dental Nursing (England and Wales)	NEBDN/City & Guilds Care, Health & Community	NEBDN City & Guilds (http://www.cityandguilds.com/uk-home.html)
The City & Guilds Level 3 Award in Dental Nursing (VRQ) (England and Wales)	NEBDN/City & Guilds Care, Health & Community	NEBDN City & Guilds
The Certificate of Higher Education in Dental Nursing	Cardiff University*	School of Postgraduate Medical and Dental Education (see p. 78 for contact details)
	Portsmouth Dental Academy (scl. admissions@port.ac.uk)	School of Professionals Complementary to Dentistry
Foundation Degree in Dental Nursing	University of Northampton (study@ northampton.ac.uk)	

*This programme has received provisional approval from the GDC Education Committee. Full GDC approval of new programmes is not granted until the first batch of students has completed their studies and examinations or assessments and the programme has been inspected by the GDC. Potential applicants should contact the provider for further information about the programme.

THE NATIONAL EXAMINATION BOARD FOR DENTAL NURSES

The National Certificate of the NEBDN (see p. 78 for contact details) provides a mix of theoretical learning and practical teaching and experience. It can be undertaken at a dental hospital or at a college of further education.

- Dental hospitals usually provide full and part-time courses.
- Colleges of further education usually provide part-time courses (mainly evening or day release).
- Full-time courses are usually work-related, and the theoretical and clinical teaching programme is combined with clinical placements in the hospital specialist departments.
- Part-time courses usually involve employment as an unqualified dental nurse in a general dental practice or equivalent in order to gain the practical experience, and attendance at part-time evening or day release classes. You will need to attend an accredited training centre to train as a dental nurse, which will cover you until registration.

The NEBDN stipulates that 24 months of verified chairside assisting (assisting a dentist or other clinician during treatment of a patient) is necessary before the qualification can be awarded. However, the national examination can be taken before these 24 months are completed.

The NEBDN syllabus has 15 sections. In addition to theoretical study, you need to complete a 'Record of Experience' in the workplace. This provides a measure of your application of skills during routine dental procedures as outlined in the syllabus. The procedures are divided into five units. For each unit, you must demonstrate competence in a prescribed number of clinical activities and provide additional evidence recorded on a 'Practical Record Sheet', which is signed and dated by a witness who holds a GDC-registerable dental qualification. You must also complete a report (case study) of no fewer than 1000 words and no more than 1500 words on one treatment session which involves provision of a fixed or removable appliance or a surgical or restorative procedure.

The national examination is held twice each year – on the third Saturday in May and November – and comprises:

- A practical test
- An oral examination (viva voce)
- Two-hour written paper, consisting of:
  - Four essay-type questions
  - Multiple-choice questions
  - Short-answer questions
  - A diagram to label with related questions
  - A dental chart (see Chapter 7) to complete.

THE CITY & GUILDS OF LONDON INSTITUTE

Vocational qualifications reflect the skills, knowledge and understanding an individual possesses in relation to a specific area of work. National Vocational Qualifications (NVQs) and Vocationally Related Qualifications (VRQs) are workplace-based. The NEBDN provides the dental expertise whereas City & Guilds is the awarding body.

The 'City & Guilds' is the main UK examining and accreditation body for vocational training. Dental nursing is also recognised as a vocational qualification.

Dental Nursing NVQ (No 3231)

You can undertake NVQs at dental hospitals and at further colleges of education. NVQs are made up of different units of competence. A portfolio of evidence is completed in the workplace, which is assessed and verified before you sit an independent assessment. The Dental Nursing NVQ (No 3231) is a Level 3 qualification and is aimed at dental nurses working in general dental practices, community dental services, dental and general hospitals, armed services, who are providing direct chairside work, patient care and support during a range of dental treatments.

To gain the full NVQ, you must complete a total of 11 mandatory units as follows:

‘Ensure your own actions reduce the risk to health and safety

Reflect on and develop your practice

Provide basic life support

Prepare and maintain environments, instruments, and equipment for clinical dental procedures

Offer information and support to individuals on the protection of their oral health

Provide chairside support during the assessment of patients' oral health

Contribute to the production of dental radiographs

Provide chairside support during the prevention and control of periodontal disease and caries, and the restoration of cavities

Provide chairside support during the provision of fixed and removable appliances

Provide chairside support during non-surgical endodontic treatment

Provide chairside support during the extraction of teeth and minor surgery.'

(City & Guilds website, http://www.cityandguilds.com/20031.html)

Dental Nursing VRQ (Vocational No 7393)

VRQ in Dental Nursing (Vocational No 7393) is another Level 3 qualification aiming to develop the knowledge required for full-time employment and/or career progression in dentistry. For full details see the City & Guilds website (http://www.cityandguilds.com/20028.html).

DENTAL NURSE REGISTRATION
Registration

The first step after qualifying as a dental nurse is to register with the GDC. The National Certificate, or the NVQ and VRQ, are required for entry in the GDC Register. GDC registration must be renewed annually.

> **KEY POINT** It is good practice to complete the appropriate paperwork beforehand so that you can send it to the Registrar at the GDC immediately on qualification.

After GDC Registration

As a registered dental professional, you must be familiar with and understand:

- Current standards and principles of dental care, and apply them at work, using your judgement in the light of the principles
- Relevant guidelines from related organisations and sources of evidence that support current standards.

As a dental nurse, you must ensure your knowledge and skills are up to date, and apply them ethically. You must also be prepared to justify your actions to the GDC. If an unsatisfactory account of the behaviour or practice is given (in line with the principles), the dental nurse's GDC registration may be at risk. In other words, a dental nurse is responsible and accountable to themselves, their colleagues, their patients and the GDC, and for continuing development of knowledge and skills. Besides the compulsory (mandatory) training, such as basic life support and infection control, which all members of the dental team are required to undergo, you will be expected to participate in continual professional development (CPD) to maintain your status on the GDC register.

Continued Professional Development

The GDC states that:

> In line with the clinicians' CPD scheme, we recommend that [Dental Care Professionals] DCPs involved in the care of patients should undertake Continual Professional Development in legal and ethical issues and complaints handling.

> Compulsory CPD maintains public confidence in the Dentists and Dental Care Professionals Registers by showing that clinicians and registered dental care professionals keep up to date so that they can give their patients a good standard of care.

Compulsory CPD means that dental nurses must complete and record 150 hours of CPD every five years, of which a third (50 hours) should be *verifiable* (Box 3.1.1). Most providers of CPD will issue a certificate for proof of attendance at the verifiable CPD event, but it is wise to check there will be CPD credits before deciding to participate in the CPD. Some CPD must be on mandatory (essential) core subjects, which are the same as for clinicians:

- Medical emergencies (10 hours per five-year cycle)
- Disinfection and decontamination (5 hours per five-year cycle)
- Radiography and radiation protection (5 hours per five-year cycle).

FITNESS TO PRACTISE

Fitness to practise generally covers issues related to:

- Misconduct
- Incompetence (poor performance)
- Adverse health conditions (medical or mental).

If there is any evidence of poor practice by a dental nurse, according to healthcare regulation, the GDC is required to undertake an investigation which will include processes to test any specific doubt that a registrant remains fit to be on the register, that is, fit to practise. These processes are called the 'fitness to practise system'.

The fitness to practise sequence has four main elements:

1. *Complaint* against, concern about or report received about a particular registrant's fitness to practise
2. *Investigation*
3. *Adjudication* (that is, an official decision), with sanctions (penalties) where these are found necessary
4. *Appeal*.

BOX 3.1.1 VERIFIABLE CPD

Verifiable CPD is defined as that which has:

- Concise educational aims and objectives
- A clear purpose or goal
- Quality controls
- Documentary proof of participation.

CAREER PATHWAYS

Following qualification and registration, gaining experience as a qualified dental nurse is paramount. It may be helpful to join the British Association of Dental Nurses (BADN), which offers guidance on matters related to dental nursing (see p. 78 for contact details).

Career pathways in dental nursing fall into three main categories: clinical, management and education. See Table 3.1.2 for examples.

Further Training

The NEBDN has several post-registration courses that could form part of a dental nurse's professional development:

- Conscious sedation
- Dental radiography
- Oral health education
- Orthodontic nursing
- Special care.

As well as a written examination, post-registration courses involve completion of a 'Record of Experience' in the workplace. This comprises:

- Log sheets verified by a registered dental professional
- Expanded case studies
- Evidence of competence.

It is essential that the dental nurse wishing to take one of the above courses works in an environment that specialises in that course. For example, for undertaking the certificate in special care, the dental nurse should be working with special care patients. The NEBDN provides a list of approved accredited centres in the UK that provide post-registration/other courses.

Other NEBDN certificated courses on offer are:

- Basic and advanced dental implants
- Infection control
- Restorative and surgical procedures.

Attending conferences also helps to gain further knowledge and information.

Employment Opportunities

A variety of employment opportunities are available in the UK for qualified dental nurses:

- Armed forces
- Bank of England
- Corporate body
- Dental access centre
- Hospital dental service
- Industry
- NHS practice
- Personal (formerly community) dental service (PDS)
- Police service
- Prison service
- Private practice
- Retail
- Specialist practice
- Temping agency
- Work overseas.

TABLE 3.1.2 Careers in Dental Nursing		
Management	**Education**	**Education and Management**
Lead Dental Nurse	Clinical Dental Nurse Trainer or Assessor	Principal/Manager of Dental Nurse Education and Training
Practice Manager	Clinical Tutor Dental Nurse	
Senior Dental Nurse	Tutor Dental Nurse	

FIND OUT MORE

Read the General Dental Council *Standards for Dental Professionals and Supplementary Guidance* (2005), which is sent by the GDC to all new registrants.

USEFUL ADDRESSES AND OTHER CONTACT DETAILS

- British Association of Dental Nurses: PO Box 4, Room 200, Hillhouse International Business Centre, Thornton-Cleveleys FY5 4QD (tel: 01253 338360; www.badn.org.uk)
- City and Guilds of London Institute, Care, Health & Community: 1 Giltspur Street, London EC1A 9DD (tel: 0207 294 2800; fax: 0207 294 2400; www.city-and-guilds.co.uk)
- General Dental Council: 37 Wimpole Street, London W1G 8DQ (tel: 020 7887 3880; www.gdc-uk.org)
- National Examining Board for Dental Nurses: 110 London Street, Fleetwood, Lancashire FY7 6EU (tel: 01253 778 417; fax: 01253 777 268; info@nebdn.org.uk; www.nebdn.org.uk)
- School of Postgraduate Medical and Dental Education, Grove Mews, 1 Coronation Road, Birchgrove, Cardiff CF14 4XY (tel: 02920 544 989; fax: 02920 617 165; jackmanjc@cardiff.ac.uk; www.dentpostgradwales.ac.uk)
- School of Professionals Complementary to Dentistry, Science Admission Centre, Science Faculty Office, St Michael's Building, White Swan Road, Portsmouth PO1 2DT (tel: 02392 84 5550; sci.admissions@port.ac.uk; www.port.ac.uk/teeth)
- Scottish Qualifications Authority, The Optima Building, 58 Robertson Street, Glasgow G2 8DQ (tel: 0845 279 1000; fax: 0845 213 5000; www.sqa.org.uk)

3.2 ETHICAL PRACTICE IN DENTAL NURSING

- Patients are increasingly better educated, much more knowledgeable, both about their rights and about healthcare in general, and have more access to information. As a consequence, many have high expectations, and want to be kept better informed and involved in decision making. The current UK government obviously supports this approach with its phrase: 'No decisions about you, without you'.

GDC GUIDANCE ON ETHICAL PRACTICE

The General Dental Council (GDC) guidance document *Standards for Dental Professionals* (2005) applies to the whole dental team. It explains the standards that the GDC expects of dental professionals – all of whom have a responsibility to work to the six key principles of ethical practice. The guidance consists of a set of documents: a core document, plus supplementary guidance documents. New registrants get a copy of all the Standards guidance when they join the GDC Register.

KEY PRINCIPLES OF ETHICAL PRACTICE (from *Standards for Dental Professionals*, GDC, 2005)

1. Putting patients' interest first and acting to protect them.
2. Respecting patients' dignity and choices.
3. Protecting patients' confidential information.
4. Co-operating with other members of the dental team and other healthcare colleagues in the interests of the patients.
5. Maintaining your professional knowledge and competence.
6. Being trustworthy.

A summary of the GDC guidance is presented below.

1. Putting patients' interest first and acting to protect them
   This sets out dental professionals' responsibility to protect patients by, for example, maintaining GDC registration, working only within the scope of their knowledge and keeping accurate patient records.

2. Respecting patients' dignity and choices
   This sets out the importance of treating patients with dignity and respect, being non-discriminatory, and recognising the patient's responsibility for making decisions, and giving them all the information they need to make decisions.

3. Protecting patients' confidential information
   This sets out the need to treat information about patients as confidential, using it only for the purposes for which it was given. Dental professionals should also take steps to prevent accidental disclosure or unauthorised access to confidential information by keeping information secure at all times.

   In some *limited circumstances*, disclosure of confidential patient information without consent may be justified in the public interest (e.g. to assist in the prevention or detection of a serious crime) or it may be required by law or by Court order. *Dental professionals should seek appropriate advice before disclosing information on this basis.* This point is covered in greater detail on pages 89–90.

4. Co-operating with other members of the dental team and other healthcare colleagues in the interests of the patients
   This states that dental professionals should work co-operatively with colleagues and respect their role in the care of patients. Dental professionals should also treat colleagues fairly and without discrimination, and communicate effectively and share knowledge and skills as necessary, in the interest of the patient.

5. Maintaining your professional knowledge and competence
   This states that dental professionals should make sure that they continuously review their knowledge, skills and professional performance, and identify and understand their limitations as well as their strengths. Dental professionals should make themselves aware of the best practice in the fields that they work in and provide good standards of care based on available evidence and authoritative guidance. They should also make themselves aware of the laws and regulations that affect their work, premises, equipment and businesses, and comply with them.

6. Being trustworthy
   This states that dental professionals should make sure that they justify the trust placed in them by their patients, the public and colleagues, by acting honestly and fairly in all their professional *and personal* dealings.

GDC Supplementary Guidance to *Standards for Dental Professionals*

The GDC has also produced a series of supplementary guidance documents that expands on how dental nurses should apply the principle 'put patients' interests first and act to protect them'.

THE GDC SUPPLEMENTARY GUIDANCE DOCUMENTS

- Principles of patient consent (June 2005)
- Principles of patient confidentiality (June 2005)
- Principles of dental team working (February 2006)
- Principles of handling complaints (May 2006)
- Principles of raising concerns (May 2006)
- Principles of management responsibility (February 2008)
- Scope of practice (November 2008)

PRINCIPLES OF PATIENT CONSENT

As a dental nurse, you must be aware of the principles of patient consent. All healthcare professionals must obtain valid consent (see p. 93) from a patient before commencing treatment, carrying out a physical investigation, or providing personal care. This is because it is the legal right of a patient to decide what happens to their body, that is, whether or not to accept a dental professional's advice or treatment. It is also a fundamental part of good practice.

This GDC guidance describes the ethical principles of obtaining patient consent in the context of dental work. If there is any doubt on the legal issues around obtaining patient consent, the clinician should ask an appropriate source – for example, a dental defence organisation – for advice. This principle is covered in greater detail on pages 93–98.

FIND OUT MORE

Check out the websites of the various dental organisations for more details about help available:

- Dental Defence Union (DDU) – http://www.the-ddu.com
- Dental Protection Limited (DP) – http://www.dentalprotection.org
- Medical and Dental Defence Union of Scotland (MDDUS) – http://www.mddus.com/mddus/home.aspx

---

PRINCIPLES OF PATIENT CONFIDENTIALITY

Dental professionals have a legal and ethical duty to keep patient information confidential and use it only in the context in which it was given. Confidential information should be kept in a secure place at all times to prevent unauthorised disclosure or accidental disclosure.

If exceptional circumstances arise in which a dental professional feels that the disclosure of confidential information is necessary for the patient's safety, they should seek appropriate advice before any action is taken.

PRINCIPLES OF DENTAL TEAMWORKING

This guidance explains how the dental team should work together in the best interests of patients.

PRINCIPLES OF COMPLAINTS HANDLING

This guidance provides a checklist that dental professionals can use to ensure that they have an effective in-house complaints procedure where they work. This principle is covered in greater detail on pages 83–85.

PRINCIPLES OF RAISING CONCERNS

This guidance explains dental professionals' responsibility to raise matters of concern about colleagues, systems and the working environment ('whistle blowing'), and how to go about this. Whistle blowing is covered in more detail on page 98.

PRINCIPLES OF MANAGEMENT RESPONSIBILITY

This guidance is about registrants' responsibilities when acting in a business capacity. Currently, all members of the registered dental team can receive payment for dental treatment, can own dental practices/dental laboratories and can employ other members of the dental team. Also, any dental practice or group of practices can become a corporate body.

Standards for Dental Professionals is also supported by the following GDC statements:

- Conducting clinical trials
- Responsible prescribing
- Child protection.

CARE PATHWAYS (CLINICAL GUIDELINES)

A care pathway is a statement that helps decision-making about appropriate healthcare for a specific clinical condition. It should be based on the available best evidence, to encourage best practice and reduce unsatisfactory variations in treatment.

No guidelines are compulsory for the clinician to follow but clinicians have a responsibility to provide best practice and will need a good argument for not following guidelines. Implementation of guidelines is the clinician's responsibility if they are self-employed, or is the responsibility of the employing NHS organisation as part of its clinical governance plan (see next section).

Several independent and government organisations in the UK have developed healthcare guidelines for use by doctors, dentists and other healthcare professionals. For example:

* National Institute for Health and Clinical Excellence (NICE) – for NHS in England and Wales
* Scottish Intercollegiate Guidelines Network (SIGN) – for NHS in Scotland
* Royal College of Surgeons of England – Faculty of Dental Surgery National Clinical Guidelines 1997.
* British Society for Paediatric Dentistry – the Paediatric Dentistry Clinical Guidelines series.
* British Society for Disability and Oral Health – relating to people with special needs.

FIND OUT MORE

Can you name the guidelines that have been produced by NICE for dentistry?

CLINICAL GOVERNANCE

Clinical governance (now increasingly called 'quality assurance' or QA) is an umbrella term for everything that helps maintain and improve the standards of patient care (Box 3.2.1). The essential features of clinical governance are:

> **KEY POINT** The care that is provided to patients should be clinically appropriate and cost-effective, and delivered with proper regard to the dignity and **autonomy** of the patient.

81

* Patient care provided should be safe and risks should be managed effectively
* Health services are accountable for the safety, quality and effectiveness of clinical care delivered to patients
* Healthcare staff should participate in shared learning and teamwork, and identify and improve any shortfalls in their knowledge and service.

Every healthcare organisation (NHS or private) is responsible for ensuring that clinical governance measures are in place. In the UK, the Care Quality Commission monitors the clinical governance arrangements of NHS organisations and rates the performance of each organisation. (Its predecessors, the Healthcare Commission, Commission for Social Care Inspection and the Mental Health Act Commission ceased to exist on 31 March 2009.)

Clinical governance can be achieved by co-ordinating its components, which are also called the 'seven pillars' of clinical governance. These are:

* *Patient and public involvement*. This includes use of patient satisfaction surveys to assess patients' views on the service being provided and the Patient Advice and Liaison Services (PALS), which exists in every NHS trust.
* *Risk management*. Risks should be assessed as a four-stage process:
  1. Identify risks using screening, checklists, etc
  2. Assess frequency and severity of risk

Term to Learn
Autonomy: the patient's right to make decisions about their medical care. Although the healthcare provider should educate and inform the patient about factors that could affect the patient's treatment, they must not try to influence the patient in their decision making or make the decision themselves.

BOX 3.2.1 CLINICAL GOVERNANCE

Clinical governance is:

- Doing the right thing
- In the right way
- At the right time
- By the right people
- To the right people
- And being able to measure it.

(after The Local Health Groups of Wales)

BOX 3.2.2 STEPS IN PERFORMING AN AUDIT

1. Prepare for audit
   - Choose a topic of concern to staff.
   - Set aside time to conduct audit.
   - Ensure support of colleagues.

   ↓

2. Select criteria
   - Select the criteria against which the issue will be compared. Clear criteria are best obtained from available guidelines or reviews of evidence (external standards).

   ↓

3. Measure performance
   - Collect data on current practice. Depending on the topic, this may be from clinical records and/or department/hospital databases. Using several data sources helps overcome problems of incomplete records.
   - Measure performance against the selected criteria.

   ↓

4. Make improvements
   - In the light of the findings, devise a plan for implementing improvements.
   - Discuss improvements with colleagues and think about potential barriers to change.

   ↓

5. Sustain improvements
   - Monitor and reinforce the improvements, and keep up to date.

---

3. Eliminate risks where possible
4. Reduce the risk, and plan for damage limitation where elimination of risk is impossible.

- *Clinical audit* (Box 3.2.2). This procedure documents what the current clinical standards are with regard to a particular issue (e.g. the quality of radiographs being taken), or a particular treatment (e.g. extraction of wisdom teeth). This is then compared with a recognised external standard, which may be a local or national standard but which is evidence based (e.g. a guideline issued by NICE), whenever this is available and appropriate. Changes are then made (if required) to ensure that the current clinical practice is in line with best available evidence. Areas that can be audited include:
  - Professional performance, that is, performance of various members of staff
  - Risk management
  - Patient satisfaction
  - Use of resources.
- *Staffing and management.* Organisations should adopt a 'quality improvement' approach to human resource management. This includes staff appraisals, and mechanisms to deal with poor performance (such as 'whistle blowing', see p. 98 for details) rather than ignoring such practices.

- *Clinical effectiveness*. This includes how each organisation implements and applies effective clinical practice (see below).
- *Continued professional development* (CPD). See Subchapter 3.1, page 76, for details.
- *Information use*. Each organisation should have information that supports clinical governance and provides information on the patient experience.

FIND OUT MORE

What are the contact details of your local Patient Advice and Liaison Services?

Clinical Effectiveness

Clinical effectiveness is about improving the quality of treatments and services. Health professionals, who provide the actual service, therefore will have the expertise, first-hand knowledge and skills, and an insight and understanding as to how the service works and how it could be improved. Their involvement in audits and improvement projects is therefore an important part of promoting good clinical practice.

Risk Management

Risk management is a standardised process to reduce injuries, errors, faults and accidents and at the same time improve quality. Up to 10% of patient care episodes result in harm to patients or staff, and half of these incidents are preventable. Clinical incidents and near-misses highlight the need to learn from such incidents and for action to reduce or manage risks.

The National Patient Safety Agency (NPSA) leads and contributes to improved, safe patient care in England and Wales. It does this by providing information, support and recommendations for safer practice to NHS organisations. It has three divisions:

- Reporting and Learning Service – this division aims to improve safety by enabling NHS organisations to learn from patient safety incidents
- National Clinical Assessment Service – this division provides confidential services to help manage any concerns about the performance of healthcare practitioners
- National Research Ethics Service – this division protects the safety and dignity of research participants by promoting ethical research.

To provide a quality health service, issues of quality, quantity and cost often compete. However, through clinical governance, the best balance can be established.

DEALING WITH COMPLAINTS

When a patient wishes to complain, depending on the nature of the complaint, they may contact:

- Their local primary care trust (PCT), Quality Care Commission or the Ombudsman for NHS care
- The Dental Complaints Service for private care
- The GDC
- The Health and Safety Executive
- The Advertising Standards Authority
- The Office of Fair Trading/Trading Standards Offices
- The police.

KEY POINT Listen to the patient's complaint, obtain all the information, and if need be, refer to a senior person, to resolve the issue quickly.

People who use healthcare services mostly understand that mistakes sometimes happen. When something goes wrong, often all the person affected wants to know is how it happened, that the persons involved are sorry, and that steps will be taken to prevent it

83

from happening again. So the way in which an organisation responds to the initial contact by a person who is unhappy about their service is important. It is crucial to obtain all the information that will allow assessment of someone's concerns correctly, resolve them quickly if possible and build a good ongoing relationship with them. Often the reason people give for being unhappy about how their complaint has been handled is *poor communication* by the services.

THINGS TO REMEMBER TO DO WHEN SOMEONE SAYS THEY ARE UNHAPPY

1. Ask the person how they would like to be addressed – as Mr, Mrs, Ms or by their first name.
2. If someone has phoned you, offer to call them back and give them the chance to meet face to face to discuss the issue.
3. Ask them how they wish to be kept informed about how their complaint is being dealt with – by phone, letter, e-mail or through a third party such as an advocacy or support service. If they say by phone, ask them for times when it is convenient to call and check that they are happy for messages to be left on their answerphone. If they say by post, make sure that they are happy to receive correspondence at the address given.
4. Check if the person has any disability or circumstances you need to take account of (for example, do they require wheelchair access, or are they on medication that can make them drowsy?).
5. Offer to meet the person at a location convenient to them.
6. Make the person aware that they can request an advocate to support them throughout the complaints process, including at the first meeting.
7. Systematically go through the reasons for the complaint with the person who is unhappy – it is important that you understand why they are dissatisfied.
8. Ask them what they would like to happen as a result of the complaint (for example, an apology, new appointment, reimbursement for costs or loss of personal belongings or an explanation). Tell them at the outset if their expectations are not feasible or realistic.
9. Agree a plan of action, including when and how the person complaining will hear back from your organisation.
10. If you think you can resolve the matter quickly without further investigation do so as long as the person complaining is happy with that and there is no risk to other service users.
11. For any complaint, remember to:
    - Check if consent is needed to access someone's personal records
    - Let the complainant know the name and contact details of the manager who will investigate their complaint
    - Let them know their rights when it comes to making a complaint.

There should be a person designated to handle complaints. It is more usual for a patient to complain verbally than in writing; in either event it is wise at this stage to communicate with the medical insurance society (e.g. the Dental Defence Union: DDU; Dental Protection: DP and Medical and Dental Defence Union of Scotland: MDDUS) and heed their advice.

IF A PATIENT COMPLAINS VERBALLY

1. A patient complaining verbally should be seen by the designated person in a private area where others cannot hear the conversation.
2. The designated person should politely listen to the complaint and make notes to ensure an accurate record of the discussion is made.
3. A copy should be given to the complainant.
4. If appropriate, a verbal apology may be offered without admitting liability or negligence.
5. The complaint must be recorded accurately in the 'patient complaints log' (Box 3.2.3). It has been compulsory for NHS organisations to keep records of patient complaints and their handling since 1996, but this should be done in any type of practice.

BOX 3.2.3 PATIENT COMPLAINTS LOG

The patient complaints log should include:

- The time and date of complaint
- How it was received
- The nature of the complaint
- How it was handled
- Correspondence, such as with lawyers etc.

IF A PATIENT COMPLAINS IN WRITING

1. If a complaint is in writing, its receipt must be acknowledged (usually by the designated person) in writing (marked private and confidential) within two working days.
2. The designated person should then investigate the complaint, keeping notes of information that is elicited.
3. The complainant must receive, within 10 working days, a written report of these investigations, but no blame should be apportioned, nor personal comments or views expressed. *An apology may be offered – this does NOT admit liability or negligence.*
4. The complainant should be given the opportunity to discuss the matter further at the practice if they choose.

Remember that all complaints offer the opportunity to review practice procedures to minimise or avoid future issues. Whilst medical/dental records must be disclosed where requested, the Complaints Log Book does not need to be disclosed.

FIND OUT MORE

Where is the patient complaints log in your workplace kept?

NHS and Adult Social Care Complaints Regulations

The NHS Constitution states that:

'any individual has the right to:

- Have any complaint they make about NHS services dealt with efficiently and have it properly investigated
- Know the outcome of any investigation into their complaint
- Take their complaint to the independent Health Service Ombudsman if they are not satisfied with the way the NHS has dealt with their complaint
- Make a claim for judicial review if they think they have been directly affected by an unlawful act or decision of an NHS body
- Receive compensation where they have been harmed by negligent treatment.'

The approach focuses on the complainant and enables NHS organisations to make a tailored response to resolve the complainant's specific concerns. It is based on the principles of good complaints handling (Box 3.2.4), published by the Parliamentary and Health Service Ombudsman and endorsed by the Local Government Ombudsman.

Dental Complaints Service

The Dental Complaints Service (DCS) is an independent dental complaints service funded by the GDC to help resolve complaints about private dental care.

> **BOX 3.2.4 PRINCIPLES OF GOOD COMPLAINTS HANDLING**
> - Getting it right.
> - Being customer focused.
> - Being open and accountable.
> - Acting fairly and proportionately.
> - Putting things right.
> - Seeking continuous improvement.

How the Caldicott Principles Affect Handling of Patient Complaints

Care must be taken at all times throughout the complaints procedure to follow Caldicott principles (see p. 87). This means that only information about the patient relevant to the investigation of the complaint should be disclosed. Further, disclosure should only be made to those who have a demonstrable need to know that information in order to investigate the complaint. Where a complaint is made on behalf of a patient who has not been able to give consent for someone to act for them, care must be taken not to disclose personal health information to the complainant.

DATA ISSUES
Freedom of Information

The Freedom of Information Act 2000 deals with the right to access official information. It gives individuals or organisations the right to request information from any public authority, companies wholly owned by public authorities in England, Wales and Northern Ireland and *non-devolved* public bodies in Scotland. Bodies and offices considered as public authorities for the purpose of the Act, are:

- Government departments
- Non-departmental government bodies – bodies to which the government has passed on certain authority, also referred to by the acronym QUANGO (quasi-autonomous non-governmental organisation)
- Parliament, the Northern Ireland Assembly and the National Assembly for Wales
- The Armed Forces (but not special forces or units working with Government Communications Headquarters)
- Local authorities
- NHS bodies
- The police
- Other bodies and offices such as regulators and advisory committees.

Some bodies are only covered for certain sorts of information, such as the BBC and Channel 4.

The Freedom of Information Act gives people the right to obtain information held by these authorities unless there are good reasons to keep it confidential. In other words, a person can ask for any information at all – but some information might be withheld to protect various interests which are allowed for by the Act. However, if this is the case, the public authority must tell the person that it has withheld information and why.

Any person can make a request for information under the Act – there are no restrictions on age, nationality, or where they live. All the person has to do is write to (or e-mail) the public authority that the person thinks holds the information they want. They should make sure that they include:

- Their name
- An address where they can be contacted
- A description of the information that they want.

Public authorities must comply with the request promptly, and should provide the information within 20 working days (around a month). If they need more time, they must write to the person and tell them when they will be able to answer the request, and why they need more time.

Data Protection

The Data Protection Act 1998 regulates how *personal* information (whether computerised data or paper records) is used by organisations and workplaces. This helps ensure confidentiality and security of personal data such as an individual's name, address, date of birth and bank details or any other information that identifies an individual. The privacy of data, especially of a personal nature, is important to most people, and there are several examples in the media of the serious loss of data – whether that be as hard copy, on USB sticks (universal serial bus flash memory devices), computer disks (CDs), personal digital assistants (PDAs) or even laptop or desktop computers. All these should be 'encrypted' or password-protected.

> **KEY POINT** If a person asks for information about *themselves*, then the request will be handled under the Data Protection Act instead of the Freedom of Information Act.

The Act classifies the following as 'sensitive' information:

- Racial and ethnic origin
- Political persuasion
- Religious or faith beliefs
- Membership of a trade union
- Physical and mental health conditions
- Criminal offences or allegations.

To use 'sensitive' information, the organisation or workplace has to meet one of a set of eight conditions (principles) to ensure the sensitive information is only used when absolutely necessary or with the individual's consent. All users of personal information are bound to comply with these principles of the Data Protection Act as outlined below.

1. Data are obtained and processed fairly and lawfully – the person understands the reason for obtaining the data and who will use it.
2. Data are processed for a limited purpose – the data can only be used for the purpose which the person understands it is for.
3. Data are adequate, relevant and not excessive – the minimum data required are obtained.
4. Data are accurate.
5. Data are kept only as required – data should be destroyed after the statutory legislation period expires.
6. Data are processed in line with the rights of an individual.
7. Data are kept physically and technically secure.
8. Data are not transferred to countries without adequate data protection legislation.

Patient Data and Confidentiality

In dentistry, personal information is essential for treating patients. Besides the patient's age, name, address and date of birth, clinicians require information about the dental, medical and social background of the person to aid diagnosis and treatment planning. All patients (including dental nurses when they may be patients) expect a high level of confidentiality, whether through verbal communication or personal records. Patient records should be restricted to those delivering the care and related administration. If possible, patient data should be saved on a secure site and not saved to a computer's hard disk.

The Caldicott Principles

In 1997, a review was commissioned by the Chief Medical Officer of England in response to concerns about ways in which patient information was being used in the NHS in England and Wales, largely due to the increasing use of IT. It was realised that electronically held information

87

could be disseminated rather widely and quite quickly. Thus it was felt that guidance was required to ensure that confidentiality was maintained appropriately. The review was chaired by Dame Fiona Caldicott and the Caldicott Report was published in December 1997. It listed six key principles (Box 3.2.5) relating to patient confidentiality and recommended ways in which the NHS could improve the handling of patient identifiable information.

A key recommendation of the report was the establishment of a network of organisational guardians (known as 'Caldicott Guardians') to oversee access to patient-identifiable information. All NHS organisations are now required to have a Caldicott guardian and a lead individual to co-ordinate a programme of work.

FIND OUT MORE

If you work in an NHS organisation, find out who is your Caldicott guardian.

BOX 3.2.5 THE CALDICOTT PRINCIPLES

Principle 1 – Justify the purpose(s)

Every proposed use or transfer of patient-identifiable information within or from an organisation should be clearly defined and scrutinised, with continuing uses regularly reviewed, by an appropriate guardian.

Principle 2 – Do not use patient-identifiable information unless it is absolutely necessary

Patient-identifiable information items should not be included unless it is essential for the specified purpose(s) of that flow. The need for patients to be identified should be considered at each stage of satisfying the purpose(s).

Principle 3 – Use the minimum necessary patient-identifiable information

Where use of patient-identifiable information is considered to be essential, the inclusion of each individual item of information should be considered and justified so that the minimum amount of identifiable information is transferred or accessible as is necessary for a given function to be carried out.

Principle 4 – Access to patient-identifiable information should be on a strict need-to-know basis

Only those individuals who need access to patient-identifiable information should have access to it, and they should only have access to the information items that they need to see. This may mean introducing access controls or splitting information flows where one information flow is used for several purposes.

Principle 5 – Everyone with access to patient-identifiable information should be aware of their responsibilities

Action should be taken to ensure that those handling patient-identifiable information – both clinical and non-clinical staff – are made fully aware of their responsibilities and obligations to respect patient confidentiality.

Principle 6 – Understand and comply with the law

Every use of patient-identifiable information must be lawful. Someone in each organisation handling patient information should be responsible for ensuring that the organisation complies with legal requirements.

Access to Health Records

The record holder of health records is the clinician.

Regulations applying:

- The Access to Medical Records Act 1991 gives patients, and patients only, the right of access to their medical and dental records. However, a written request is needed.
- If any one else wishes to access a patient's medical reports, this is governed by the Access to Medical Reports Act 1988.
- Access to the health records of living patients is governed by the Data Protection Act 1998.
- Access to the health records of a deceased person is governed by the Access to Health Records Act 1990.

Any request for dental records must be made in accordance with the Data Protection Act 1998 (section 7), and the clinician must supply the patient with dental notes, records and any dental X-rays. A fee, currently £50 maximum, can be charged for their supply. Note that only the record holder (the clinician) can grant access to records; *other staff including the dental nurse must not hand over records without the express permission of the clinician.* The record holder (the clinician) must respond to a request within 40 days. If the clinician does not do this, he or she will be breaking the Data Protection Act 1998. This means that the patient can make an application to the court for a judge to order disclosure of the dental records. The patient may also make a complaint to the GDC about the non-disclosure of dental records. Circumstances where the clinician is legally allowed not to disclose some or all of the records are:

- Where the record disclosure would cause serious harm to the patient
- Where another person is referred to in the records and they have not given their consent to disclosure (this does not apply to where that person is a healthcare worker involved in the patient's care)
- Where the records have a note to say that access is not to be granted in the event of a patient's death.

The written permission of the patient must be obtained before anyone else can have access to their records. The clinician must check the identity of the person making the disclosure request before releasing the records. The patient's name, address, date and size of debt can be given to a debt collector employed by the practice to collect debts.

> **KEY POINT** A dental nurse can be dismissed if they breach confidentiality or the Data Protection Act.

CLINICAL RECORDS

It is crucial for dental nurses to maintain confidentiality and to comply with the local requirements for the safe storage of clinical and other records. Patients' record cards or other similar data should not be left anywhere else. Even at work, a patient's record card should be placed face down. Clinical records are best never removed from the workplace but, if they must be, a lockable case or box is desirable to ensure they do not get lost or stolen. If they are transported in a car they must be safely locked away out of sight.

CLINICAL IMAGES

Clinical images automatically form part of the patient record and, as such, they are protected by the Data Protection Act 1998. Consent should be obtained, whatever use is proposed for a patient photograph.

COMPUTER RECORDS

The Data Protection Act 1998 requires that there should be no unauthorised access to the data on a computer. Laptop computers and portable hard-drives or USB 'sticks' are too frequently lost or stolen, so they must ALWAYS be password-protected ('encrypted').

TABLE 3.2.1 Retention Times for Records

Purpose	Retention Times
Adult clinical records	General Dental Services: 2 years (but 11 years is much safer!) Hospital: 8 years Community: 11 years
Audit records	5 years
Children's clinical records	Hospital: retain until the patient's 25th birthday or 26th if young person was 17 at conclusion of treatment, or until 8 years after death. If the illness or death could have potential relevance to adult conditions or have genetic implications for the family of the deceased, the advice of clinicians should be sought as to whether to retain longer Community: 11 years or up to their 25th birthday, whichever is the longer
Patient information leaflets	6 years after the leaflet has been superseded
Phone messages	2 years
Photographs (clinical)	30 years where images present the primary source of information for the diagnostic process
Staff CPD records	8 years
X-rays and other imaging	8 years after conclusion of treatment

When any computer or hard drive is disposed of they must be carefully cleaned (e.g. using software such as File Shredder (http://www.fileshredder.org), preferably by a specialist contractor, or destroyed or securely stored as part of the clinical record, since documents on any hard drive are retrievable by using forensic techniques, even though the user may have thought they had 'deleted' them.

Retention of Records

As mentioned in the previous section, the record holder of dental records is the clinician. *Records are best kept as long as possible, but there are certain minimal retention times* after which records can be destroyed (Table 3.2.1) – but always under confidential conditions.

All clinical records must be kept for 11 years or until the patient is aged 25, whichever is the longer. This includes records for patients who have not attended, moved to another clinician, or died. They can then be disposed of, ensuring the information is rendered unreadable. To ensure this, the records should be incinerated.

EMPLOYEE DATA

Employees' personal information should be up to date, confidential and kept in a secure place.

KEY POINT Under the Data Protection Act 1998 and Computer Misuse Act 1990 it may also be a criminal offence to breach confidentiality of data.

OTHER DATA

This could include financial data or service and suppliers' contracts, and should be kept in a secure site or place. A dental nurse may well come across data such as these. It is vital the information is kept confidential and not shared. Information should not be sought out if it does not concern or involve you. There are usually local and professional regulations that relate to this.

ENSURING DATA SECURITY

- The best policy is to treat all information as if it were your own.
- Manual records must be kept secure.
- Filing cabinets and drawers must be kept locked and the keys kept in a locked place.
- If possible, the clinic, office and or department should be locked and the alarm activated when not in use. It is advised to change key codes and locks annually.

E-mails

Always remember that anything sent by e-mail is as open to view as anything written on a postcard. Take great care.

There are rules precluding patients' names and personal details being used on e-mails unless encrypted. Many employers also have protocols for use to:

- Reduce the risk of offending other staff
- Ensure that the employer's money and time is not squandered
- Reduce the risk from computer viruses.

If the terms of employment require employees to adhere to such a code defined by their employer, there may be grounds for disciplinary action if this requirement is broken.

Security Breaches

If you discover data has been tampered with or lost, report it immediately to your line manager, or if appropriate, the security information officer. The report should include:

- Date and time
- Identification of data
- Action taken
- Reason for the loss or tampering
- Any follow-up action.

The report should be noted in the practice **incident book**.

CLOSED CIRCUIT TELEVISION (CCTV)

Businesses that use a CCTV system must display notices to that effect. They may also need to register with the Information Commissioner (see p. 98 for contact details).

> **Term to Learn**
> **Incident book:** a book in which all injuries, crimes, and other incidents related to patient or staff safety are recorded.

91

DISABILITY DISCRIMINATION

Legislation applying:

- Disability and Discrimination Act 2005
- Equality Bill.

Employers' Duties

- *Employment.* Employers must not treat a disabled employee or job applicant less favourably than someone else.
- *Accessing goods and services.* Employers must make sure that disabled people are not treated less favourably and that they can access any services provided. This may require an employer to make physical changes to their premises.

The Equality and Human Rights Commission has further information on duties under the Disability and Discrimination Act 2005. The Equality Bill aims among other things to:

- Further address socio-economic inequalities
- Re-state the greater part of the enactments relating to discrimination and harassment on the grounds of certain personal characteristics.

Employment

Anyone employing staff must comply with employment legislation including:

- The National Minimum Wage Act
- The Working Time Regulations
- The Employment Rights Act.

FIND OUT MORE

There are many helpful booklets available on employment issues. Try to obtain some from your local Jobcentre.

EVIDENCE-BASED DENTISTRY (EBD)

Ever-increasing amounts of published literature means there is a large amount of evidence available for various dental treatments. However, the research and the evidence is sometimes of questionable quality; therefore, practice has traditionally been based on 'authority', that is experience of authoritative figures in the field. This is sometimes called 'eminence-based healthcare'.

EVIDENCE-BASED HEALTHCARE

- Is the use of the best available evidence to make a decision regarding healthcare.
- Optimises the effective use of available literature.
- Allows clinicians to keep up to date with rapid changes.
- Raises patient and professional expectations.
- More effectively regulates competing pressures on resources.

Evidence-based healthcare can be defined on different levels: an organisation such as NICE produces national clinical guidelines that are relevant to all, a hospital department can review the literature to produce a specific protocol it feels is needed, or a clinician can undertake their own review to help guide specific clinical decisions. The steps in doing a review for the benefit of applying evidence-based healthcare are the same whatever the scale of the review.

When evaluating the literature for the above purpose, the 'strength' or 'level' of the evidence from a particular study or review of studies will be largely influenced by the methods used to conduct the study or review. There is a well-established hierarchy of the different types of study that can be done and thus the level of evidence they provide. The smaller the number in the hierarchical table, the greater is the strength of the evidence (Box 3.2.6).

The Cochrane Collaboration conducts systematic reviews of evidence from RCTs and the specific Cochrane Oral Health Group has conducted reviews in many aspects of dentistry.

FIND OUT MORE

Where is the Cochrane Oral Health Group based? (See http://www.ohg.cochrane.org)

Terms to Learn

RCT: randomised controlled trial; a study in which people are allocated in a random order to receive one of two or more treatments. Usually, one of the treatments will be the current standard treatment or it may be a placebo or nothing at all (control).

Cohort study: a study which includes people who are similar in most ways but different in one main characteristic (for example, all university graduates who play sport but may be smokers or non-smokers) are included to study a particular outcome of a caries treatment.

Case–control studies: A study that helps to identify risk factors for developing a disease or condition. It does this by comparing two groups of people: those with the disease or condition (cases) with those (from the same population) who do not have that disease or condition (controls).

Case study: a published report of a single example of a disease or treatment, for example the description of the characteristics and perhaps treatment of one person with a rare disease.

BOX 3.2.6 LEVELS OF EVIDENCE

The five levels of evidence:

1a. Evidence from a systematic review of several **randomised controlled trials** (RCTs) – this is a special kind of analysis involving complex statistical methods that considers together the results of several studies, specifically RCTs

1b. Evidence from one well-designed RCT

2a. Evidence from a systematic review of **cohort studies**

2b. Evidence from one cohort study, or low-quality RCT

3a. Evidence from a systematic review of **case–control studies**

3b. Evidence from one case–control study

4. Evidence from non-analytical studies (**case studies**)

5. Opinions of expert committees or respected authorities

MEDICAL DEVICES

All GDC registrants who prescribe, manufacture or fit dental appliances have a role to play in protecting patients from harm and in providing a safe and effective standard of care. All dentists, dental technicians and clinical dental technicians should understand and know they are responsible for the decisions they make when commissioning or manufacturing dental appliances or other medical devices.

In the context of dentistry, medical devices are devices that can be used for diagnosis, prevention, monitoring or treatment of a dental condition (e.g. a mouth-guard or a removable brace), or for compensation of an injury or handicap. They may also be used for investigation purposes or replacement or modification of the anatomy (e.g. an **obturator**) or of a physiological process (e.g. appliances to help stop habitual mouth breathing or **sleep apnoea**).

The Medicines and Healthcare products Regulatory Agency (MHRA) is the regulatory body that is responsible for ensuring the safety of all medical devices used in the UK. If a manufacturer breaches MHRA regulations, they are usually given the opportunity to correct the breach of the regulations voluntarily. If this proves not possible or there is an immediate threat to public safety, the MHRA has the power under the Consumer Protection Act to remove the device from the market and prosecute the errant manufacturer. Penalties imposed on prosecution can be a fine of up to £5000 per offence or six months' imprisonment.

Medical devices are classified as given in Annex IX of the European Union Council Directive 93/42/EEC. There are basically four classes, based on the level of risk of injury to staff or patients due to failure or misuse of the device:

- Class I (including Is and Im) – devices with the lowest risk, e.g. dental impression materials
- Class IIa – e.g. dental filling materials
- Class IIb – e.g. permanent dental implants
- Class III – devices with the highest risk, e.g. absorbable sutures.

In the EU all certified medical devices should have the 'CE' mark on the packaging, insert leaflets, etc. The packaging should also show the standard pictograms and 'EN' logos to indicate essential features such as instructions for use, expiry date, manufacturer, sterile, do not reuse, etc. Some dental appliances, e.g. that do not need to be sterilised, can be self-certified by the manufacturer. Others will need to be validated by an accredited body.

A dental appliance that is specifically made for a particular patient is defined as a custom-made device, and the requirements of Annex VIII of the Medical Devices Directive applies to those who wish to manufacture these products. A statement should accompany the individual device confirming that the device conforms to the essential requirements specified in Annex I of the Medical Devices Directive 93/42/EEC, which are incorporated into UK law.

> **Terms to Learn**
> **Obturator:** a dental appliance that is used to close an opening, for example in patients with a cleft palate or a surgical defect, to stop foods and liquids going into the nose.
> **Sleep apnoea:** a disorder in which a person stops breathing for a short time (usually more than 10 seconds) while asleep.

FIND OUT MORE

Look at a couple of appliances that have just come in from a dental laboratory and read the statement confirming that the appliance conforms to the regulations.

PATIENT CONSENT

Consent in relation to dentistry is the expressed or implied agreement of the patient to undergo a dental examination, investigation or treatment. The law in relation to consent is evolving and there are significant variations between countries. However, the principles are essentially the same:

- Before a health professional examines, treats or cares for competent adult patients they must obtain the patient's consent.

- Adults are always assumed to be competent unless demonstrated otherwise. If there are doubts about their competence, the question to ask is: 'Can this patient understand and weigh up the information needed to make this decision?' Unexpected decisions do not prove the patient is incompetent, but may indicate a need for further information or explanation.
- Patients may be competent to make some healthcare decisions, even if they are not competent to make others.
- Giving and obtaining consent is usually a process, not a one-off event. Patients can change their minds and withdraw consent at any time.

In the UK, all competent adults, namely a person aged 18 and over who has the capacity to make their own decisions about treatment, can consent to dental treatment. They are also entitled to refuse treatment, even where it would clearly benefit their health. At age 16, a young person is regarded as an adult and can be presumed to have the capacity to consent to treatment. Consent regarding children is discussed on page 97.

Informed Consent

'Informed' consent means that the patient agrees to treatment based on the assumption that they are fully aware of the treatment they will undergo, including its intended benefits, its possible risks and the level of these risks. In particular, patients must be warned about:

- Any preparation that may be required before treatment (e.g. giving an anaesthetic before a tooth extraction)
- Possible adverse effects of the treatment (e.g. prolonged numbness in the lip and cheek after a wisdom tooth extraction)
- Possibility of any effects that may occur straight after a procedure (e.g. swelling, bruising, pain)
- Where they will be during their recovery
- Possible use of intravenous infusions or other invasive treatments.

Valid Consent

To give valid consent, patients must receive sufficient information about their condition and proposed treatment. It is the dentist's responsibility to explain all the relevant facts to the patient, and to ascertain that they understand them. The information given to patients must, as a minimum, include:

- The nature, purpose, benefits and risks of the treatment
- Alternative treatments and their relative benefits and risks
- All aspects of the procedure expected to be carried out
- The **prognosis** if no treatment is given.

Term to Learn
Prognosis: a prediction of how a disease or patient's condition may worsen or improve over time, with or without treatment.

If the patient is not offered as much information as they reasonably need to make their decision, and in a form they can understand, their consent may not be valid. For example, information for those with visual impairment may be provided in the form of audio tapes, Braille, or large print.

Form of Consent

Consent can be written (Figure 3.2.1), oral or non-verbal. It must be obtained from all patients having an operation. The possible benefits of the treatment must be weighed against the risks and are always discussed by the person carrying out the procedure, or, if for some reason this is not possible, a delegated person with the appropriate expertise to do so. A signature on a consent form does not itself prove the consent is valid – the point of the form is to record the patient's decision, and also, increasingly, the discussions that have taken place.

FIND OUT MORE

Does your workplace have a policy setting out when the dentist needs to obtain consent in writing?

94

Tests of Consent

There are ways of legally testing whether the consent given by a patient was valid or not. The 'Bolam test' is one such way. The Bolam test states that a doctor who:

- Acted in accordance with a practice accepted as proper by a responsible body of medical men skilled in that particular art is not negligent if he is acting in accordance with such a practice, merely because there is a body of opinion which takes a contrary view.

Patient agreement to investigation or treatment

Patient details (or pre-printed label)

Patient's surname/family name ....

Patient's first names ....

Date of birth ....

Responsible health professional ....

Job title ....

NHS number (or other identifier) ....

☐ Male   ☐ Female

Special requirements ....
(eg other language/other communication method)

To be retained in patient's notes

FIGURE 3.2.1

Standard form for patient agreement to investigation or treatment including the confirmation of consent by the patient. This form is accompanied by detailed guidance for health professionals. These are also available at: www.dh.gov.uk/en/ Publichealth/Scientificdevelopment geneticsandbioethics/Consent/Consent generalinformation/index.htm.

Continued

Patient identifier/label

Name of proposed procedure or course of treatment (include brief explanation if medical term not clear)

....

....

....

Statement of health professional (to be filled in by health professional with appropriate knowledge of proposed procedure, as specified in consent policy)

I have explained the procedure to the patient. In particular, I have explained:

The intended benefits ....

....

Serious or frequently occurring risks ....

....

Any extra procedures which may become necessary during the procedure
☐ blood transfusion
☐ other procedure (please specify)

....

I have also discussed what the procedure is likely to involve, the benefits and risks of any available alternative treatments (including no treatment) and any particular concerns of this patient.

☐ The following leaflet/tape has been provided ....

This procedure will involve:
☐ general and/or regional anaesthesia   ☐ local anaesthesia   ☐ sedation

Signed: ....   Date ....

Name (PRINT) ....   Job title ....

Contact details (if patient wishes to discuss options later) ....

Statement of interpreter (where appropriate)

I have interpreted the information above to the patient to the best of my ability and in a way in which I believe s/he can understand.

Signed ....   Date ....

Name (PRINT) ....

Top copy accepted by patient: yes/no (please ring)

2

FIGURE 3.2.1, cont'd

However, a judge may on certain occasions choose between two bodies of medical opinion, if one is to be regarded as that which cannot be logically defended (Bolitho principle). The main alternative to the Bolam test is the 'prudent-patient test', which is widely used in North America. According to this test, doctors should provide the amount of information that a 'prudent patient' would want.

Confirmation of Consent

Confirmation of consent (see last part of Figure 3.2.1) should be completed by a health professional when the patient is admitted for the procedure, if the patient has signed the form in advance.

Statement of patient   **Patient identifier/label**

Please read this form carefully. If your treatment has been planned in advance, you should already have your own copy of page 2 which describes the benefits and risks of the proposed treatment. If not, you will be offered a copy now. If you have any further questions, do ask – we are here to help you. You have the right to change your mind at any time, including after you have signed this form.

I agree to the procedure or course of treatment described on this form.

I understand that you cannot give me a guarantee that a particular person will perform the procedure. The person will, however, have appropriate experience.

I understand that I will have the opportunity to discuss the details of anaesthesia with an anaesthetist before the procedure, unless the urgency of my situation prevents this. (This only applies to patients having general or regional anaesthesia.)

I understand that any procedure in addition to those described on this form will only be carried out if it is necessary to save my life or to prevent serious harm to my health.

I have been told about additional procedures which may become necessary during my treatment. I have listed below any procedures **which I do not wish to be carried out** without further discussion.

Patient's signature .... Date ....
Name (PRINT) ....

A witness should sign below if the patient is unable to sign but has indicated his or her consent. Young people/children may also like a parent to sign here (see notes).

Signature .... Date ....
Name (PRINT) ....

Confirmation of consent (to be completed by a health professional when the patient is admitted for the procedure, if the patient has signed the form in advance)

On behalf of the team treating the patient, I have confirmed with the patient that s/he has no further questions and wishes the procedure to go ahead.

Signed: .... Date ....
Name (PRINT) .... Job title ....

Important notes: (tick if applicable)

☐ See also advance directive/living will (eg Jehovah's Witness form)

☐ Patient has withdrawn consent (ask patient to sign /date here)

3

FIGURE 3.2.1, cont'd

Consent for Children

Children under the age of 16 years and minors aged 16 and 17 may have capacity to consent provided they are 'Gillick competent'. This means they have the ability to understand the nature, purpose and possible consequences of the proposed investigation or treatment, as well as the consequences of non-treatment. Such children may consent to treatment without their parents' authorisation, although their parents should ideally be involved. Legally, a parent can consent if a competent child refuses, but it is likely that taking such a serious step will be rare.

Where a child under 16 is not deemed competent to consent, a person with parental responsibility (e.g. their mother or guardian) may authorise investigations or treatment which are in the child's best interests. Generally, however, formal assent to treatment from a legal parent or guardian is sought for treatment of all children under 16 years.

Consent for Adults without Capacity

Adults without capacity cannot give consent to treatment. Currently, in England and Wales, no one can authorise treatment on behalf of an adult. However, patients without capacity to consent may receive dental treatment if it is in the patient's *best interests*, with the views of relatives and carers taken into account.

In contrast, the Adults with Incapacity (Scotland) Act 2000, which came into effect in 2002, allows a competent adult to nominate a person, known as a welfare attorney or proxy, to make medical decisions on their behalf if and when they lose the capacity to make those decisions for themselves. The Act also provides for a general power to treat a patient who is unable to consent to the treatment in question. In order to bring that power into effect, the medical practitioner primarily responsible for treatment must have completed a certificate of incapacity before any treatment is undertaken, other than in an emergency.

The Mental Health (Care And Treatment) (Scotland) Act 2003 allows for medical/dental intervention to prevent serious deterioration in the patient's mental health condition or to prevent the patient from harming themselves.

The Mental Capacity Act (England and Wales) (MCA) is central to the legal issues around treating patients over the age of 16 who lack capacity to consent to treatment. The Act is particularly significant in two ways relevant to consent to medical management:

- It allows consent to be given or withheld, for the medical treatment of patients who lack capacity, by another person (typically a close relative).
- It provides statutory recognition of 'advance directives'. These are statements made by a person while competent (i.e. while having legal capacity) about the treatment that they would want, or not want, in specified situations, in the future were they to lack capacity at the time the treatment would be relevant.

The above information provided is from UK law. Remember that the legal situation with regard to consent varies around the world and is subject to continued debate and development.

WHISTLE BLOWING

It is important to act to protect patients when there is reason to believe that they are threatened by a colleague's conduct, performance or health. The safety of patients must come first at all times and should override personal and professional loyalties. A dental nurse has an obligation to act pro-actively if they believe a colleague is acting in such a way that patients are being harmed or put at risk. It is important that dental staff do not attempt to complain about a colleague unjustifiably, but if you become aware of any situation which puts patients at risk, you should discuss the matter with any one of the following:

- A senior colleague
- Local dental adviser
- Consultant in Dental Public Health to the patient's PCT
- An appropriate professional body, such as the NEBDN.

USEFUL CONTACTS

Information Commissioner: Office of the Information Commissioner, Wycliffe House, Water Lane, Wilmslow, Cheshire SK9 5AF.

Care Quality Commission: Citygate, Gallowgate, Newcastle upon Tyne, NE1 4PA; tel: 03000 616161; website: http://www.cqc.org.uk.

National Patient Safety Agency, 4–8 Maple Street, London W1T 5HD; tel: 020 7927 9500; website www.npsa.nhs.uk.

CHAPTER 4

Anatomy and Physiology

CHAPTER POINTS

- This chapter covers the requirements of the NEBDN syllabus Section 4: Anatomical structures and systems relative to dental care. The chapter is divided into two subchapters:

  4.1: General Anatomy and Physiology

  4.2: Dental Anatomy and Physiology

4.1 GENERAL ANATOMY AND PHYSIOLOGY

- This chapter covers the requirements of the NEBDN syllabus Section 4: Anatomical structures and systems relative to dental care, part 4.1.

99

DEFINITIONS

- *Anatomy* is the study of the structure of the body.
- *Physiology* is the study of the working of the body – how it functions.

THE STRUCTURE OF THE BODY

Everything in the body has a structure and a function or purpose. Virtually all body parts are necessary for health but organs such as the brain, heart, lungs and small intestine, in particular, are essential to life. *Organs* are complex structures that are made up of various *tissues*. The tissues themselves are further built up from millions of *cells*, which are the smallest units of life.

The Cells

There are many different cell types, but the basic design is the same for all cells (Figure 4.1.1):

- The *cell* or *plasma membrane* (the outer membrane) – which controls the movement of water, nutrients and waste material into and out of the cell.
- The *cytoplasm* – which forms the main part of the cell and contains many important structures, especially mitochondria (single: mitochondrion) – the power houses of the cell. Mitochondria produce the energy needed by the cell to function. The most important molecule that is involved in energy production is called adenosine triphosphate (ATP).
- The *nucleus* – the control centre of the cell. The nucleus is essential to everything the cell does, and contains the key to life itself, the DNA.

FIGURE 4.1.1
The basic parts of a single cell.

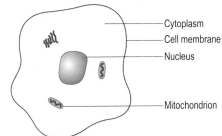

Cytoplasm
Cell membrane
Nucleus

Mitochondrion

100

DNA stands for 'deoxyribonucleic acid', and makes up the genes that form the **chromosomes**. The genes co-ordinate the formation (synthesis) of all proteins in the body. Proteins are essential for virtually all body structures and functions. Genes are inherited from the parents and, because they control **protein** synthesis, they are responsible for many of the differences between individuals (including differences in the susceptibility or resistance to disease). Gene abnormalities are the cause for many diseases.

Humans have 23 pairs of chromosomes, one pair of which are the sex chromosomes (X and Y). The sex chromosomes determine whether a baby will be male or female; females have only X chromosomes (XX) and males have an X and a Y chromosome. Chromosomal abnormalities can cause conditions such as Down syndrome.

Cell function and growth are controlled by signals that are sent to the cell from, for example, hormones (chemical messengers). The molecules that carry the signals bind to *receptors* on the cell membrane, triggering molecules on the inner side of the cell membrane to carry the signal deep into the cytoplasm and to the nucleus. In this way the cell carries out the activities it is instructed to do.

Many, but not all, cells grow and divide to produce daughter cells. Careful control of growth is essential for not just the health of the cell but the health of the entire individual. If the normal pattern of growth is disturbed, it may lead to diseases such as **cancer**.

The Tissues

Cells group together to form larger structures called tissues. The four main types of tissue in the human body, each of which performs particular functions, are:

- *Epithelium* – this makes up the outer layer of the skin and surface of the lining of the mouth (the *mucosa*), gastro-intestinal and genitourinary tract.
- *Connective tissue* – this makes up the supporting structures of the body, which include the tendons, ligaments, cartilage, bone and fat.
- *Muscle* – this tissue can contract and relax to produce movement. This includes movement of the body as a whole or just a part of the body (e.g. food is taken from one part of the digestive system to the next by the pushing movement produced by contraction and relaxation of the muscles of the digestive tract).
- *Nerve tissue* –this is made of special cells such as the neurones, which direct other cells in the body to perform certain functions by generating and passing on messages (signals) to them.

FIND OUT MORE

What is the difference between: (a) tendons and ligaments; (b) cartilage and bone?

The Organs

An organ is a structure that contains at least two different types of tissue that work together for a common purpose (Figure 4.1.2). Organs include the brain, heart, liver, kidneys, skin and others.

The Systems

The main functions of the body such as breathing, circulation of blood, digestion of food require several organs to work together. Organs that function together form a system: for example the heart and blood vessels form the circulatory system, which is responsible for circulating blood throughout the body.

TERMS USED IN ANATOMY

The special terms used in anatomy to describe the relationship of one part of the body to another are shown in Table 4.1.1. To help describe the position of structures in the body relative to each other and also the movement of various parts of the body in relation to each other, the body can be divided into anatomical planes (Figure 4.1.3) that correspond to the vertical and horizontal planes of space (Table 4.1.2).

THE CIRCULATORY SYSTEM

The blood is circulated around the body to all organs, tissues and cells by the circulatory system. This system consists of:

- The blood – which carries oxygen and nutrients to all the cells of the body and removes waste products; thus its circulation is vital for survival
- The blood vessels (arteries and veins) – the network of blood vessels in which the blood circulates all around the body
- The heart – the pump that makes the blood flow in the blood vessels.

Blood

The blood is a special kind of tissue that consists of a variety of cells suspended in a solution called *plasma*.

BLOOD CELLS

There are three types of blood cell:

- *Red blood cells* (*erythrocytes*): these transport oxygen from the lungs to the various body tissues and organs. The oxygen binds to a pigment inside these cells called *haemoglobin*. When this happens the haemoglobin becomes 'oxygenated' and turns red in colour, so blood carrying oxygen is bright red in colour. After most of the oxygen is given off to the tissues, the haemoglobin becomes 'de-oxygenated' and it (and also the blood) becomes darker red in colour. If there is very little oxygen in the blood, it may even become bluish in colour (called *cyanosis*), and this makes certain parts of the body also appear blue, such as the lips, tongue and tips of fingers. De-oxygenated blood carries the waste carbon dioxide from the tissues back to the lungs, from where the carbon dioxide is exhaled into the air.

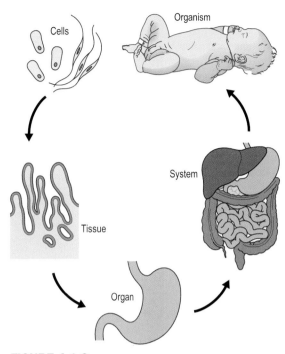

FIGURE 4.1.2
Development of the human organism: from cells to tissues, tissues to organs, organs to systems and from systems to a complete body.

101

TABLE 4.1.1 Terms Used in Anatomy	
Term	**Definition**
Superficial	Closer to the surface
Deep	Further from the surface
Anterior	Closer to the front of the body
Posterior	Closer to the back of the body
Superior	Closer to the top of the head
Inferior	Closer to the soles of the feet
Medial	Closer to the midline of the body
Lateral	Away from the midline of the body
Proximal	Closer to the point of origin of a structure
Distal	Further from the point of origin of a structure

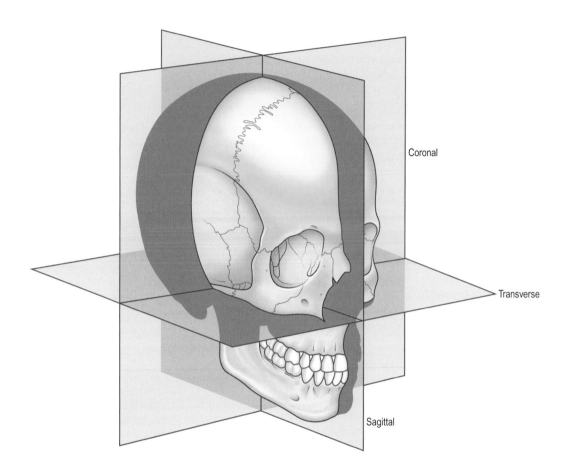

FIGURE 4.1.3
The anatomical planes.

- *White blood cells* (*leucocytes*) – these cells are part of the body's defence and help fight against the micro-organisms that can cause infections.
- *Platelets* – these play an important part in haemostasis (see Box 4.1.1).

TABLE 4.1.2 Anatomical Planes

Anatomical Plane	Spatial Plane	Body is Divided by Plane into Portions
Coronal	Vertical	Anterior and posterior
Transverse	Horizontal	Superior and inferior
Sagittal	Vertical	Right and left

BOX 4.1.1 HAEMOSTASIS AND WOUND HEALING

Haemostasis

When a blood vessel is damaged, the process that normally stops the blood escaping is called haemostasis. Haemostasis occurs in several steps:

1. Almost immediately the blood vessel constricts, which slows down the bleeding (vasoconstriction).
2. The platelets start to stick to the blood vessel walls around the damaged area to form a 'platelet plug'.
3. The blood coagulation factors are activated, leading finally to the formation of a blood clot (haematoma).
4. Later, the clot is removed as part of wound healing.

Continued...

BOX 4.1.1 HAEMOSTASIS AND WOUND HEALING—continued

Wound Healing

Wound healing starts after the formation of the blood clot. It involves special cells called macrophages. The macrophages produce substances called 'growth factors' that trigger the formation of a special healing tissue called granulation tissue. Granulation tissue consists of macrophages and also another type of cell called the fibroblast. The fibroblasts produce the fibrous tissue that replaces the damaged tissue.

Within hours of an injury, the epithelium in the damaged area starts to regenerate as the surface cells of the skin or mucosa (called keratinocytes) migrate across the wound to cover it. Later, as the **fibrous tissue** grows stronger it produces the scarring that is seen in place of the wound.

Term to Learn
Fibrous tissue: this is a specialised tissue that contains tightly woven strands of a fibrous protein called collagen. Besides occurring normally in the body, it is found in scar tissue.

PRODUCTION OF BLOOD CELLS

The blood cells are produced in the bone marrow, found inside many bones. Blood cell production requires many substances called *haematinics*, such as iron, and vitamins – folic acid (folate) and vitamin B12. These substances are present in the food we eat and therefore a good diet is essential for blood cell production. A person who does not eat a diet that contains all the substances required for blood production may not have enough red cells and haemoglobin and the person is said to have **anaemia**.

Blood cell production also requires a healthy bone marrow. People whose bone marrow is damaged (e.g. because they have had **radiotherapy** or **chemotherapy** for a cancer) may lack all types of blood cells. They can then have anaemia and they also have a tendency to catch infections due to a lack of white blood cells for defence (see Box 4.1.2 below) and they can also have a tendency to bleed (since platelets are also damaged).

A hormone produced in the kidney called erythropoietin (EPO) stimulates the bone marrow to produce red cells. People with kidney disease may lack EPO and also develop anaemia. Some athletes use commercially available EPO to increase the oxygen-carrying capacity of their blood – but this is illegal.

> **KEY POINT** A lack of oxygen supply to the brain (called hypoxia) can cause severe brain damage and can kill a person within three minutes.

Term to Learn
Anaemia: when the cells do not get enough oxygen; symptoms include feeling tired easily.

103

Terms to Learn
Chemotherapy: the use of strong chemicals (drugs) to treat cancer. Chemotherapy drugs aim to kill the cancerous cells but also have many side-effects on other normal parts of the body.
Radiotherapy: the treatment of disease (especially cancer) by exposure to an ionising radiation beam (see Chapter 14) or to a radioactive substance.

THE PLASMA

The blood plasma is made up of many kinds of protein, for example proteins called the blood coagulation factors – these work with the platelets to help form a clot to stop bleeding. Other proteins in the blood work with the white blood cells in defending the body against micro-organisms. These are called antibodies.

> **KEY POINT** People with diseases (e.g. haemophilia) that affect the production or action of the platelets and the blood coagulation proteins can have serious bleeding after operations including tooth extraction. Therefore it is very important to find out whether a dental patient may have such a condition.

The Blood Vessels

There are three types of blood vessel:

- *Arteries* – these take the blood (usually oxygenated) away from the heart to the tissues.
- *Veins* – these return the blood (usually de-oxygenated) to the heart.
- *Capillaries* – these are the smallest branches of the blood vessel network and link the arteries to veins. These are also the vessels where the blood gives off the oxygen and takes up carbon dioxide from the cells (see p. 106).

The pulmonary artery and vein are the opposite of the rest of the arteries and veins, since the pulmonary artery carries de-oxygenated blood from the heart to the lungs and the pulmonary vein carries the oxygenated blood from the lungs to the heart (see Figure 4.1.5 below).

The Heart and the Flow of Blood around the Body

The heart is the organ that is found in the centre of the chest (the *thorax*). It has four chambers: two large *ventricles* and two smaller *atria* (Figure 4.1.4).

The heart pumps de-oxygenated blood to the lungs via the pulmonary arteries. In the lungs the blood releases the carbon dioxide and becomes oxygenated. It then travels in the pulmonary veins back to the heart entering it at the left atrium (Figure 4.1.5). From the left atrium blood is pumped into the left ventricle. The opening between these two chambers is controlled by a valve called the *mitral valve*.

FIND OUT MORE

How does the valve control the flow of blood – does it allow the blood to flow in only one direction or both?

Term to Learn
Aorta: the main artery of the body.

Blood is pumped out of the left ventricle into the **aorta**. The aortic valve controls the opening to the aorta. The aorta and its branches take the blood to all tissues and cells in the various parts of the body. Therefore the left ventricle is the most powerful heart chamber as it has to move blood all around the body. Because of this, the heart beat, which is the sound of the pumping action of this chamber, is heard and felt to the left side of the chest rather than in the centre.

104

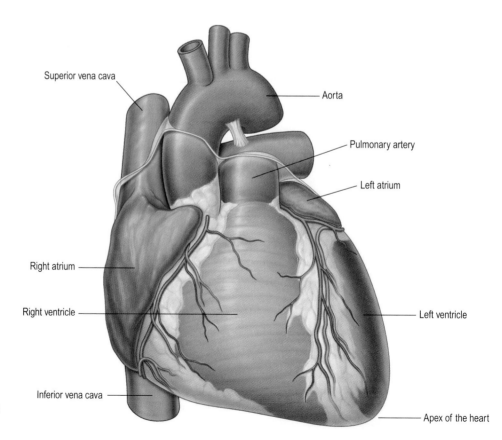

FIGURE 4.1.4
The chambers of the heart and main blood vessels.

Superior vena cava

Aorta

Pulmonary artery

Left atrium

Right atrium

Right ventricle

Left ventricle

Inferior vena cava

Apex of the heart

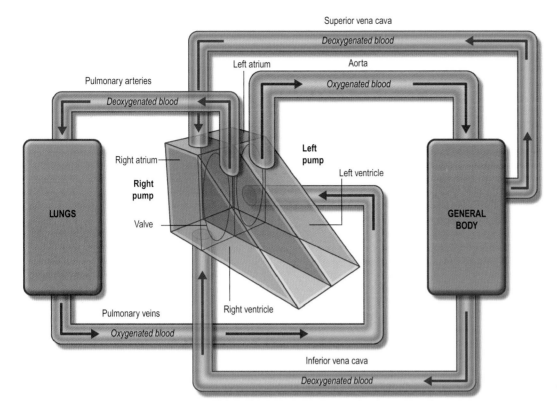

Superior vena cava
Deoxygenated blood
Left atrium
Aorta
Pulmonary arteries
Oxygenated blood
Deoxygenated blood
Left pump
Right atrium
Left ventricle
Right pump
LUNGS
Valve
GENERAL BODY
Pulmonary veins
Right ventricle
Oxygenated blood
Inferior vena cava
Deoxygenated blood

FIGURE 4.1.5
The circulatory system.

From the arteries, the blood enters the capillaries. It is in the capillaries that the oxygen is released to the tissues and the carbon dioxide collected as a waste product. The space between the capillaries and the cells of a tissue is filled with a substance called the interstitial fluid and the gases and nutrients travel through this (see Figure 4.1.7 below).

The de-oxygenated blood then returns to the heart at the right atrium via the **superior and inferior venae cavae**. Blood then flows from the right atrium to the right ventricle, controlled by the tricuspid valve. Blood leaves the right ventricle through the pulmonary artery (where the pulmonary valve controls flow) to the lungs.

> **KEY POINT** Oxygenated blood reaches the tissues of the heart itself by way of branches of the aorta called the coronary arteries (Figure 4.1.6). If the coronary arteries get blocked, this stops the oxygen supply to the heart and causes the condition called angina or a heart attack (also called myocardial infarction or coronary thrombosis; see Chapter 2 and Chapter 17.1).

105

The rate at which the heart pumps blood is called the *heart rate* and the strength with which it pumps blood is the *heart beat*. The heart rate and heart beat are controlled by the brain and hormones (especially adrenaline, which increases both the rate and beat). Adrenaline release is stimulated by anxiety and exercise.

> **KEY POINT** Anxiety and exercise can increase the heart rate and the force of the heart beat.

Terms to Learn
Superior vena cava:
the large vein that collects the blood from the parts of the body above the heart.
Inferior vena cava:
the large vein that collects the blood from the parts of the body below the heart.

The Lymphatic System

The lymphatic system (Figure 4.1.7) is the part of the circulatory system that cleanses it of impurities. It also forms an important part of the immune system (Box 4.1.2). The lymphatic system consists of the following parts:

- The *lymph* – this is the fluid that circulates within the lymphatic vessels. It is formed by interstitial fluid within the tissues (Figure 4.1.7).

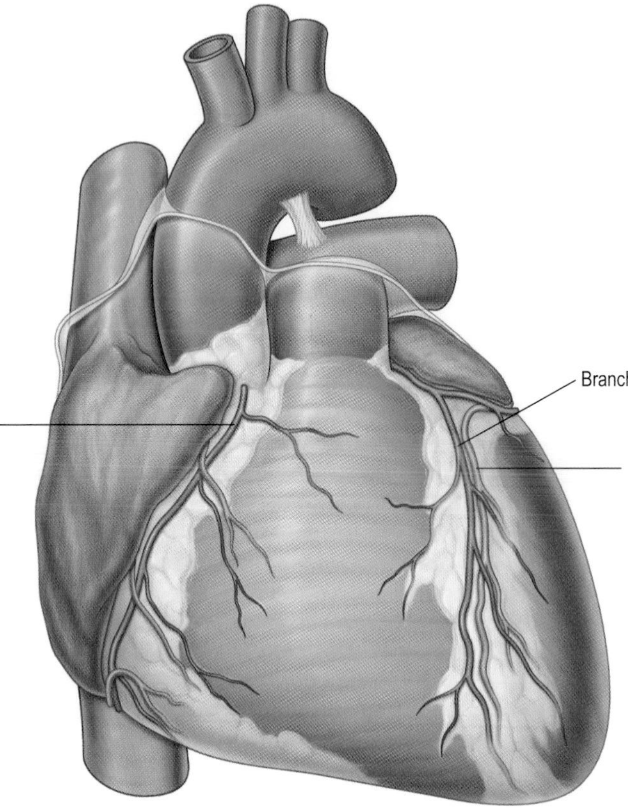

FIGURE 4.1.6
The blood supply of the heart.

Right coronary artery

Branch of left coronary artery

Great cardiac vein

- The *lymphatic vessels* – these are the vessels that transport the lymph.
- The *lymph nodes* – the knob-like structures that are usually found in clusters along the lymph vessels. They filter the passing lymph to catch its impurities (e.g. pathogens and other foreign material, stray cancer cells). The cells in the lymph nodes are called lymphocytes and form part of the body's immune defence system (see Box 4.1.2).

The lymph is not actively pumped through the body like blood. It is moved mostly by virtue of muscle contractions. The lymph vessels carry the lymph to the neck where it then enters the veins and eventually becomes part of the blood.

THE RESPIRATORY SYSTEM

The respiratory system (Figure 4.1.8) has two parts:

- *Upper respiratory tract* – this is located in the head and neck and consists of the nose, paranasal sinuses (see p. 117), pharynx and larynx.
- *Lower respiratory tract* – located mainly inside the chest, this consists of the airways (trachea, bronchi and bronchioles) and the lungs.

Defence Mechanisms in the Respiratory Tract

The defence mechanisms in the respiratory tract include those discussed in Box 4.1.2 as well as:

- The *mucociliary lining*: the mucosa of the respiratory system is covered by a layer of thick slippery fluid called mucus. In addition, the cells also have tiny hair-like projections called cilia. Particles or micro-organisms that are inhaled while breathing are trapped in mucus and driven by the cilia into the pharynx to be swallowed or coughed out.

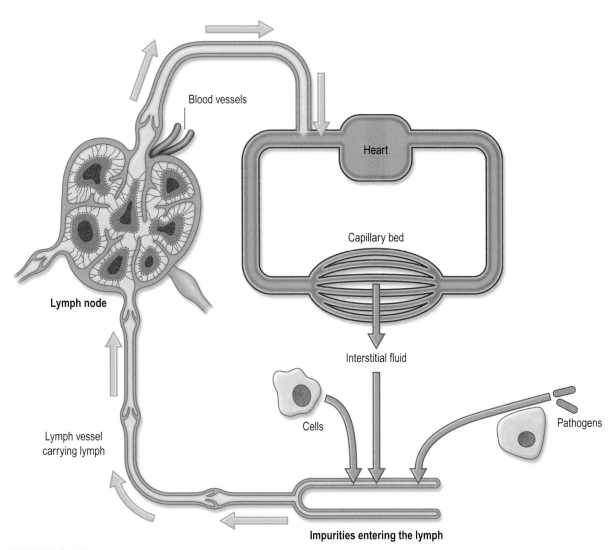

Blood vessels

Heart

Capillary bed

Lymph node

Interstitial fluid

Lymph vessel carrying lymph

Cells

Pathogens

Impurities entering the lymph

FIGURE 4.1.7
The lymphatic system.

107

BOX 4.1.2 IMMUNITY AND INFLAMMATION

The immune system is responsible for protecting the body against potentially harmful substances that may cause damage or infection. The body's response to such an attack is called the immune response or immunity.

The first line of defence is the intact skin and mucosa (the lining of internal body cavities). When the skin or mucosa is cut or damaged, there is haemostasis, and then inflammation is induced. Inflammation consists of increased blood flow to the area (with heat and redness), leakage of the plasma proteins from the inflamed blood vessels into the tissues (with swelling), and the release of pain-inducing chemicals from cells. Inflammation is thus recognised by the presence of:

- Heat
- Redness (erythema)
- Swelling
- Pain.

Following inflammation, special cells called macrophages and a kind of white blood cell called neutrophils are activated. These recognise, eat and kill bacteria (*phagocytosis*) and cleanse foreign matter from the injured site. This is the body's second line of defence.

Continued...

BOX 4.1.2 IMMUNITY AND INFLAMMATION—continued

The other white blood cells involved in defence are the lymphocytes:

- B lymphocytes – these protect the body against bacteria by producing antibodies
- T lymphocytes – these protect mainly against viruses and fungi.

Central to the immune response are also organs such as the spleen and lymph nodes, which are together called the lympho-reticular or reticulo-endothelial system (RES)). The lymph nodes are basically collections of lymphocytes and macrophages. These cells catch and deal with pathogens or other foreign materials that have escaped from the blood into the tissues and then entered the lymph (Figure 4.1.7).

The white blood cells also release a number of proteins called *cytokines*, which trigger the various events involved in inflammation and healing.

108

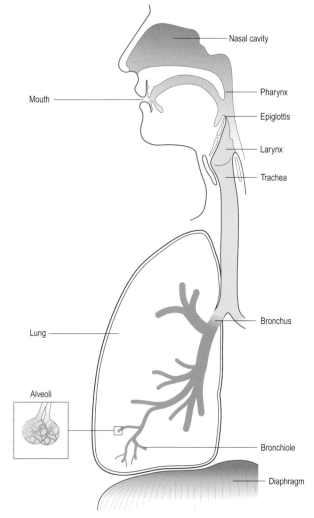

FIGURE 4.1.8
The respiratory system.

- The *cough reflex* – this is crucial in preventing food, drink and other material from entering the larynx (see below) and thence the lungs. If coughing is impaired (when a person is under general anaesthesia (GA) or conscious sedation for dental treatment) the person may inhale (aspirate) foreign material into the airways and the lungs. This can lead to a lack of oxygen or it can lead to a dangerous lung infection. Lack of oxygen can be because of difficulty breathing due to blocked airways or damage to the alveoli.

> **KEY POINT** If the respiratory system's defences are impaired (as they are by general anaesthesia), foreign material can enter the lungs and block the airways or cause infections.

FIND OUT MORE

Why do people with asthma have difficulty breathing?

The Nose

Air enters the nose through the openings in the face called the anterior nares. It exits the nose into the pharynx which connects to the lungs via the larynx, trachea and bronchi (Figure 4.1.8). The mucosal lining of the nose is rich in blood vessels and glands that produce protective mucus. The plentiful blood warms the inspired air. The nose also has special cells that enable us to smell. The functions of the nose thus include:

- Olfaction (smelling)
- Warming incoming air (via the blood)
- Filtering incoming air (via the mucociliary lining)
- Humidifying incoming air
- Collecting and disposing of secretions of various cells in the upper respiratory tract.

The Pharynx

The pharynx (the throat) extends from the nose and serves as a passage for air into the larynx and trachea. It also carries the food from the mouth into the oesophagus and so is also part of the digestive system. The pharynx can thus be divided into three parts: the nasopharynx, oropharynx and laryngopharynx.

The Larynx

The larynx has three important functions:

- It is part of the respiratory passageway
- It has a flap (epiglottis) that covers the airway during swallowing to prevent food from entering the airway
- Its walls contain the vocal cords that produce the sounds during speaking.

The larynx is also close to a very important gland called the thyroid gland (see p. 116). The larynx can be visualised in the neck as the 'Adam's apple'. The larynx leads into the trachea (the windpipe).

> **KEY POINT** The shape and area of the opening between the two vocal cords changes continuously during speech and respiration. This helps, for example, to modulate the voice.

The Trachea and Bronchi

The trachea is the windpipe and divides into the right and left main bronchi, which carry air to the right and left lungs, respectively. The bronchi divide into smaller tubes called bronchioles.

> **KEY POINT** The right main bronchus is shorter, wider and more vertical than the left. Thus, if, for example, a small dental instrument or a part of a tooth or a filling is inhaled, it tends to enter the right bronchus because it is wider and more directly continuous with the trachea. The use of rubber dam (p. 217) should prevent such catastrophic accidents.

The Lungs

The lungs are made of the alveoli, which are clusters of cells at the tip of the terminal branches of the bronchioles. This is where the oxygen and carbon dioxide exchange in the blood occurs.

People with lung disorders may not be able to have treatment under GA and conscious sedation as their breathing may be compromised.

THE DIGESTIVE SYSTEM

The digestive system (Figure 4.1.9) starts at the mouth and ends at the anus. It is responsible for:

- Chewing, digestion and absorption of food
- Removal of waste food and other waste matter.

Swallowing

After being chewed (*masticated*) and mixed with saliva, food is swallowed. Swallowing (also called *deglutition*) helps carry the food into the *pharynx* and then into the *oesophagus* (the food pipe) and finally into the stomach. Swallowing is a complex process co-ordinated by the brain, which sends messages through several nerves. Swallowing is divided into three phases:

- Phase 1 is *voluntary* – it involves the collection of the chewed food into a bolus and the first part of the swallowing of the food bolus.
- Phase 2 – this is the passage of food through the pharynx into the oesophagus. It is *involuntary*.
- Phase 3 – this is also involuntary and involves the passage of food from the oesophagus into the stomach.

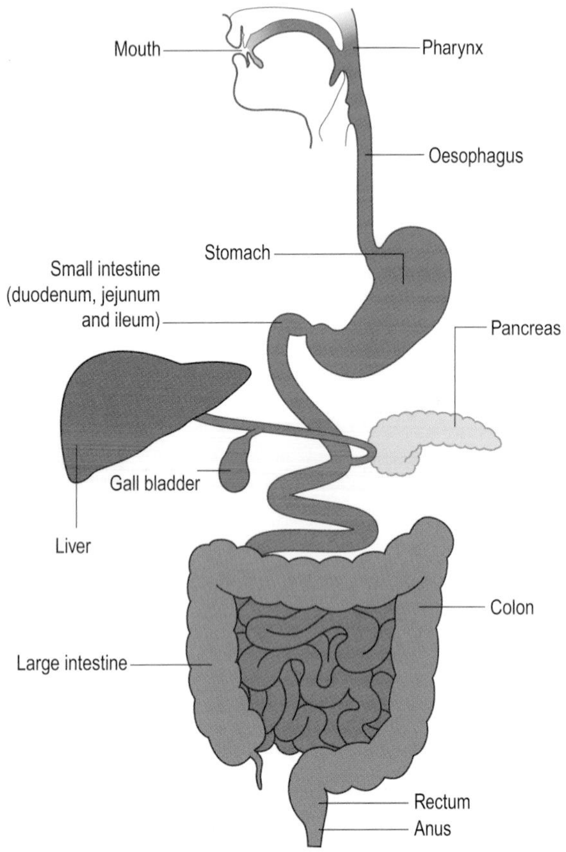

Mouth — Pharynx

Oesophagus

Stomach

Small intestine
(duodenum, jejunum
and ileum)

Pancreas

Gall bladder

Liver

Colon

Large intestine

Rectum
Anus

FIGURE 4.1.9
The digestive system.

110

> **KEY POINT** Obstruction to the
> pharynx or oesophagus can cause **dysphagia**. Cancer
> is an important cause of such obstruction.

Stomach

It is in the stomach that most digestion begins. The cells in the stomach walls produce a variety of substances (e.g. hydrochloric acid and pepsin) that help break down the food by chemical reactions. The secretion of these substances is regulated by complex hormonal and nerve (vagal nerve) mechanisms. The stomach cells also produce mucus and bicarbonate to neutralise the acid, which can damage the lining of the stomach itself. The stomach is not crucial to life but intrinsic factor, produced there, is essential for vitamin B12 absorption in the small intestine. The stomach is a common site for cancer and ulceration.

The Small Intestine

The small intestine is a very long tube (approx 7 m) made of three parts: duodenum, jejunum and ileum. It is the main site of digestion and absorption of food and is crucial to life. Food that has started to be digested in the stomach is fully digested in the small intestine with the help of intestinal and pancreatic **enzymes**. The nutrients – fats, carbohydrates and proteins – thus released are absorbed into the blood in the small intestine. The blood then takes the nutrients to other parts of the body for use or for storage.

Diseases of the small intestine cause **malabsorption** and **diarrhoea** or **steatorrhoea**. This can lead to feelings of tiredness and weakness, loss of weight and anaemia.

The Pancreas

The pancreas produces several of the digestive enzymes (e.g. amylase and lipase) and also secretes hormones (insulin and glucagon) that regulate the amount of sugar (glucose) in the blood.

The Large Intestine

The large intestine has two functions:

- Recovery of water and electrolytes (sodium and chloride) from the digestive tract
- Formation and storage of faeces.

Lying between the small intestine and the anus, the large intestine consists of:

- The *caecum* – this is a blind-ended pouch that carries a worm-like extension (the appendix) that can become inflamed (appendicitis)
- The *colon* – this forms most of the length of the large intestine
- The *rectum* – this is the short last segment, continuous with the anus.

The large intestine is not crucial to life, and it is a common site for cancer.

Liver

The liver is located in the right part of the upper abdomen. Its functions are:

- Turning extra glucose into glycogen, which is then stored in the liver. Glycogen is converted back into glucose when required, maintaining stable blood glucose levels. Excess **carbohydrates** and protein are converted to fat, which can also be converted to glucose when required.
- Making proteins, for example most of the blood clotting factors.
- Making bile, which is essential for fat digestion and absorption of some vitamins. Bile is stored in the gall bladder between meals and when a person eats, it is discharged into the duodenum.
- Producing or storing several vitamins (A, D, E, K, folate, vitamin B12), and storing minerals (e.g. copper and iron).
- Breaking down worn out haemoglobin, **cholesterol**, proteins and many drugs.

> **KEY POINT** Haemoglobin consists of two parts, haem and globin. In the liver, haem is broken down into biliverdin and bilirubin, which are bile pigments and give colour to the urine and faeces. If bilirubin builds up in the blood it can cause the body, especially the white of the eyes, to appear yellow (jaundice). The urine also appears darker in jaundice.

OTHER BODY SYSTEMS
The Urinary System

This system produces urine and therefore regulates the water content of the body and removes many waste products. The main organs in this system are (Figure 4.1.10):

- *Kidneys* – these form the urine
- *Ureters* – these carry the urine from the kidneys to the urinary bladder
- *Urinary bladder* – this is where the urine is stored until it is passed out from the body.

The kidneys also produce a number of important hormones (e.g. erythropoietin (p. 114), and renin, which helps in the regulation of blood pressure).

The Integumentary System

The integumentary system consists of the skin and mucosa. Its functions include:

- Providing the first line of defence (see Box 4.1.2)
- Heat regulation (via sweating)
- Providing sensation (touch, pressure, pain).

The mucosae are the moist linings that line the inside of body cavities, such as that in the mouth and upper respiratory tract, eyes, gastro-intestinal tract and genitals. It is similar to skin but it is designed to cope with constant exposure to moisture.

The Musculoskeletal System

The musculoskeletal system consists of the skeleton and muscles. The skeleton consists of bones, cartilage and the joints between them. The main bones of the human skeleton are shown in Figure 4.1.11.

BONES

Bones are the hardest structures in the body besides the teeth. The functions of bone include:

- Supporting the body
- Protection (the skull protects the brain, the rib cage protects the lungs and heart)
- Movement
- Storehouse for calcium
- Red blood cell production (in the bone marrow).

Terms to Learn
Carbohydrate: a major class of food, an important structural component of cells and a vital source of energy.
Cholesterol: a fatty, wax-like substance that is a component of the fats found in the blood, cell membranes, some hormones and vitamin D. The body makes all the cholesterol it requires but it is also present in foods such as meat and whole milk so it is important not to eat excessive amounts of cholesterol-containing foods. There are two types of cholesterol: the high-density lipoproteins (HDL), the 'good' cholesterol that protects the heart, and low-density lipoproteins (LDL), the 'bad' cholesterol which causes heart disease and other conditions.

111

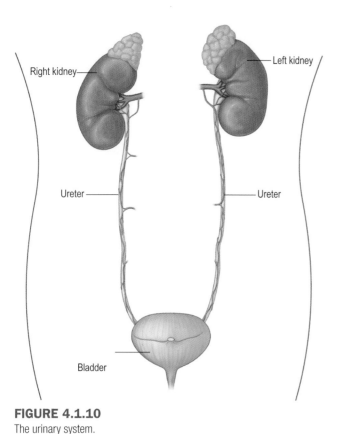

FIGURE 4.1.10
The urinary system.

112

> **KEY POINT** The health of the bone depends on adequate availability of calcium and vitamin D and some other hormones and substances such as bone morphogenetic proteins (BMPs). BMPs are sometimes used in dentistry, e.g. to repair defects in the tissues that support the teeth.

FIGURE 4.1.11
The human skeleton.

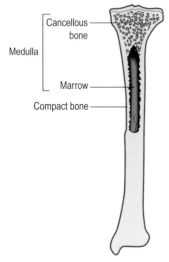

FIGURE 4.1.12
Structure of bone.

Bones consist of a dense outer layer called the *cortex* (a tube of compact bone that confers most of the strength to the bone), and a softer, spongy textured inner layer called *cancellous bone*. Some bones have bone marrow within the cancellous bone (Figure 4.1.12), where blood cells are produced.

The *periosteum* is a dense white fibrous membrane that covers the bone. Muscle tendon fibres interlace with periosteal fibres to anchor to bone.

Calcium is important to ensure strong bones and teeth, and it also helps muscles and nerves to work properly. Good dietary sources are dairy foods (milk, yogurt and cheese) and calcium-enriched orange juice. Vitamin D is found in fish, liver and egg yolk and sunlight (absorbed through the skin). Good sources are fortified foods and beverages such as milk, soya drinks and margarine. Vitamin D is required for bone development and growth in children, bone maintenance in adults and prevention of **osteoporosis** and fractures in older people. Exercise also promotes bone formation, whereas smoking may impair it.

After a fracture or surgery such as a tooth extraction it is normal for bone to undergo repair. This is a type of wound healing, where bone rather than scar tissue ultimately replaces the defect.

THE FOUR PHASES OF BONE REPAIR

1. Formation of a blood clot (called haematoma). Fractures always lead to bleeding (haemorrhage).
2. Growth of new, soft bone (callus) at the fractured ends.
3. Shaping (modelling) of the new bone to match the shape of the original bone.
4. Hardening of the soft new bone to form normal bone that can withstand the usual stresses, e.g. body weight.

CARTILAGE

Cartilage is a less rigid form of hard tissue than bone and is found in areas that require greater flexibility, e.g. bridge of the nose and the ear.

JOINTS

A joint forms the connection between any of the rigid body parts of the skeleton (bones or cartilage).

MUSCLES

Muscles consist of fibres which can contract. Voluntary contraction is used to move the limbs and other parts of the body. The muscles that can contract voluntarily are called *skeletal muscles*. These are attached to bones, usually via an intermediate structure called *tendons*. A few are attached elsewhere, for example into skin (such as the muscles used for facial expressions).

The heart and gut muscles are called *involuntary muscles* (or *smooth muscles*). They are controlled by specialised parts of the brain. Contraction of heart muscle drives the heart beat and contraction of the gut causes **peristalsis**.

The Nervous System

The nervous system (and the endocrine system) control and co-ordinate the body's activities. In this way, we can do several things at once, for example, running, breathing and listening to music. The *neurones* are the special cells of this system and form a network in the brain and throughout the body and transmit information to and from the brain and the other organs. Each neurone has a body and several projections (Figure 4.1.13). The main one is called the *axon* and the neurone sends out signals through the axon. The smaller *dendrites* receive the signals from the axons of other neurones across a gap called the synapse via chemicals called neurotransmitters. The axons are also called *nerve fibres* and many nerve fibres together form a cord called the nerve.

There are three types of nerves, depending on the type of fibres that they have:

- *Motor* (or *efferent*) – these carry messages from the brain to the muscles to make them contract or relax.

FIGURE 4.1.13
A neurone.

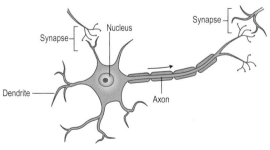

- *Sensory* (or *afferent*) – these carry messages to the brain and spinal cord about sensations of touch, temperature and pain, as well as special senses (smell, taste, vision, hearing).
- Other nerves (*interneurones*) send messages between the brain and other nerve cells.

FIND OUT MORE

Can nerves have both sensory and motor nerve fibres?

The nervous system has three parts:

- The central nervous system
- Peripheral nervous system
- Autonomic nervous system.

CENTRAL NERVOUS SYSTEM (CNS)

This consists of the brain and the spinal cord. Located in the head and protected by the skull, the brain is the organ of thought, and controls:

- The senses
- Movement
- The endocrine (hormone) glands (see below)
- Body functions such as:
  - ○ Heart rate
  - ○ Blood pressure
  - ○ Fluid balance
  - ○ Body temperature.

PERIPHERAL NERVOUS SYSTEM

This is made up of the **cranial** and **peripheral** (spinal) **nerves.**

Sensory nerves carry information to the brain and motor nerves carry information away from the brain. These nerves act as lines of communication between the CNS and the skin, joints and the skeletal muscles in the rest of the body.

There are 12 pairs of cranial nerves and each has a:

- Name – related to its function or appearance.
- Number – from I to XII from the order in which they leave the brain from front to the back, usually written in Roman numerals.

See Table 4.1.3 for the list of cranial nerves and functions.

THE AUTONOMIC NERVOUS SYSTEM

This supplies the circulatory, respiratory, digestive, urinary and reproductive systems, all the glands, and all other smooth (involuntary) muscles. It is further subdivided into:

- The *sympathetic* nervous system – which prepares the body for emergencies (anxiety, pupils dilate, increase in heart rate and breathing)
- The *parasympathetic* nervous system – which basically has the opposite effects and aims at conserving and restoring energy.

The Endocrine System

The endocrine organs are called glands (Figure 4.1.14) and they secrete chemicals called *hormones* that travel in the blood to help regulate functions in other organs of the body. Some of the important hormones and what they control are given below.

Terms to Learn
Cranial nerves: the nerves with neurones whose cell bodies lie in the brain.
Peripheral nerves: the nerves with neurones whose cell bodies lie in the spinal cord.

114

TABLE 4.1.3 The Cranial Nerves (Those marked with * are relevant to the dental nurse)

Nerve	Number	*Functions*
Olfactory	I	Supplies the nose and controls the sense of smell
Optic	II	Supplies the eyes and controls the sense of vision
Oculomotor	III }	Supply the eye muscles and control the movement of the
Trochlear	IV }	eye in various directions (motor supply) along with cranial nerve VI
Trigeminal*	V	This has three parts and contains both motor and sensory nerves. Ophthalmic division (V1: controls the sensory sensations (touch, temperature and pain) in the upper face) Maxillary division (V2: controls the sensory sensations in the middle face (including maxillary sinuses, nose, upper lip and teeth, hard and soft palates, and the tonsils)) Mandibular division (V3: is sensory to lower face, temporomandibular joint, lower lip and teeth, mucosa of cheek, and anterior two-thirds of tongue. It also has the motor nerves that supply the muscles of mastication)
Abducens	VI	Motor to eye muscle
Facial*	VII	Taste (gustatory): from the anterior two-thirds of tongue, floor of mouth and palate; motor to muscles of facial expression
Vestibulocochlear	VIII	Controls hearing and balance by supplying the ear
Glossopharyngeal*	IX	Sensory to posterior third of the tongue and pharynx (sensation of taste)
Vagus	X	This is mixed like cranial nerve V and supplies several structures including: • Sensory to: the posterior part of the skull and its contents • Motor to: muscles of the pharynx, larynx and oesophagus
Accessory	XI	Motor to muscles of the pharynx, and the neck muscles (sternomastoid and trapezius muscles)
Hypoglossal*	XII	Motor to the tongue muscles

Adrenaline and Noradrenaline

- *Origin*: Adrenal glands
- *Functions*: Constricts blood vessels; stimulates breakdown of glycogen to glucose when more energy is required, e.g. the flight or fight response.

FIND OUT MORE

What is the flight or fight response?

Growth Hormone

- *Origin*: Pituitary gland
- *Function*: increases protein synthesis and so is important for growth.

Insulin

- *Origin*: Pancreas

FIGURE 4.1.14
The endocrine glands are spread out throughout the body.

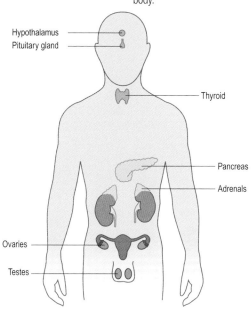

Hypothalamus
Pituitary gland
Thyroid
Pancreas
Adrenals
Ovaries
Testes

- *Functions*: Helps the cells take up glucose by cells for storage as glycogen; enhances protein, and fatty acid synthesis.

Thyroid Hormone
- *Origin*: Thyroid gland
- *Function*: Increases the rate of use of energy and basal metabolic rate.

Parathyroid Hormone
- *Origin*: Parathyroid gland
- *Function*: Controls amount of calcium in the bones and blood.

4.2 DENTAL ANATOMY AND PHYSIOLOGY

- This chapter covers the requirements of the NEBDN syllabus Section 4: Anatomical structures and systems relative to dental care, part 4.2.

INTRODUCTION
The oral cavity is the area the dental team is most concerned with. Therefore it is essential that dental nurses have a thorough understanding of the relevant knowledge of the head and neck.

THE SKULL
The skull (cranium) protects the brain. It **articulates** by way of paired *joints* (the temporomandibular joints or TMJs) with the mandible (the lower jaw). It consists of 21 bones that are bound together by **fibrous joints** called *sutures*. The *periosteum* covering the outer surface of the skull is called the pericranium and that covering its inner surface is called the dura mater. Skull fractures may often be associated with brain damage. Figure 4.2.1 shows the main bones of the skull and the mandible.

Terms to Learn
Articulation: the bones in the body connect with each other at particular points called joints. Thus the bones *articulate* with each other at joints.
Fibrous joints: these are the virtually immovable joints, where no movement usually occurs.

116

FIND OUT MORE
Can you point out the TMJ on Figure 4.2.1?

THE FACE
The face is the region bordered by the forehead, chin and the ears. Its shape is determined by:

- The bones that support it (the skull, the right and left maxillae (singular: maxilla; the upper jaw), zygomatic bones (cheek bones), the nasal bones (nose bones) and the mandible)
- The *facial muscles*
- The fat pads (*buccal pads*) within the cheeks.

KEY POINT Damage to the facial nerve (as after trauma or a stroke) can cause facial palsy, which is an inability to smile, whistle or shut the eye, and drooping at the angle of the mouth on the affected side leading to tears and saliva trickling from the eye and mouth, respectively.

The facial muscles are commonly called the *muscles of facial expression* and their contraction and relaxation is controlled by the seventh cranial nerve (the facial nerve). Figure 4.2.2 shows the main muscles of facial expression.

THE JAWS
There are two jaws, the upper (*maxilla*) and lower (*mandible*) jaws. Each bears an extension called the *alveolar process*, in which the teeth develop and are anchored.

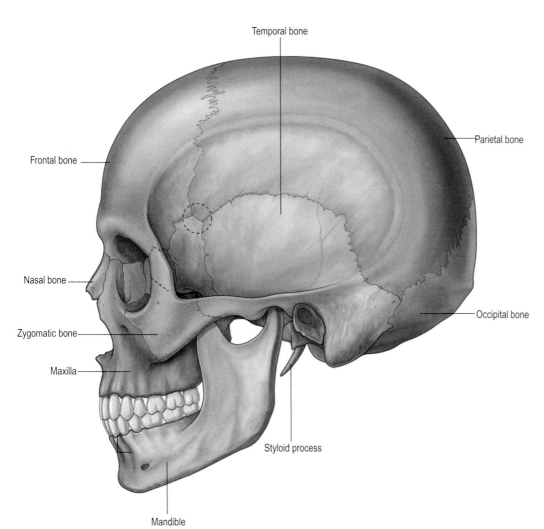

Temporal bone

Parietal bone

Frontal bone

Nasal bone

Zygomatic bone

Maxilla

Occipital bone

Styloid process

Mandible

117

FIGURE 4.2.1
The bones of the skull.

The Maxilla

The maxilla (see Figure 4.2.1) is fixed to the skull and is hollow. It contains one of the paranasal sinuses (Figure 4.2.3) called the maxillary sinus or antrum. The maxilla supports a variety of structures that are essential to normal vision (eyes), respiration (nose), olfaction (nose), mastication (chewing; mouth), deglutition (swallowing) and speech.

PARANASAL SINUSES

The bones of the skull that surround the nasal cavity are hollow and the spaces within them are called the paranasal sinuses. These sinuses are lined with mucosa. They are important in that they permit these bones to be lighter, they produce mucus, which drains into the nose, and they give speech its special qualities. Hence, when a person has sinusitis, their head feels heavy as the sinuses are filled with mucus, which discharges through the nose and the quality of their voice changes.

The roots of the maxillary (upper) teeth are close to the floor of the maxillary antrum. Therefore pain from the upper posterior (back) teeth can be **referred** to the maxillary sinuses and vice versa.

During tooth extraction and implant placement the clinician has to be careful not to penetrate the sinus. If this happens, it results in a communication between the antrum and the roof of the mouth called an oro-antral fistula. Alternatively a tooth or root can get pushed into the sinus.

Term to Learn
Referred pain: a pain that is felt in one part of the body but actually originates in another part.

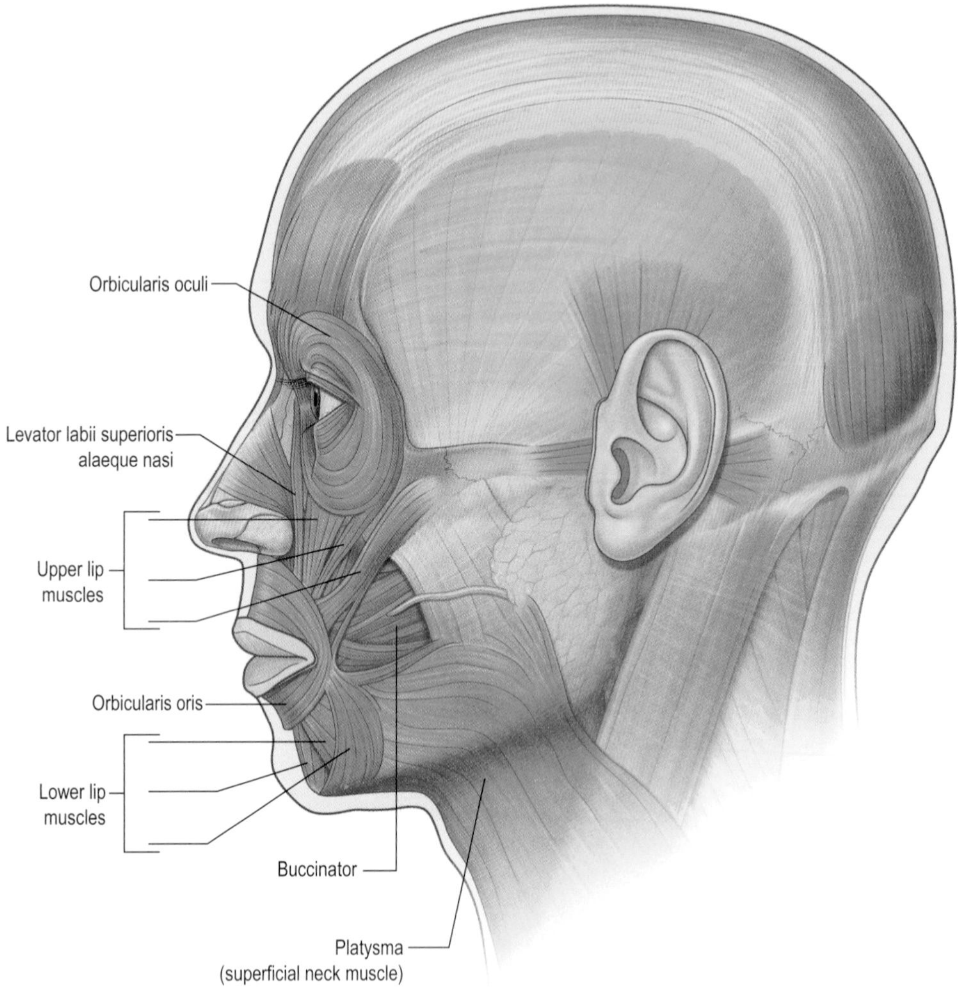

118

FIGURE 4.2.2
The muscles of facial
expression, surrounding the
eyes, nose, mouth and ears,
and forming the cheeks,
forehead, scalp and neck.

The Mandible

The mandible is virtually solid, containing no sinuses. It consists of (Figure 4.2.4):

- A horizontal body
- The two angles between the horizontal and vertical parts (ramus, plural rami)
- The coronoid processes
- The mandibular condyles – these articulate with the temporal bone of the skull at the glenoid fossa via the temporomandibular joints (TMJs).

The mandible is essential to chewing (mastication) and to speech and swallowing.

THE TEMPOROMANDIBULAR JOINTS

There are two TMJs, one on either side of the face. Each TMJ is formed from two bones, the skull bone called the temporal bone, above, and the mandible below (Figure 4.2.5). To reduce the friction between the two bones, there is a disc of cartilage tissue between the two, called the articular disc. This disc divides the joint into an upper and lower cavity. The TMJ is one of the most frequently used joints in the body, permitting speech, chewing, yawning, swallowing and sneezing. The movements that are possible at this joint are given in Table 4.2.1.

> **KEY POINT** The TMJs are the two most frequently used joints in the body.

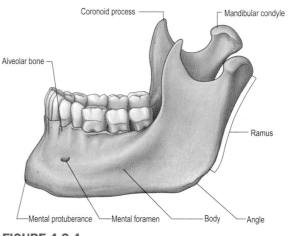

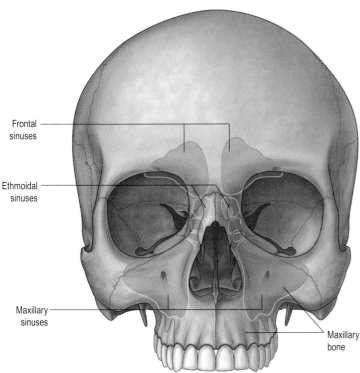

FIGURE 4.2.4
The mandible.

FIGURE 4.2.3
The main paranasal sinuses.

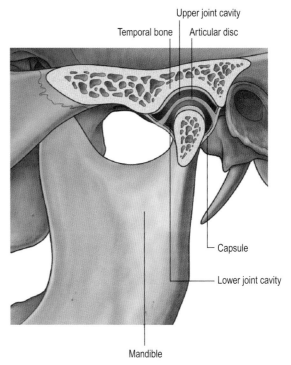

119

THE MUSCLES OF MASTICATION

Mastication or chewing is the process by which food is crushed and ground by the teeth. The muscles of mastication help in chewing of food by moving the mandible in relation to the maxilla (Table 4.2.1) at the TMJs. The maxilla is fixed and does not move. The muscles of mastication (Figure 4.2.6) are:

- *Temporalis* – this is attached to the side of the skull at the temporal bone and to the mandibular coronoid process
- *Masseter* – this is attached to the skull at the zygomatic bone (Figure 4.2.1) and to the body of the mandible
- *Medial pterygoid* – this is attached to the skull and to the medial side of the body of the mandible
- *Lateral pterygoid* – this is attached to the skull and to the capsule around the condyle of the mandible.

FIGURE 4.2.5
Detailed view of the temporomandibular joint.

TABLE 4.2.1 **The Mandibular Movements**

Movement	Function
Jaw opening (depression)	Separation of the biting (occlusal) surfaces of the teeth
Jaw closing (elevation)	Bringing the mandibular and maxillary teeth together into occlusion*
Jaw sideways movements (lateral motion)	From occlusion*, sliding the teeth from side to side while maintaining tooth contact
Pushing jaw forwards (protrusion)	Bringing mandibular incisors anterior to maxillary incisors
Pulling jaw back (retrusion)	From protruded position moving mandibular incisors posterior to (behind) the maxillary incisors

*Centric occlusion is when the maxillary and mandibular teeth are in maximal contact.

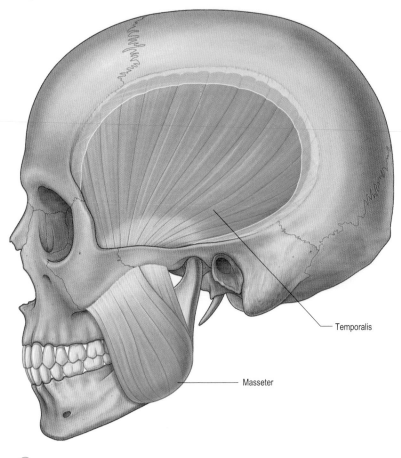

(A)

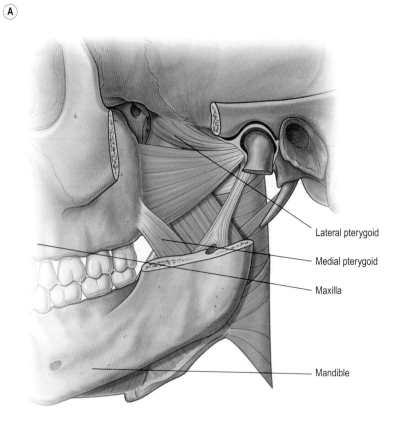

(B)

FIGURE 4.2.6
Muscles of mastication. (A) masseter and temporalis; (B) medial and lateral pterygoids.

All these muscles of mastication are paired, with one each on the right and left sides. Their nerve supply is from the cranial nerve called the trigeminal nerve (see Table 4.1.3). Other muscles such as those in the tongue and cheeks may also help in mastication.

Disorders affecting the masticatory muscles may cause **trismus** and interfere with speech and swallowing.

> **KEY POINT** During mastication, food is first cut mainly using the incisor teeth or torn with the canines, and then positioned by the cheek and tongue between the premolars and molars for grinding (p. 127). After chewing, the food (then termed a bolus) is swallowed.

THE ALVEOLAR PROCESSES

The alveolar processes of the jaws are the parts that form the sockets (alveoli; singular alveolus) for the teeth (Figure 4.2.4). The bone lining an alveolus is called bundle bone. This is because the periodontal ligament fibres (see p. 128) which attach the tooth roots to the bone are attached to this bone. On X-rays, this layer appears as a more radio-dense (lighter) line (that is, it appears distinctly white) called the *lamina dura*.

Term to Learn
Trismus: the condition of limited mouth opening.

IDENTIFY AND LEARN
Find a couple of intra-oral X-rays in your workplace and ask your supervisor to point out the lamina dura.

THE SALIVARY GLANDS

Saliva is produced by the salivary glands and released into the mouth where it is essential to oral health, and for speaking, tasting, eating and swallowing. The functions of saliva include:

> **KEY POINT** A lack of the lamina dura appearance on the X-ray is considered a sign of disease.

- Lubrication – for taste, speech, and swallowing
- Digestion – the saliva contains an enzyme called salivary amylase, which starts to digest the starches in the food
- Protection – the maturation of tooth enamel (p. 132), its health and remineralisation are all helped by the mechanical washing effect of saliva. Other protective mechanisms of the saliva are: general immune-protective mechanisms (the saliva has anti-microbial enzymes and other substances that help fight infections) and buffering (preventing acidity).

The salivary glands can be classified as:

- *Major salivary glands* – these glands communicate with the oral cavity (mouth) through tubes called the salivary ducts
- *Minor salivary glands* – these open directly into the oral cavity.

There are three paired major salivary glands (Figure 4.2.7):

- *Parotid gland* – this is located just in front of the ears
- *Submandibular gland* – this is located just beneath the mandible
- *Sublingual gland* – this is located under the tongue.

The many minor salivary glands include:

- *Lingual glands* – in the tongue
- *Labial glands* – in the lower lip especially
- *Buccal glands* – in the cheek mucosa
- *Palatal glands* – in the roof of the mouth (mainly in the soft palate).

Saliva from the minor salivary glands, the sublingual glands and the submandibular glands contains the lubricating substances called mucins and is largely sticky and mucous in nature. Parotid saliva is usually principally watery (serous).

121

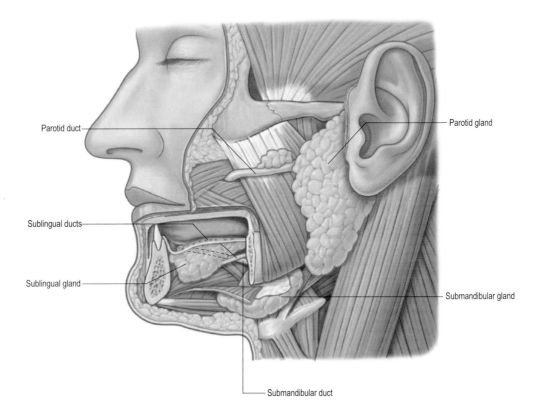

FIGURE 4.2.7
The salivary glands.

Nerve Supply of the Salivary Glands

The salivary glands are controlled by the nerves of the autonomic nervous system (p. 113) and the nerves consist of both sympathetic and parasympathetic nerve fibres. Parasympathetic stimulation increases the quantity of saliva. Sympathetic stimulation causes cessation of salivation.

FIND OUT MORE

Have you noted your mouth goes dry when you are anxious? Which nerves are stimulating the salivary glands at this time?

The nerves to salivary glands run alongside the lingual, facial and glossopharyngeal nerves and along the blood vessels.

Reduced salivation or *hyposalivation* (also called dry mouth or *xerostomia*) can also be caused by:

- Drugs that interfere with saliva formation (e.g. anti-depressant or anti-hypertensive drugs)
- Loss of fluid (as in dehydration and diabetes)
- Damage to the salivary glands by radiotherapy (e.g. as treatment for cancer) or diseases such as Sjögren syndrome.

Hyposalivation can cause difficulties with taste, chewing, swallowing and speech. It also predisposes to *dental caries* and tooth wear, and infections in the mouth (*candidosis*) and salivary glands (*sialadenitis*). These conditions are all described in detail in Chapter 5.

THE ORAL CAVITY

The term oral cavity is used by healthcare workers to describe what is commonly called the mouth. However, strictly speaking, the mouth is the entrance to the oral cavity – that is,

Term to Learn
Sjögren syndrome:
the disease in which a person has dry eyes and a dry mouth.

it is the hollow space between the lips. The oral cavity consists of the:

- Lips and cheeks
- Vestibule (the space between the teeth and the lips and cheeks)
- Teeth
- Oral cavity proper (which is the area bounded by the upper and lower teeth on the sides, by the palate above and by the floor of the mouth below).

The tongue lies within the oral cavity proper (Figure 4.2.8). The oral cavity is the entrance to the gastro-intestinal (digestive) tract. Its functions include the following.

- It acts as the receptacle for food and drink.
- It is the passageway to/from the gastro-intestinal tract (and an alternative to the nose as a passage to the respiratory tract; e.g. when the nose is blocked due to infection, people breathe through their mouth).
- It is the place where digestion starts:
  - ○ The food is chewed in the oral cavity (mastication)
  - ○ Food is mixed with the saliva, which lubricates it for ease of swallowing, and also starts the breakdown of the food with its digestive enzyme called salivary amylase
  - ○ It takes part in the first phase of swallowing (deglutition).
- It is the main site of taste.
- It works in concert with the larynx in the production of speech (the lips, tongue and palate are essential to normal speech because they are required to make certain sounds).

Diseases of the oral cavity can thus interfere with eating (mastication, swallowing, taste) and speaking.

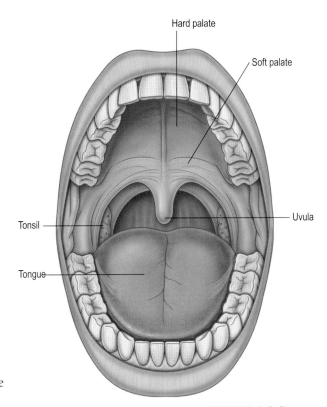

FIGURE 4.2.8
The oral cavity proper.

123

Dental Terminology

Clinicians use a range of terms to describe the position of the structures within the oral cavity (Table 4.2.2).

TABLE 4.2.2 Dental Terminology

Terminology	Meaning
Apical	Towards the tooth apex
Buccal/facial	Facing the cheek (posterior teeth) (also used to describe structures in the cheek mucosa)
Cervical	Towards the neck or cervix of a tooth (also used when talking about structures in the neck itself)
Coronal	Closer to the crown of a tooth
Distal	Further from dental arch midline
Gingival	Toward the gingival margin
Labial/facial	Facing the lips (anterior teeth)
Lingual	Facing the tongue (lower dental arch) (also used to describe structures on the tongue)
Mesial	Closer to dental arch midline
Palatal	Facing the palate (upper dental arch) (also used to describe structures in the palate)
Periapical	Close to the tooth apex
Periodontal	Of the periodontium (see p. 127)

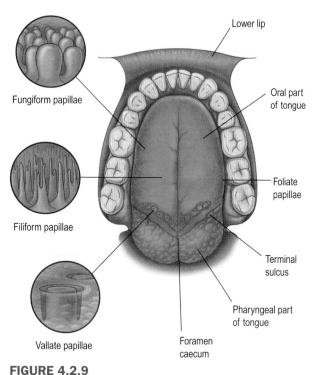

Fungiform papillae

Filiform papillae

Vallate papillae

Lower lip

Oral part of tongue

Foliate papillae

Terminal sulcus

Pharyngeal part of tongue

Foramen caecum

FIGURE 4.2.9
The tongue.

124

The Lips

The lips (*labia*) surround the opening (*orifice*) to the oral cavity: the red part of the lips is called the *vermilion*. The angles of the mouth are called the *commissures*. The upper lip starts just below the nose and ends at the oral orifice. The lower lip starts in the groove on the chin (called the labiomental groove) and ends at the oral orifice. The lip muscles are involved in facial expression and they are controlled by the facial nerve. The sensation of touch and pain in the lips is conveyed by the trigeminal nerve.

The Tongue

The tongue (Figure 4.2.9) is a very muscular organ and is needed for:

- Speech
- Taste
- Swallowing (deglutition).

The anterior two-thirds, the 'oral tongue', lies in the oral cavity. A V-shaped groove called the terminal sulcus separates the oral part of the tongue from the posterior one-third, which lies in the pharynx (pharyngeal part). Each arm of the terminal sulcus begins in the centre of the tongue at the foramen caecum and continues anteriorly and laterally to end on the sides in two arches called the palatoglossal arches. The surface of the tongue is rough due to the presence of papillae. There are four types of papillae (Figure 4.2.9):

- Filiform – on the top (dorsum) of the anterior two-thirds
- Fungiform – on the top (dorsum) of the anterior two-thirds
- Foliate – on the sides (lateral borders) posteriorly
- Circumvallate – on the top (dorsum) separating the anterior from posterior tongue.

These papillae increase the ability of the tongue to grasp objects and they may also have taste buds.

THE TASTE BUDS

The taste buds help detect salt, sweet, sour and bitter tastes, and are found on the top (dorsum) and sides of the tongue, and also on the soft palate and the epiglottis. Normal saliva production is necessary to taste food, as food substances must dissolve in saliva to reach the taste buds. People with dry mouths thus often complain of taste disturbances.

The posterior third of the tongue also has a rough appearance due to the presence of the *lingual tonsil*. The tonsils form part of a protective ring of lymphatic tissue around the opening to the pharynx (*Waldeyer's ring*), which also includes the palatine tonsils (Figure 4.2.8) and adenoids (in the nasopharynx).

NERVE SUPPLY OF THE TONGUE

- The tongue muscles are controlled mainly by the hypoglossal nerve.
- The taste sensation from the anterior two-thirds is conveyed via the trigeminal nerve, and from the posterior third via the glossopharyngeal nerve.
- The main sensory nerve to the tongue is the lingual nerve, which is a branch of the mandibular division of the trigeminal nerve. Damage to this nerve can cause a feeling of

'pins and needles' (paraesthesia), slight numbness (hypoaesthesia) or complete numbness (anaesthesia) in the side of the tongue, as well as disturbed taste.

> **KEY POINT** The lingual nerve runs close to the mandibular third molar (wisdom tooth). Thus it can be easily damaged during lower third molar extractions, or during jaw surgery.

BLOOD SUPPLY TO THE TONGUE

The main artery that supplies blood to the tongue is the lingual artery; the de-oxygenated blood (venous drainage) flows to the lingual or facial veins. The tongue also has lymph vessels and these drain into the several lymph nodes in the neck (cervical lymph nodes). The lymph from the anterior part of the tongue flows into the anterior neck (submental) lymph nodes.

> **KEY POINT** Infections and cancer in the mouth and related areas can be spread via the lymphatics to the cervical lymph nodes, which may become swollen (*lymphadenopathy*).

The Palate

The palate is composed of:

- *Hard palate* (anterior two-thirds)
- *Soft palate* (posterior one-third).

The hard palate forms the roof of the mouth and the floor of the nasal cavity. The mucosa of the hard palate is firmly bound to the underlying bone. Anteriorly, at the tip of the palate is a papilla called incisive papilla. Lateral to the incisive papilla the mucosa is thrown into folds which make the surface of the palate rough. These are called the transverse palatine folds or rugae.

The soft palate is suspended from the posterior edge of the hard palate and is therefore mobile. It is made of muscle and also has nerves, blood vessels, mucous glands and lymphatic tissue. A conical midline projection, called the *uvula*, hangs from its free inferior border. At the sides of the mouth, the soft palate merges with the tongue and wall of the pharynx to form the palatoglossal and palatopharyngeal arches (*fauces*). The lingual tonsil lies between these arches. The palatoglossal arch represents the border between the oral cavity and oropharynx. It is commonly called the oropharyngeal isthmus or the isthmus of the fauces.

The sensory nerve supply to the hard palate and most of the soft palate is via the trigeminal nerve, and to the posterior part of the tongue is via the glossopharyngeal nerve (this nerve also controls most of the muscles in this region).

> **KEY POINT** Touching the posterior palate or tongue can readily cause retching (gagging).

125

IDENTIFY AND LEARN
Can you identify the uvula on Figure 4.1.8?

NERVE SUPPLY TO THE FACE AND THE ORAL CAVITY

The sensory supply (sensation) to the face and oral cavity structures is provided mainly by the trigeminal nerve, the fifth cranial nerve. The trigeminal is primarily a sensory nerve, but it also has some motor nerve fibres (these control the functions of biting, chewing and swallowing).

The name trigeminal nerve comes from the fact that the nerve has three (tri-) major divisions or branches. The **dermatomes** supplied by the three branches are distinct with relatively little overlap (Figure 4.2.10; unlike the dermatomes in the rest of the body, which show considerable overlap).

> **Term to Learn**
> **Dermatome:** an area of skin which is usually supplied by a single spinal nerve. By checking the sensations felt in a particular area of the skin, doctors can know whether the nerves supplying that area are functioning normally or not.

Foramina

The three divisions of the trigeminal nerve leave the skull through various foraminae (Figure 4.2.11). The mnemonic; standing room only' (SRO = Superior orbital fissure; Rotundum; Ovale) can be used to remember where the divisions leave the skull:

1. *Ophthalmic nerve* – this leaves the skull through the Superior orbital fissure and is purely sensory. It carries sensory information from various areas including the scalp and forehead, the upper eyelid, part of the eye, the nose (including the tip of the nose), and the nasal mucosa.
2. *Maxillary nerve* – this leaves the skull through the foramen Rotundum and is purely sensory. The maxillary nerve also carries sensory information from various areas in the face including the lower eyelid and cheek, the opening of the nose (nares) and upper lip, the upper teeth and gingiva, the nasal mucosa, the palate and roof of the pharynx, and the maxillary antrum.

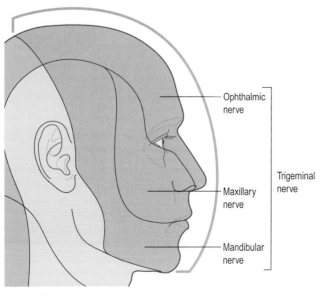

FIGURE 4.2.10
Sensory nerve supply to the face and oral cavity: the three divisions of the trigeminal nerve.

3. *Mandibular nerve* – this leaves the skull through the foramen Ovale and has both sensory and motor nerve fibres. The mandibular nerve carries touch/position and pain/temperature sensation from the mouth, and from parts of the ear. It does not carry taste sensation, but one of its branches, the lingual nerve, does. (This is because nerve fibres from other nerves come and join the lingual nerve.) The mandibular nerve also supplies muscles of mastication, and one middle ear muscle (tensor tympani) and one palatal muscle (tensor palatini).

The main branch of the mandibular nerve is the *inferior alveolar (dental) nerve* (Figure 4.2.11), which carries sensory information from the lower lip, the lower teeth and gingiva, the chin and jaw (except the angle of the jaw). The inferior alveolar nerve starts lingual to the mandibular

126

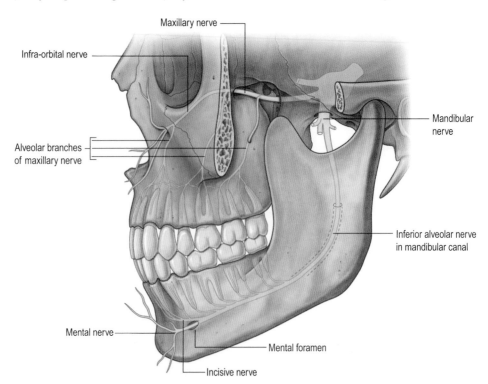

FIGURE 4.2.11
Nerve supply to the mandible and maxilla and the teeth.

BOX 4.2.1 LOCAL ANAESTHESIA SITES IN THE MOUTH

- *ID block injection*: this injection aims to block the inferior alveolar (dental) nerve and thus anaesthetise the teeth on that side of the lower jaw.
- *Mental nerve block injection*: this will anaesthetise anterior teeth only, mainly the lower canine and incisors on that side.
- *Lingual nerve block injection*: this causes numbness in the areas supplied by the lingual nerve.

Administration of local anaesthetic near the mandibular foramen causes blockage of the inferior alveolar nerve and the nearby lingual nerve which is why the numbing of the lower jaw during dental procedures causes the patient to lose sensation on that side in:

- Lower teeth (inferior alveolar nerve block)
- Lower lip and chin (mental nerve block)
- Tongue (lingual nerve block).

Often an injection called *buccal infiltration* is also given to anaesthetise the buccal nerve, which is another branch of the mandibular nerve and supplies the buccal mandibular gingiva posteriorly.

---

ramus, where it enters the mandible through the mandibular foramen to run within the inferior alveolar canal, giving off branches to all the mandibular teeth on that side. At about the level of the mandibular second premolars, the nerve gives off the mental nerve, which exits the mandible via the mental canal to supply the lower lip and chin on that side. The lingual nerve arises from the mandibular nerve above the mandibular foramen, and runs close lingual to the mandibular molar teeth to enter the tongue.

KEY POINTS The ophthalmic and maxillary nerves provide sensory information.

The mandibular nerve provides sensory and motor information.

Injection of a local anaesthetic can result in the complete loss of sensation from well-defined areas of the face and mouth (Box 4.2.1).

THE TEETH AND THEIR SUPPORTING STRUCTURES (THE PERIODONTIUM)

Functions of Teeth

Teeth are specialised structures and form the hardest tissues in the body. They contribute towards:

- Facial appearance (aesthetics)
- Chewing (mastication)
- Speech
- Defence.

Functionally, teeth may be divided into two types:

- Anterior teeth (incisors and canines (or cuspids)) – these are used for seizing food (or in defence)
- Posterior teeth (molars and premolars (or bicuspids)) – these are used to grind food and, with the help of saliva, prepare the food bolus for swallowing.

The teeth are firmly anchored in the alveolar processes of the upper and lower jaws via the periodontal ligament, which along with their hard, robust structure helps them carry out their functions.

Tooth Structure

Each tooth has two parts: the *crown*, which is visible in the mouth; and the *root*, which is the part that lies within the bone (Figure 4.2.12). The crown is covered by a very hard structure

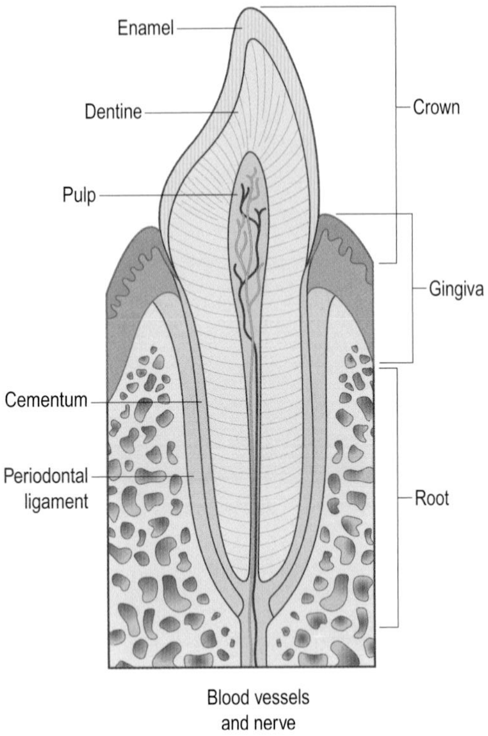

Enamel

Dentine

Pulp

Cementum

Periodontal ligament

Crown

Gingiva

Root

Blood vessels and nerve

FIGURE 4.2.12
Parts of a typical tooth.

128

Term to Learn
Interproximal area: area between the proximal surfaces of neighbouring teeth.

called *enamel*. Under the enamel is slightly softer, sensitive tissue called *dentine*. Within the dentine, in the middle of the tooth is the living tissue called the *pulp* (sometimes called the 'nerve'). It has nerves and blood vessels which pass out through an opening at the tip of the root, called the apical foramen, to connect with the nerves and vessels in the alveolar bone.

The tooth root does not have any enamel covering. Instead it is covered by another tissue called *cementum*.

The tooth is suspended in its socket by a specialised tissue called the *periodontal ligament*. The fibres of this ligament attach to the cementum on one side and the alveolar bone on the other. This joint is unique in the body and is called *gomphosis* – the only joint in which a bone does not join another bone, as teeth are not technically bone.

The junction between the crown and root of a tooth is called the neck or cervix of the tooth (*cervical margin*). Where a tooth is partially erupted into the mouth, only part of the full (anatomical) crown is visible. This is called the *clinical crown*. The rest is covered by a soft tissue called the *gingiva* (plural gingivae; also called gums). Healthy gingivae appear pink, and have a stippled surface (like the peel of an orange) and are tightly bound to the tooth crown, forming a close fitting cuff around the cervix. The rest of the gingivae cover the alveolar bone. Between the gingiva and tooth crown is a shallow gingival crevice.

The Dentitions

The teeth erupt into an arch form called the dental arch. The U shape of the dental arch is a result of the combined pressures from the tongue on the lingual/palatal side and the buccal and facial musculature on the other side. Within each arch, the teeth are in contact with their neighbouring teeth. These are called the contact areas and the area is called the **interproximal area**.

Humans have two dentitions, which appear in sequence and allow for growth of the face and jaws from childhood to adult.

THE DECIDUOUS DENTITION

The first or primary set of smaller teeth (also called deciduous, milk, or baby teeth) include four incisors, two canines and four molars in each jaw (total 20 teeth). These are successively replaced by the secondary (permanent) dentition.

PERMANENT DENTITION

The normal permanent (adult) set of teeth includes four incisors, two canines, four premolars, and up to six molars in each jaw (32 teeth).

The dentitions are described in greater detail later in the chapter.

Tooth Development

All the deciduous teeth and some of the permanent teeth start developing in the fetus. The first signs of tooth development can be seen at about one month of pregnancy.

TOOTH FORMATION (ODONTOGENESIS)

Teeth develop from the epithelium in the mouth of the developing fetus. This epithelium first shows a horseshoe-shaped thickening (called the *dental lamina*) that corresponds to the future dental arches of the maxilla and mandible. Bulb-like thickenings then grow at intervals along the length of the dental lamina (Figure 4.2.13A). These are called the tooth germs, and eventually form a tooth. At the same time, bone starts to grow around the tooth germs so they come to be enclosed within crypts in the future alveolar bone of the jaw.

The tooth germ is also called the enamel organ. Figure 4.2.13 shows that the enamel organ has several distinct layers of cells including:

- Outer enamel epithelium
- Inner enamel epithelium.

The cells of the outer enamel epithelium, called the *ameloblasts*, produce the enamel.

The dental papilla contains cells that develop into *odontoblasts*, which form the dentine, and other cells that form the dental pulp. The dental follicle surrounds the enamel organ and gives rise to:

- Cementoblasts, which form cementum
- Osteoblasts, which form the alveolar bone
- Fibroblasts, which form the periodontal ligament.

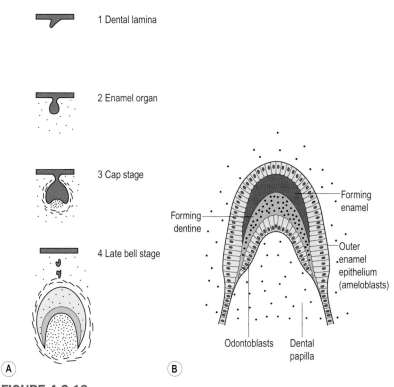

FIGURE 4.2.13
(A, B) Stages of tooth formation.

There are six stages of tooth formation (stages 2–4 are so called because of the shape of the enamel organ at that stage, Figure 4.2.13A):

1. Initiation
2. Bud
3. Cap
4. Bell
5. Apposition (laying down of enamel and dentine)
6. Maturation (mineralisation of the enamel and dentine)

The enamel and dentine when first formed are soft tissues. As the tooth develops, the cells deposit minerals (primarily calcium), which harden the soft tissue. This is called mineralisation. All teeth are mineralising by birth. Mineralisation of the permanent incisor and first molar teeth begins at, or close to, the time of birth, with mineralisation of other permanent teeth starting later. Table 4.2.3 lists the approximate times of development of the teeth.

Tooth eruption in both dentitions occurs after crown formation and mineralisation are largely complete but before the roots are fully formed.

Tooth eruption is chronicled in Table 4.2.4. Roughly speaking, the teeth erupt three years after crown formation.

KEY POINT The 'rule of 3s' is that tooth crowns develop three years before eruption.

Disturbances in Tooth Formation

Disturbances in tooth formation can lead to tooth abnormalities as follows:

- *Anodontia* – this refers to the lack of teeth: anodontia may be complete (very rare) or partial (hypodontia or oligodontia – not uncommon).

TABLE 4.2.3 Summary of Tooth Development

Tooth	Tooth Germ Formed (Time of Intrauterine Life*)	Crown Mineralisation Begins (Time of Intrauterine Life)	Crown Mineralisation Complete (Time after Birth)	Tooth Appears in Oral Cavity (Time after Birth**)	Root Complete (Number of Years after Eruption)
Deciduous Teeth					
Incisors	17th week	4 months	2–3 months	6–9 months	1–1.5 years for all
Canines	18th week	5 months	9 months	16–18 months	
1st molars	19th week	6 months	6 months	12–14 months	
2nd molars	19th week	6 months	12 months	20–30 months	
Permanent Teeth					
Incisors	30th week	2–4 months (10–12 for maxillary lateral incisor)	4–5 years	6–8 years (mandibular)	2–3 years for all
Canines	30th week	4–5 months	6–7 years	7–9 years (maxillary) 9–10 years (mandibular)	
Premolars	30th week	1.5–2.5 years (after birth)	5–7 years	11–12 years (maxillary) 10–12 years (mandibular)	
1st molars	24th week	At birth	2.5–3 years	6–7 years	
2nd molars	6 months	2.5–3 years	7–8 years	11–13 years	
3rd molars	6 years after birth	7–10 years	12–16 years	17–21 years	

*Intrauterine life: this is the period of life before birth, within the uterus.
**First appearance; see Table 4.2.4 for full eruption times.

TABLE 4.2.4 Tooth Eruption Times

Deciduous (Primary) Teeth	Upper Months of Age	Lower Months of Age
Central incisors	8–13	6–10
Lateral incisors	8–13	10–16
Canines	16–23	16–23
First molars	13–19	13–19
Second molars	25–33	23–31

Permanent Teeth	Upper Years of Age	Lower Years of Age
Central incisors	7–8	6–7
Lateral incisors	8–9	7–8
Canines	11–12	9–10
First premolars	10–11	10–12
Second premolars	10–12	11–12
First molars	6–7	6–7
Second molars	12–13	11–13
Third molars	17–21	17–21

- *Supernumerary* – additional teeth.
- *Microdontia* – small teeth; this commonly affects permanent maxillary incisors or third molars.
- *Macrodontia* – large teeth; rare.
- *Dens invaginatus* (dens in dente) – this refers to a deep pit on the lingual surface of a permanent maxillary incisor. Such teeth are more vulnerable to decay.
- *Enamel or dentine dysplasia* – this refers to faulty development of either enamel or dentine.

Tooth Morphology

The deciduous dentition (Figure 4.2.14) has no premolars. The morphology of the other teeth is similar to the permanent teeth although there are some differences:

- They are typically smaller than their permanent counterparts
- They are whiter in colour
- They have a comparatively larger crown and shorter roots, larger pulps and broader contact points

Table 4.2.5 lists the essential features of the deciduous teeth.

Permanent teeth (Figure 4.2.15) are larger than deciduous teeth and are mainly different from one another because of the differences in crown shape, the number of cusps (see Table 4.2.6) and the number of roots (Table 4.2.7). The shapes of individual teeth are related to function of each tooth type (cutting, shredding or grinding food) (Table 4.2.6 and Figure 4.2.15). Root shape is highly variable.

The Mature Dental Tissues

The mature dental tissues are:

- Teeth
  - ○ Enamel
  - ○ Dentine

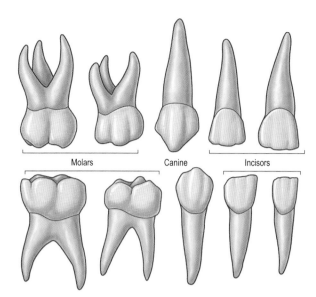

Molars   Canine   Incisors

FIGURE 4.2.14
The deciduous teeth.

KEY POINT Teeth may have one, two, three or occasionally more, roots (Table 4.2.7). This knowledge is particularly important in endodontics (Chapter 9) and tooth extraction, where each root has to be accounted for separately.

131

TABLE 4.2.5 Features of the Deciduous Teeth			
Tooth	**Function**	**Position in Dental Arch**	**Morphology**
Incisors	Cutting	These are the eight front teeth	Flat crown surfaces, a straight sharp horizontal edge and a single, conical root
Canines	Tearing and shredding	These are the four pointed corner teeth	Conical crown that projects beyond the level of the other teeth, single, conical root
Molars	Chewing and grinding (*mola* is Latin for mill)	The eight molars form the back teeth	The largest of the deciduous teeth. Each molar has a flat, large **occlusal (upper) surface**, with four pyramidal-shaped projections called cusps, and two to three roots

Term to Learn
Occlusal surface: the chewing surface of the molars and premolars.

FIGURE 4.2.15
A, B The permanent teeth.

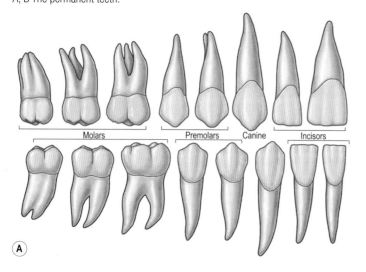

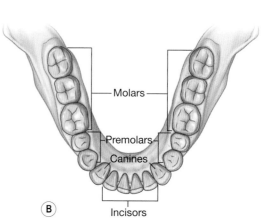

Ⓐ

Ⓑ

TABLE 4.2.6	Features of the Permanent Teeth		
Tooth	**Function**	**Position in Dental Arch**	**Morphology**
Incisors	Cutting	These are the eight front teeth	Flat crown surfaces, a straight sharp horizontal edge and a single long, conical root
Canines (upper canines may be called eye teeth)	Tearing and shredding	These are the four pointed corner teeth	Large, conical crown that projects beyond the level of the other teeth and a single conical root, longer than the roots of all other teeth in the arch
Premolars	Chewing	There are eight premolars, and they are located lateral to and just behind the canines	The crowns have two cusps each and they have one to two roots each
Molars (third molars are also called wisdom teeth)	Chewing and grinding (*mola* is Latin for mill)	There are 12 molars, and these are the back teeth	The largest of the permanent teeth, with large and flat **occlusal (upper) surface** and several cusps, and two to four roots

TABLE 4.2.7 Usual Number of Roots on Permanent Teeth

Tooth		1	2	3	4	5	6	7	8
Number of roots	Maxillary	1	1	1	2	1	3	3	Varies
	Mandibular	1	1	1	1	1	2	2	Varies

- ○ Pulp
- ○ Cementum
- Periodontal ligament

ENAMEL

Enamel is produced by cells called ameloblasts and is the most highly mineralised tissue of the body. It is composed of:

- Mineral (calcium phosphate or hydroxyapatite)
- Protein matrix (amelogenin).

Where enamel is thicker, less light passes through and the tooth appears whiter. As enamel thickness varies across the surface of a tooth so does the tooth colour. The very highly mineralised nature of enamel makes teeth extremely resistant to destruction. It is not surprising therefore that dental remains may be the only identifiable remains useful for identification in **forensic dentistry** or in archaeological research.

The high mineral content makes enamel susceptible to 'de-mineralisation' by acids. In the mouth, acids are formed by bacteria that usually live in the mouth. Demineralisation makes the tooth vulnerable to dental caries (decay). Acids from foods, drinks and the stomach can also demineralise and erode enamel (see Chapter 5).

DENTINE

Produced by odontoblasts within the outermost layer of the pulp (see Figure 4.2.13), dentine is a living tissue, very sensitive and softer than enamel but harder than bone. To a certain extent, some dentine (called secondary dentine) can continue to form for years. Dentine is made up of 70% inorganic material, chiefly hydroxyapatite, 20% organic (mainly proteins called collagen) and 10% water. Dentine has a variable yellowish colour that gives teeth their colour. Dentine is readily damaged by dental caries (see Chapter 5). Where a tooth pulp has become diseased, it may lead to discoloration of dentine and such teeth have crowns that then appear darker. The mechanism whereby dentine is so exquisitely sensitive is still unknown. Whatever stimulus is applied to dentine, whether it is thermal, mechanical, osmotic or electrical, the only sensation perceived is that of pain.

DENTAL PULP

Dental pulp is a vascular (lot of blood vessels), very sensitive, soft connective tissue that is the source of nourishment for a tooth and its vitality. Pulp tissue contains:

- Odontoblasts (cells that produce dentine)
- Fibroblasts (produce and maintain **collagen** fibres and **ground substance**)
- Defence cells.

Term to Learn
Forensic dentistry: the branch of dentistry concerned with the identification and examination of dental evidence in relation to crimes and the law.

KEY POINT Enamel has a dynamic relationship with the oral environment, particularly saliva. This means that while the enamel can dissolve in acids, it can also take up certain minerals from the saliva (remineralisation). This property of enamel is made use of in the prevention (prophylaxis) of caries with topical fluoride application. In this, a layer of fluoride containing varnish or gel is applied to the surfaces of the teeth. The fluoride ion makes the enamel mineral product, hydroxyapatite, more resistant to acid dissolution; it also helps the re-precipitation of hydroxyapatite.

Terms to Learn
Collagen: the main protein of the connective tissue, which provides strength, resilience and support to various parts of the body, such as the skin, ligaments and tendons.
Ground substance: the matrix in which the cells in a tissue are embedded.

133

The pulp space within the crown is termed the pulp chamber and the parts that lie within the cusps are called *pulp horns*. The pulp space within the root(s) is called the *root canal system*. The nerves and vessels that serve the pulp enter principally through each root's apical foramen (Figure 4.2.12). But accessory, lateral connections between the pulp and the periodontal ligament may also exist.

Secondary dentine develops after root formation is complete and is produced throughout the life of a tooth at an extremely slow rate. This progressively reduces the pulp space.

FIND OUT MORE

How does secondary dentine create difficulties in endodontics?

PERIODONTIUM

The periodontium (from the Greek *peri-*, meaning 'around' and *-odont*, meaning 'tooth') is the collective term for the specialised tissues that surround and support the teeth, maintaining them in the jaw bones. The periodontium consists of the:

- Cementum
- Periodontal ligament.
- Alveolar bone
- Gingiva.

Cementum

Cementum (or cement) is a specialised mineralised tissue that covers the tooth root. It is produced by the cementoblasts. Cementum is less mineralised than enamel or dentine, yellowish in colour and softer and thickest at the root apex. The main role is to anchor the tooth in its socket, via the periodontal ligament. Excess cementum (hypercementosis) can make tooth extraction difficult.

Periodontal Ligament

The periodontal membrane or ligament (PDL) anchors the root (via the cementum) in the alveolar bone of the tooth socket. The PDL is a fibrous connective tissue consisting of collagen fibres which, when not under stress, have a relaxed and wavy course across the width of the periodontal space. A healthy PDL is able to withstand the not inconsiderable forces applied to teeth during use, yet provides flexibility that prevents them shattering. The functions of the PDL are:

- Supportive – anchoring the tooth.
- Sensory – via sensitive periodontal **mechanoreceptors**. The slightest interference that causes even minimal tooth displacement is consciously felt by an individual. It is immediately followed by reflex muscle activity to try to correct the problem. For example, if an individual bites on something hard unexpectedly the mouth immediately opens.

Periodontal disease (see Chapter 5) progressively destroys the PDL and, eventually, the remaining tissue is unable to withstand normal chewing forces so that the tooth becomes **mobile** (loose).

Gingiva

The gingiva is the mucosa overlying the alveolar bone, to which it is tightly bound to resist the friction of food passing over. Healthy gingiva is usually coral pink, but it may be pigmented. This is normal. The gingiva surrounds the cervical margin of the teeth in the area of the *amelo-cemental junction* (junction between the enamel and cementum), where it provides a seal. There is a shallow sulcus or crevice between the margin of the gingiva and tooth crown just above the seal. The gingiva is divided anatomically into:

- Marginal – the gingiva overlying the gingival sulcus
- Attached – the gingiva attached to the tooth and bone
- Interdental – the gingiva in the spaces between the teeth.

The attached gingiva blends into the oral mucosa in the vestibules.

Accumulation of **plaque** on the tooth cervical regions may result in inflammation of the gingival margin (called gingivitis or marginal gingivitis). With age, especially when toothbrushing is incorrectly performed, the amount of tooth visible in the mouth is greater than the anatomical crown due to recession of the gingiva. The root surface below the cervical margin becomes exposed as the gingiva recedes and sometimes, if the dentine is exposed, the patient complains of pain (hypersensitivity), especially with cold fluids or food.

> ### KEY POINTS
> Teeth start to develop *in utero* (before birth).
> Root formation is completed after eruption.
> The full primary set of teeth has 20 teeth in total.
> The full permanent set of teeth has 32 teeth in total.
> Anterior teeth have one root only.
> Lower molar teeth usually have two roots and upper molar teeth have three.

Term to Learn
Mechanoreceptor: a receptor that senses mechanical pressure or distortion.
Mobile tooth: a loose tooth; mobility can be of various degrees.

Terms to Learn
Plaque: a biofilm composed of mucus and bacteria that forms on tooth surfaces, particularly the **interproximal surfaces** and along the gingival margins of teeth (cervically), and in the fissures and pits on the occlusal surface.
Interproximal surface: the surfaces of adjacent teeth that face each other. In a healthy dentition, the interproximal surfaces touch each other at the *contact point*.

135

CHAPTER 5

Oral Disease

CHAPTER POINTS
- This chapter covers the requirements of the NEBDN syllabus Section 5: Oral disease and pathology.

INTRODUCTION

The oral diseases described in this chapter are seen routinely in the dental surgery. Therefore as a dental nurse, you are required to have background knowledge about them.

Diseases may be *congenital* (present at birth) or *acquired* (develop at some stage after birth). Most dental (**odontogenic**) disease is acquired and caused by the build-up and activity of micro-organisms (mainly bacteria) on the tooth surface within the dental bacterial plaque.

Plaque is a film containing bacteria (a biofilm) that builds up rapidly and is usually removed by toothbrushing and other mechanical oral hygiene aids. If plaque is not removed it eventually hardens into calculus because of the deposition of calcium salts. Chemicals in certain mouthwashes and toothpastes can inhibit the build up of plaque, and some inhibit *calculus* (tartar) formation. These oral healthcare products are discussed in Chapter 8.

The activity of the micro-organisms in plaque is responsible for, or may aggravate, a variety of oral diseases, in particular *dental caries* (tooth decay) and inflammatory periodontal disease (*gingivitis* and *periodontitis*), which are the most common oral diseases.

Terms to Learn
Odontogenic: of dental origin.

137

DISEASES OF THE TEETH

Table 5.1 shows the main dental diseases.

Tooth Eruption Problems

TEETHING PROBLEMS

Just before primary teeth erupt, the gingiva may show a bluish colour and become swollen. This is usually because of transient bleeding into the gingiva, which stops spontaneously.

An infant who is teething may show irritability, disturbed sleep, flushed face, drooling, a small rise in temperature and/or a rash. Teething does not cause diarrhoea or any other disease (but these may occur coincidentally).

DELAYS IN ERUPTION

Teeth can erupt up to 12 months late – this is usually of little significance. Longer delays in tooth eruption are often caused by local factors such as the tooth becoming impacted against another tooth as it travels through the bone. The teeth that most often get impacted are the third molars (wisdom teeth), premolars and canines, because these are usually the last teeth to erupt.

TABLE 5.1 The Main Dental Diseases

Disease	Main Micro-organism Responsible	Prevention	Treatment
Caries	*Streptococcus mutans* Lactobacilli *Actinomyces*	Minimise dietary sugar intake Use fluoride toothpastes and mouth washes	Restorative dentistry (fillings)
Periodontitis	*Porphyromonas gingivalis* Many other bacteria	Improve oral hygiene, minimise or avoid tobacco use or smoking	Scaling, polishing, root planing, periodontal care (see Chapter 8, p. 206)

If tooth eruption is delayed for more than one year the dentist will often take an X-ray to check the reason.

FIND OUT MORE

Look at some X-rays of impacted teeth – how many of them were third molars and canines?

Dental Caries (Tooth Decay)

Dental caries is a very common disease. The main plaque micro-organism that causes dental caries is the bacterium *Streptococcus mutans* (also called *viridans streptococci*). Other bacteria such as *Lactobacillus* and *Actinomyces* may also play a role. The bacteria act by converting the sugars in the diet to acids (especially lactic acid). The acids destroy (decalcify) the enamel and dentine of the teeth (Figure 5.1).

Sugars are mainly found in the diet as sugar (lactose) in milk and non-milk sugars. Lactose is less cariogenic than the other sugars.

138

FIGURE 5.1

(A) Carious cavities in upper anterior teeth. (B) X-ray showing an abscess at the base of the carious second molar.

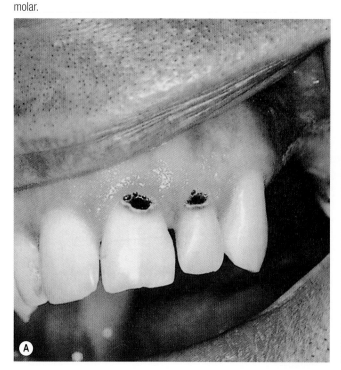

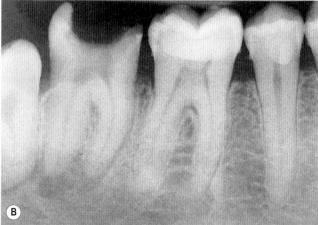

TABLE 5.2 Cariogenic Sugars

Pure Sugars	Mixtures
Dextrose	Brown sugar
Fructose (except in fresh fruits and vegetables)	Golden syrup
Glucose	Honey
Hydrolysed starch	Maple syrup
Invert sugar	Treacle
Maltose	
Sucrose	

The non-milk sugars include the common table or cane sugar (sucrose), glucose, and fruit sugar (fructose). Sugars are also added to many foods and drinks, in particular to refined carbohydrates such as starch and foods such as cakes and biscuits. Non-milk sugars (Table 5.2) are the most **cariogenic**. Dietary starch is also broken down slowly by salivary enzymes to glucose and maltose. Concentrated fruit juices and dried fruits also have a high concentration of sugars such as fructose and are therefore also cariogenic. Fresh fruits and vegetables are not cariogenic.

Term to Learn
Cariogenic: a factor that can cause caries.

CARIES PREVENTION

- Saliva protects against caries. In people who produce a good amount of saliva the chances of developing caries is far less than in those who have a dry mouth or hyposalivation (see p. 150).
- Teeth can be remineralised by fluorides, or solutions of calcium and phosphate (e.g. Tooth Mousse). The number of people developing caries has been declining for some years, mainly because of the protective effect of fluoride in toothpastes.

THE CARIES DISEASE PROCESS

139

The sugars in the diet are converted to lactic acid. When the acidity increases to a particular level (i.e. the pH falls), minerals such as calcium and phosphate are released from the tooth (called demineralisation or decalcification) causing dental caries (decay). The level of acidity is measured by finding out the pH, which is low when the acid level is high. If the pH in the mouth falls below 5.5 (the *critical pH*) the tooth starts to decalcify. The longer the pH remains low in the mouth, the greater the decalcification and damage. Thus eating sticky sugars (e.g. toffees), repeatedly eating or drinking sugary foods, or sucking sweets for hours, leads to a long drop in the pH, and a lot of damage. Even more damage occurs if the sugars are eaten just before going to sleep, because saliva production falls during sleep, and therefore the natural cleaning of the mouth is reduced.

The least tooth damage is done by:

- Avoiding consuming sugars completely
- Minimising non-milk sugar intake
- Eating sugar-containing products all at once only and over a short period of time
- Not eating sugars as the last thing at night.

Decalcification produces opaque whitish areas on the tooth, which are painless. Decalcification is also reversible to a point if the person changes their diet and reduces intake of more cariogenic carbohydrates.

The critical pH for dentine demineralisation is higher at around 6.5 (so less acid needed) and the dentine is softer than enamel, so caries spreads more rapidly once it reaches dentine. It may then spread to the pulp causing infection, inflammation and pain (pulpitis).

Table 5.3 summarises the key points you need to know about dental caries.

KEY POINT Sugars, particularly non-milk sugars in food and drink, are major cariogenic factors.

TABLE 5.3	Facts You Should Know About Dental Caries
Cause	Plaque bacteria, especially *Streptococcus mutans*, which acts on sugars to produce lactic acid, which decalcifies (demineralises) the teeth
Plaque	This biofilm tends to form in pits and fissures, interproximally at contact areas; and at the cervical margins (sites where caries begins)
Main sugars implicated in caries	Sucrose, glucose
Sugars and sweeteners rarely implicated in caries	Fructose, lactose, sorbitol, aspartame
Acidity (critical pH) below which enamel decalcification occurs	5.5
Methods of detection	Visual examination Bitewing radiographs (see Chapter 14) Transillumination (shining a light through the tooth) Electronic caries detectors Using a probe (but this may cause further damage; see Chapter 7)
Preventive measures	Consuming less sugars in the diet Using fluorides, e.g. fluoridated toothpastes Using amorphous calcium phosphate

IF CARIES IS NOT TREATED

If the carious process is allowed to progress, it destroys the enamel, causing a cavity to form in the tooth. Eventually it reaches the dentine. Once caries reaches the dentine, the carious process speeds up. Also, the patient may feel pain on stimulation with sweet/sour or hot/ cold. This pain is similar to the pain that occurs when dentine is exposed due to loss of enamel for other reasons such as trauma, erosion or abrasion (see p. 141). The pain subsides within seconds of removing the stimulus. The pain may be poorly 'localised', that is, it may be difficult for the patient to say where exactly it is. Often pain is localised only to an approximate area within two to three teeth of the affected tooth.

The inflammation causes swelling of the pulp but, since the pulp is confined within the rigid pulp chamber, the pressure builds up. Thus there is severe and persistent pain in the tooth. The swelling also stops the blood flow into the pulp – which then dies. The pain may then subside for a while. However, the dead pulp is infected with bacteria from the mouth. So the infection can then spread through the tooth root apex and cause *apical periodontitis*. This is very painful, especially when the tooth is touched or the patient bites on it. Such a tooth must be root treated (endodontics) or extracted (exodontics) in a timely fashion. Otherwise a dental **abscess** (Figure 5.1B), *granuloma* or **cyst** (see below) will eventually form.

Term to Learn
Cyst: an abnormal sac-like structure that is usually filled with fluid.
Abscess: a collection of pus.

PAIN AND DENTAL CARIES

Early caries, that is when there is only enamel decay, is painless. When the caries reaches the dentine, the person may get transient pain with sweet, hot or cold stimuli. When the caries approaches the pulp, the person may feel more prolonged pain, which may sometimes be spontaneous. Once caries reaches the pulp it becomes inflamed, causing spontaneous and severe pain (toothache).

TREATMENT OF CARIES

Caries is removed by the clinician (dentist or dental therapist). Then the tooth is restored (filled) (see Chapter 9).

140

Periapical Abscess (Dental Abscess)

A dental abscess often follows **pulpitis** caused by caries or trauma. The pulp, and so the affected tooth, is dead (non-vital). Therefore although the tooth cannot itself cause pain, the inflammation travels to the bone surrounding the tooth apex. This is called apical periodontitis. If the inflammation persists, it may cause an abscess (apical or dental abscess) both of which produce pain. A dental abscess will cause pain and also result in a swelling, typically in the labial or buccal gingiva (Figure 5.2). Sometimes the face can swell up too (Figure 5.3) and the patient may also develop lymph node swelling and a fever.

Analgesics and **antibiotics** may be needed in the short term to alleviate the patient's symptoms. Eventually, extraction or root canal treatment of the affected tooth will be required to remove the source of infection, or the problem will return.

If the tooth is not correctly treated, a cyst (periapical, radicular or dental cyst) can develop. Again, either root canal treatment or root end surgery (*apicoectomy* or *apicectomy*) will then be needed (see Chapter 9).

Trauma

Trauma to the teeth is commonly seen in sports, road accidents, violence, epilepsy, and in restorative dentistry! Tooth trauma is seen mainly in boys or young men. It usually affects the maxillary incisors. Because of the impact of trauma, a tooth can be lost from the mouth or dislodged within its socket (Figure 5.4), fractured (the crown or root), or it can die. (See also Chapter 16). Dental trauma is also seen in children who have been abused. In all forms of trauma, there can also be damage to the jaws or soft tissues. Thus it is important for the clinician to take a careful history and do a thorough examination to ensure there are no injuries elsewhere in the body, especially head or chest injuries (which can be fatal), or damage to the neck – which can lead to paralysis or death.

> **Term to Learn**
> **Pulpitis:** the condition in which the tooth pulp is inflamed; it is commonly due to progression of dental caries inside the tooth.

> **Terms to Learn**
> **Analgesic:** a pain-killing drug, e.g. paracetamol (also called acetaminophen).
> **Antibiotics:** drugs that stop the growth of or kill micro-organisms.

141

FIND OUT MORE

What instruments would the dentist require to examine a patient who has presented after trauma to the teeth?

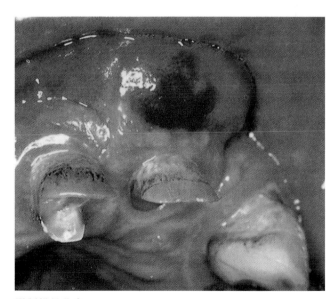

FIGURE 5.2
Dental abscess.

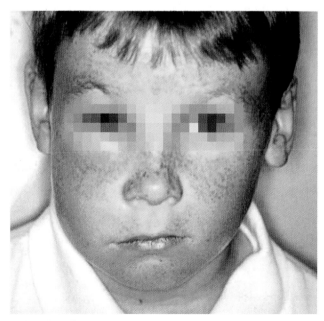

FIGURE 5.3
Severe infection in the canine region.

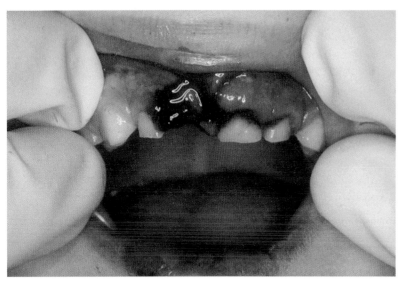

FIGURE 5.4
Palatal luxation of upper left deciduous central incisor.

> **Terms to Learn**
> **Incisal edge:** the thin surfaces of the incisors that are used for biting.
> **Cusp:** the triangular elevations on the occlusal surfaces of molars and premolars and the pointed tip of the canine.

Attrition

Attrition is a form of tooth surface loss. It is the wearing away of a tooth's biting (occlusal) surfaces due to chewing (mastication). It is most obvious in people who have a coarse diet. Attrition can also occur in people with a habit such as bruxism (grinding of teeth). The **incisal edges** of the anterior teeth and the **cusps** on the occlusal surfaces of the premolars and molars wear down. Once the enamel is breached, the softer dentine is lost faster than the enamel, which results into a flat or hollowed surface (Figure 5.5). The tooth may need a restoration (see Chapter 9).

Abrasion

Abrasion is another form of tooth surface loss – the wearing away of the hard tissues at the neck of the tooth by a habit such as toothbrushing with a hard brush and coarse toothpaste. The gingiva recedes but is otherwise healthy. The cementum and dentine wear down but the harder enamel survives, resulting in a notch (Figure 5.6). The exposure of dentine also means the tooth may become sensitive to hot and cold. There may also eventually be tooth fracture. The tooth may need a restoration (see Chapter 9). Use of desensitising toothpastes and fluoride application may also help.

Erosion

Erosion is tooth surface loss caused by dissolution of the tooth minerals by acids other than those produced in caries. Fruits or fruit drinks, cola (and other carbonated drinks) and stomach (gastric) acid are the main causes of erosion. In most patients there is little more than a loss of normal enamel contour but, in more severe cases, dentine or pulp may be involved. Patients who have a habit that causes erosion should be counselled to stop the habit. The teeth may need to be restored (see Chapter 9).

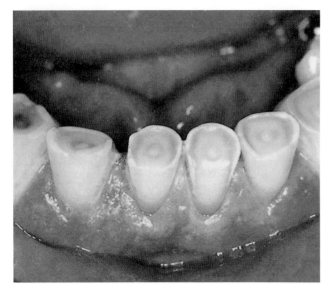

FIGURE 5.5
Attrition.

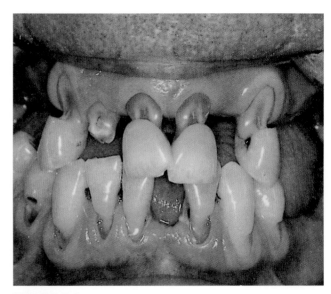

FIGURE 5.6
Abrasion.

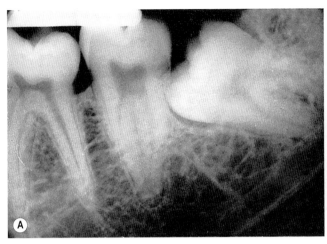
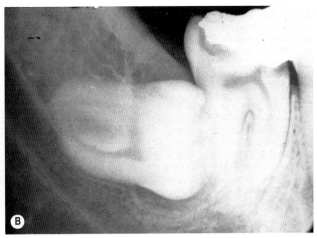

FIGURE 5.7
(A) A mesio-angular impacted lower left third molar and (B) a horizontally impacted lower right third molar.

Impacted Teeth

Teeth can fail to erupt fully because of insufficient space in the dental arch. The teeth most commonly affected are the third molars (wisdom teeth, lower third molars most common), second premolars and canines (Figure 5.7).

Impacted teeth may well be **asymptomatic**, but occasionally they can cause pain. This is usually because of the caries or pericoronitis that develops. Impacted teeth may also lead to cyst formation. There is no evidence that they contribute to **malocclusion**.

Treatment may include orthodontics to guide the impacted tooth to its correct position and sometimes surgery. The latest guidelines of the National Institute for Health and Clinical Excellence (NICE) recommend removal of impacted teeth only if they are causing problems such as recurrent pericoronitis or caries.

Pericoronitis

Pericoronitis is the inflammation of the gingival flap (operculum) over an erupting or impacted tooth. Usually this happens around the lower third molar (see Subchapter 17.1).

Variations in Tooth Number

HYPERDONTIA (TOO MANY TEETH)

In the **mixed dentition period** it is not uncommon to see what appear to be two rows of teeth in the lower incisor region. Additional teeth may be seen occasionally in otherwise healthy individuals, occasionally in those with rare disorders.

- Extra teeth of normal shape (supplemental teeth; Figure 5.8) are uncommon, but most frequently seen in the maxillary lateral incisor, and in the premolar and third molar regions of either jaw.
- Extra teeth of abnormal form (supernumerary teeth) are also uncommon, usually small and/or conical in shape and are seen particularly in the midline of the upper arch (mesiodens).

HYPODONTIA (TOO FEW TEETH)

Reasons for teeth missing from the dental arch include:

- The tooth may have failed to erupt
- It may not have developed
- It may have been lost prematurely.

> **Terms to Learn**
> **Asymptomatic:**
> a condition that is not producing any symptoms.
> **Malocclusion:** when the teeth in the upper and lower arches do not 'bite' normally, for example because they are very crowded or some teeth are missing.

143

> **Term to Learn**
> **Mixed dentition period:** this is when the permanent teeth start erupting, which is before all the deciduous incisors have been lost (exfoliated) so that there are both permanent and deciduous teeth in the mouth at the same time.

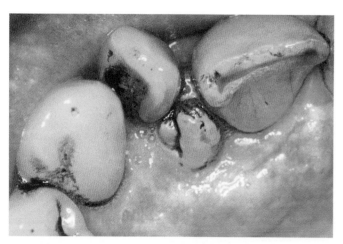

FIGURE 5.8
A supernumerary incisor.

Hypodontia is not uncommon. It is most often genetic, and most frequently affects the third molars, the second premolars and the maxillary lateral incisors. Occasionally hypodontia can occur as part of a generalised (systemic) disorder such as *ectodermal dysplasia*. Rarely, all the teeth are absent (anodontia).

In hypodontia, when the permanent successor is missing, it is common for the deciduous tooth to be retained long after it should have been shed. The patient may need a restoration (see Chapter 9).

Anomalies of Tooth Size, Shape and Structure

Although the delicate process of tooth development is generally well protected in the developing baby or child, it may be affected by diseases, radiotherapy, drugs or infections.

ENAMEL HYPOPLASIA

Between birth and 6 years of age, the permanent incisors and canines are developing (see Subchapter 4.2). If the developing tooth bud is damaged, it can produce a cosmetic problem, because the damage will be evident on smiling. Enamel hypoplasia is when the tooth crown appears opaque, or yellow-brown or deformed. Infections such as German measles (rubella), cancer treatments or jaundice may cause this type of hypoplasia. The defects correspond to the site of tooth enamel formation at the time of the insult ('chronological' hypoplasia).

DISCOLOURED TEETH

Discoloration of several teeth is usually because of superficial (extrinsic) staining that results from:

- Poor oral hygiene
- Use of substances such as tobacco, betel nuts, khat tea, coffee, red wine or chlorhexidine,
- Caries
- Trauma
- Tooth filling material.

Such superficial tooth discoloration affects mainly the interproximal and cervical surfaces of the teeth (where plaque also accumulates) and can be removed by the dental clinician.

Generalised 'intrinsic' tooth staining of a brown or grey colour is caused by the use of the drugs called tetracyclines by a pregnant or lactating mother or children under the age of 8 years. Tetracyclines can cross the placenta and then enter breast milk and are taken up by developing teeth and by bone. Intrinsic staining cannot be removed by the dental clinician. However, because of this problem, tetracyclines are not recommended for pregnant women and infants any more. Staining may also be because of hypoplasia or some rare inherited tooth defect (amelogenesis imperfecta or dentinogenesis imperfecta).

Discoloration of a single tooth is usually intrinsic, that is from within the tooth and happens because the tooth is:

- Non-vital
- Heavily filled or
- Carious.

Non-vital teeth progressively darken more with time, sometimes to a brownish colour (Figure 5.9), and also become more brittle.

FIND OUT MORE

What are betel and khat? Which ethnic communities are they commonly associated with?

Fluorosis

Fluoride in the correct amount usually protects the tooth against caries by hardening the enamel, which is why patients are encouraged to use fluoridated toothpaste/mouthwash and drink fluoridated water. But excessive intake of fluoride can cause fluorosis, which also causes discoloration of the teeth. Depending on the amount of fluoride, defects can range from white flecks or spotting or diffuse cloudiness to yellow-brown or darker patches and staining and 'pitting' of the enamel (Figure 5.10).

High levels of fluoride in drinking water are uncommon in the developed world, but are common in parts of the Middle East, India and Africa. Swallowing large amounts of fluoride toothpastes or mouthwashes, or overdose of fluoride supplements can also cause fluorosis.

Teeth with severe fluorosis are restored with veneers or crowns (see Chapter 9).

Tooth (Dentine) Hypersensitivity

Tooth hypersensitivity is often the result of abrasion from over-enthusiastic toothbrushing (see above). Exposure of the dentine to cold air, water or fruit drinks can cause pain. Use of a good toothbrush with an effective method of tooth cleaning minimises the risk of tooth hypersensitivity. Carious teeth can also be hypersensitive.

If a person has tooth hypersensitivity they should see a dental clinician to ensure there are no cavities and whether they require any treatment. Application of a fluoride varnish (see Chapter 8), and use of desensitising toothpastes can help relieve hypersensitivity.

Malocclusion

See Chapter 11.

> **KEY POINT** Tooth cleansing, whitening and restorative options such as veneers or crowns (see Chapter 9 for definitions) may be used to improve or correct cosmetic defects.

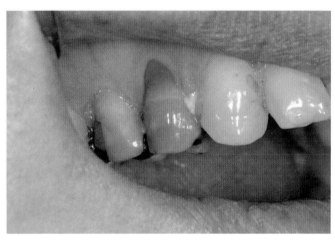

FIGURE 5.9
A non-vital tooth.

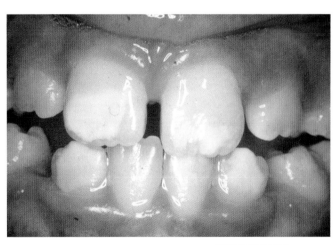

FIGURE 5.10
Fluorosis.

145

PERIODONTAL DISEASE (GINGIVITIS AND PERIODONTITIS)
Inflammatory Gingival and Periodontal Disease

Plaque accumulation may, because of the bacteria in the biofilm, cause inflammation of the gingiva (gingivitis).

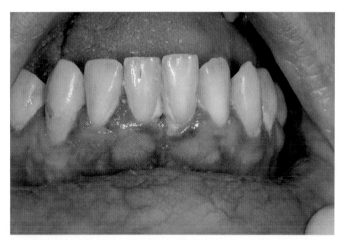

FIGURE 5.11
Generalised gingivitis.

Gingivitis is painless but may lead to bleeding of the gingiva, particularly when brushing the teeth or eating hard foods such as apples. The most common features of gingivitis (Figure 5.11) are:

- Bleeding
- **Halitosis** (oral malodour)
- **Erythema**
- Swelling
- Bleeding on **probing** by the clinician.

Without proper oral care, gingivitis may progress and cause inflammation in the periodontal membrane (periodontitis), with pocket formation, tooth loosening and finally tooth loss.

WHAT IS CALCULUS (TARTAR)?
Plaque must be regularly removed at least once each day, or it will irritate the gingiva, causing gingivitis. With time plaque calcifies to form hard calculus (tartar) above (supra-gingival) and below (sub-gingival) the gingival margin. At the same time, the bacteria destroy the periodontal ligament attachment of the teeth to the jaw bones (periodontitis; pyorrhoea is an old term). Calculus cannot be removed by brushing – only by a clinician.

146

Risk Factors for Periodontal Disease
- Lifestyle factors such as cigarette smoking, and diseases such as diabetes and HIV/AIDS make the person more vulnerable to more rapidly progressive gingival and periodontal disease.
- An exaggerated inflammatory reaction to plaque in pregnancy can also lead to gingivitis. Pregnancy gingivitis usually develops around the second month and reaches a peak in the eighth month.

Management
Treatment is basically improvement in oral hygiene and scaling by the dental clinician to remove any calculus. Since plaque is the main cause of gingivitis, use of anti-plaque agents and increased toothbrushing are important to minimise the problem.

KEY POINT Although periodontal disease is caused by bacterial infection, systemic antibiotics have no place in its treatment. Rather, it is improvement in oral hygiene that is essential.

In periodontitis, plaque accumulates below the gingival margin, so between the tooth and the gingiva. These areas are called periodontal pockets. Patients with periodontal pockets require a special kind of surgery called periodontal surgery to remove the pocket wall and diseased tissue so that the patient can clean the area better. Nowadays, regeneration of lost periodontal tissue (with techniques such as guided tissue regeneration (GTR)) may be required (Chapter 9).

People with atherosclerosis, hypertension, coronary heart disease, cerebrovascular disease, and other general diseases and also **low birth-weight babies** are thought to be at greater risk of developing periodontal disease and there is speculation that periodontal disease may contribute to these general disorders.

Acute Necrotising Ulcerative Gingivitis

This is also called acute ulcerative gingivitis, acute necrotising gingivitis, AUG, ANG, ANUG, Vincent's disease and trench mouth.

ANUG is a rare, non-contagious gingival infection, which typically affects teenagers and young adults. It especially affects those living in institutions, or in the armed forces, that is in conditions where many young people are living together. Other predisposing factors include smoking, viral infections and immune defects such as HIV/AIDS.

Characteristic features of ANUG are:

- Severe gingival soreness
- Profuse gingival bleeding
- Halitosis
- Bad taste.

The **interdental papillae** are ulcerated.

MANAGEMENT

ANUG is managed by oral **debridement**, improving oral hygiene and use of antibiotics to control the infection.

Desquamative Gingivitis

Desquamative gingivitis is usually seen in people with skin diseases, especially lichen planus or pemphigoid. The main problem that the patient has is persistent gingival soreness, which is worse when eating acidic foods such as tomatoes and citrus fruits. The treatment consists of improving oral hygiene and use of topical corticosteroids.

Tooth Loss

Teeth can be lost due to an injury, such as while playing sports, or if a person is assaulted or has a fall, or is involved in a road traffic accident. Teeth can also be lost due to the extraction that is required if caries has destroyed the tooth to the point that it cannot be restored. People with periodontal disease can lose teeth because of the loss of attachment.

MUCOSAL PROBLEMS
Infections

Many oral diseases apart from caries and periodontal disease can also be caused by infection.

CANDIDOSIS

Candidosis is also called candidiasis. It is caused by the fungus *Candida albicans*, which normally lives in the mouth. If the oral environment is changed (e.g. by wearing a dental appliance, use of drugs or dryness due to lack of saliva, or if there is compromised immunity (e.g. HIV/AIDS), the fungal growth is uncontrolled. This leads to inflammation.

Candidosis is also common, for example, underneath upper dentures (denture-related stomatitis).

DENTURE-RELATED STOMATITIS (DENTURE SORE MOUTH)

Wearing of dentures and other dental appliances can produce several ecological changes in the mouth. This includes accumulation of plaque on and in the fitting surface of the appliance and the underlying mucosa. Dental appliances (mainly upper dentures), especially when worn throughout the night, or in a dry mouth, are the major predisposing factors. Fungi such as *Candida albicans* are found in up to 90% of persons with denture-related stomatitis.

Clinical signs are redness of the mucosa which is not sore. Angular cheilitis may occur. Patients with denture-related stomatitis are usually otherwise healthy.

Terms to Learn
Interdental papillae: the triangular areas of the gingiva that fill in the gaps between adjacent teeth.
Debridement: In general medicine, this refers to cleaning of wounds by surgical removal of dead tissue or foreign material. This promotes healing by preventing infection. In dentistry, debridement also refers to the removal of plaque and calculus.

147

Management

Since the denture-fitting surface is infested with micro-organisms, usually with *Candida albicans*, dentures should be taken out at night, cleaned and disinfected, and stored in an antiseptic denture cleanser such as chlorhexidine gluconate (Corsodyl) or hypochlorite (Milton).

ANGULAR CHEILITIS

Angular cheilitis is inflammation at the angles of the lips (the commissures). It often occurs on both sides. There is erythema followed by fissuring or ulceration. Angular cheilitis is also called angular stomatitis, cheilosis or perleche.

In people wearing full dentures, denture-related stomatitis can further lead to angular cheilitis. In such cases, the offending micro-organism is commonly *Candida albicans*. So treatment with anti-fungal medications (e.g. miconazole (Daktarin)) is usually effective. Sometimes new dentures may be required if the patient's lips are drooping too much.

FIND OUT MORE

What happens at the corners of the mouth when the lips droop too much?

COLD SORES (HERPES LABIALIS)

> **Term to Learn**
> **Ganglion:** a collection of nerve cells.

Herpes labialis is blistering at the lips caused by the herpes simplex virus (HSV). After the primary infection (herpetic stomatitis), usually in a child, HSV remains dormant in the trigeminal nerve **ganglion** (see Chapter 4). However, it can be reactivated when the body's resistance is lowered by:

- Fever
- Sunlight
- Trauma
- Immune system compromise (immunosuppression).

In most patients, healing occurs within one week to 10 days. But the condition is both uncomfortable and unsightly. Therefore antiviral treatment may be indicated (e.g. with aciclovir (Zovirax) or penciclovir (Denavir)).

Cancer

> **Terms to Learn**
> **Risk factor:** something that is likely to increase the chances that a particular event or disease will occur.
> **Lesion:** a patch of a body tissue that has become abnormal or diseased.

Mouth cancer (oral squamous cell carcinoma) is among the 10 most common cancers worldwide. It mostly affects older men, but is increasingly seen in younger adults too. There are several lifestyle factors that increase the risk of developing oral cancer:

- Tobacco use
- Alcohol use
- Betel nut use.

Some researchers believe that cannabis use could also be a **risk factor**. Micro-organisms such as *Candida*, the syphilis bacterium, and human papillomaviruses (HPV) may have a role too. Eating a diet rich in fresh fruits and vegetables and in vitamin A may have a protective effect.

Some other diseases also have the potential to become malignant (precancerous) **lesions**, which then progress to cancer. For example:

- Erythroplasia (erythroplakia): a red patch in the mouth
- Leukoplakia: a white patch in the mouth

Most oral cancer occurs at the lateral border of the tongue and/or the floor of the mouth.

> **KEY POINT** If a single lesion lasts over three weeks, it may be a cancer. A biopsy will usually be required.

CLINICAL SIGNS OF CANCER

Cancer may appear in different ways, such as a persistent:

- Ulcer with fissuring or raised edges
- Red patch
- White patch
- Mixed white and red patch
- Lump
- Non-healing extraction socket
- Ulcer
- Lymph node enlargement.

MANAGEMENT

Planning of cancer treatment requires a multidisciplinary team (MDT) consisting of a range of specialists: dentist, surgeon, anaesthetist, oncologist, nursing and other dental staff, nutritionist, speech therapist and physiotherapist etc.

Oral cancer is treated largely by surgery and/or radiotherapy.

- After surgery, there may be some cosmetic, sensory and functional problems.
- After radiotherapy, there may be functional problems such as xerostomia (dry mouth) and difficulty in opening the mouth (trismus).
- These also increase the risk of caries and infections such as candidosis and sialadenitis (salivary gland inflammation).
- The mouth becomes sore (mucositis) and the jaws may be liable to infection (osteoradionecrosis).

Cleft Lip and Palate

Clefts are the result of problems during formation of the face in the developing baby. There is a familial tendency in cleft lip and palate: when one parent is affected, the risk of their child also having it is about 1 in 10 live births.

Cleft lip and palate together is more common than having a cleft lip alone (see Figure 11.8). Cleft lip and palate are, in about 20% of affected people, associated with head and neck, genital and/or heart defects.

Fordyce Spots

Fordyce spots are oil glands similar to those found in skin. They are seen as creamy-yellow dots (Fordyce spots) along the border between the vermilion and the oral mucosa. They are not associated with hair follicles. Fordyce spots are **benign** and very common but a few patients become concerned about them. No treatment is indicated, other than reassurance.

Geographical Tongue

Geographical tongue is a common harmless condition in which the filiform papillae on the tongue (see Subchapter 4.1) are lost temporarily in the presence of irregular map-like red areas. The pattern of redness changes from day to day and even within a few hours. It may cause soreness. Geographical tongue is also called erythema migrans, benign migratory glossitis and migratory stomatitis.

No effective treatment is available, so the patient just needs to be reassured.

Leukoplakia

Leukoplakia is the name given to white patches on the oral mucosa. It may occur as a single, localized lesion or multiple and diffuse widespread lesions. Mostly these are smooth plaques

Term to Learn
Benign: a lesion that is not a cancer, but which can grow or spread locally.

149

(homogeneous leukoplakias) seen on the lip, buccal mucosa or gingiva; others are irregular (non-homogeneous). Of these some are warty (verrucous leukoplakia).

> **KEY POINT** Leukoplakia is a potentially malignant disorder: that is, in up to a third of patients, it can eventually turn to cancer.

Biopsy is required to exclude cancer. Persons with leukoplakia should be advised to stop any tobacco/alcohol/betel habits, and to consume a diet rich in fruit and vegetables. The lesion is also usually removed by surgery.

Lichen Planus

Lichen planus is a chronic disorder of uncertain cause. It affects the mouth, genital areas and/or skin. The mouth lesions are typically white lesions in the buccal (cheek) mucosa on both sides.

The usual treatment is with corticosteroids. Like leukoplakia, lichen planus is a potentially malignant disorder.

Ulcers

Mouth ulceration is not a specific disease, rather it is the outcome of one of a range of disorders or causes. Local causes such as trauma, and recurrent aphthous stomatitis (RAS) are the most common, but ulcers in the mouth can also arise in patients with systemic (general) disease (especially blood diseases, infections, gastro-intestinal and skin disorders), cancer, or drug reactions.

RAS consists of multiple ulcers occurring throughout the mouth. It usually starts in childhood. Local treatments with corticosteroids may be used.

SALIVARY PROBLEMS
Drooling

Drooling is a problem for many children with cerebral palsy, intellectual disability, and other neurological conditions. It also happens in adults, particularly those who have Parkinson's disease or have had a stroke. Drooling is caused either by increased saliva flow (sialorrhoea), or by poor oral and facial muscle control (secondary sialorrhoea). For management of drooling, physiotherapy, drugs or surgery may be needed.

Xerostomia (Dry Mouth)

Dry mouth, also called xerostomia or hyposalivation, often occurs as a side-effect of some drugs or as a result of radiation to the salivary glands during cancer treatment. Sjögren syndrome, diabetes, or occasionally HIV infection, also cause dry mouth.

Dryness of the mouth is uncomfortable for the patient because it may cause:

- Mouth soreness
- Burning sensation
- Difficulty eating dry foods such as biscuits (the cracker sign)
- Difficulty controlling dentures
- Speech problems
- Difficulty swallowing.

Term to Learn
Sialadenitis: inflammation of the salivary glands or their ducts.

Complications of dry mouth include: caries, candidosis or **sialadenitis**. Complications can be avoided or managed by:

- Avoiding sugary foods
- Keeping the mouth clean

150

- Using fluorides
- Using chlorhexidine mouthwashes
- Stimulating salivation.

Salivation may be stimulated by:

- Chewing gum (containing xylitol or sorbitol, not sucrose)
- Eating diabetic sweets
- Using drugs that stimulate salivation (sialogogues).

Use of artificial saliva (mouth wetting agents) may also help.

Mucocele

This is a small blister that arises when a small amount of saliva gets into the tissues or is trapped in a gland. Mucoceles may resolve themselves or require surgery for removal.

Mumps

Mumps is an acute infectious disease caused by the mumps virus. It is also called acute viral sialadenitis or epidemic parotitis. Typically the patient has a painful swelling in the region of the parotid gland, usually on both sides, with trismus, fever and malaise. Complications of mumps include:

- Orchitis in boys (inflammation of the testes; ensuing infertility is rare).
- Pancreatitis (inflammation in the pancreas)
- Encephalitis (inflammation of the brain).

No specific anti-viral drugs are available to treat mumps. So treatment is aimed at relieving the symptoms, and giving fluids and analgesics. Mumps is seen more now because of the reduced uptake of the MMR vaccine in recent years.

151

FIND OUT MORE

Why have some parents been worried about giving the MMR vaccine to their child in recent years?

Salivary Duct Obstruction

Salivary duct obstruction is not uncommon. It is usually caused by a 'stone' (calculus) and is commonly seen in the submandibular duct. This is called *sialolithiasis*.

> **KEY POINT** Aspirin should not be given to children as it may cause a dangerous reaction in the liver (Reye syndrome).

Typically the patient will give a history of painful salivary gland swelling just before, or at, mealtimes. Calculi are usually yellow or white and can sometimes be seen in the duct. X-rays can be taken to check as the stone can be **radiopaque**. The stones are usually removed by surgery, or destroyed by breaking them with sound waves (lithotripsy).

> **Term to Learn**
> **Radiopaque:** a substance through which X-rays do not pass, so it appears white on the X-ray film.

Anything that hinders the production of saliva can predispose the mouth to bacterial infection (sialadenitis); e.g. salivary stones may cause sialadenitis. The parotid glands may be affected after radiotherapy. Acute parotitis presents as a painful parotid enlargement, tender to touch. Prompt antibiotic treatment and surgical drainage are needed.

DISEASES OF THE JAWS (BONE)
Dry Socket

If the blood clot in an extraction socket breaks down, then the socket is 'dry'. This is also called alveolar osteitis. Symptoms of a dry socket are:

- Fairly severe pain two to four days after extraction
- Bad taste in the mouth
- Halitosis.

To aid healing, the socket is irrigated to flush out any debris and a dressing is applied.

Osteonecrosis of the Jaws

> **Term to Learn**
> **Necrosis:** when a tissue or cell dies prematurely due to, for example, trauma or infection.

Jaw **necrosis** can be caused by radiation for cancer treatment or as a side-effect of some drugs (e.g. bisphosphonates). Osteoradionecrosis is the term used when jaw necrosis follows radiotherapy. The cause is often trauma, such as tooth extraction, or oral infection or ulceration from a denture. These patients usually present with painful, exposed and necrotic bone. Treatment includes antibiotics and analgesics, and surgery may be needed.

Bisphosphonates: these are powerful drugs that inhibit cells that should dissolve the bone (osteoclasts) as part of general bone maintenance. This action needs to be prevented in some patients after cancer treatment and to prevent osteoporosis in older people.

Temporomandibular Pain Dysfunction Syndrome

Temporomandibular pain dysfunction syndrome includes features such as:

- Recurrent clicking in the temporomandibular joint (TMJ)
- Limitation of jaw movement
- Pain in the joint and surrounding muscles.

This is seen predominantly in young women. It almost certainly is considered a psychological response to stress. That is, with jaw clenching under stress, there is increasing muscle tension in the muscles of mastication (mainly the temporalis, masseter, and pterygoid muscles).

TMJ dysfunction does not seem to lead to long-term joint damage. Some patients get better spontaneously, thus treatment is not always indicated. Conservative measures such as use of plastic splints on the occlusal surfaces of teeth (occlusal splints) are usually at least partially successful.

Torus Palatinus and Torus Mandibularis

Tori are bony lumps typically seen in the midline of the palate or lingual to the mandible (Figure 5.12). They are benign and usually require no treatment.

PAIN

Pain in the orofacial region is common. Mostly there are obvious local causes for the pain, relating to the teeth (odontogenic pain) (Table 5.4). Occasionally pain is:

- Neuralgia (nerve pain)
- Migraine
- More imagined than real, especially in patients with psychological problems
- Referred to the mouth from elsewhere such as the heart (angina).

Pain can vary in:

- Nature (e.g. throbbing, burning, dull, stabbing)
- Frequency of occurrence
- Severity or intensity.

The diagnosis is usually made from the history and the pain features. For example, odontogenic pain

152

FIGURE 5.12
A mandibular torus.

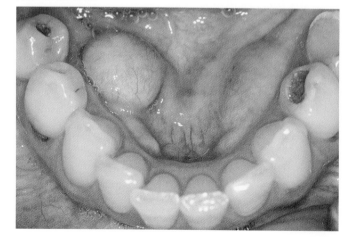

TABLE 5.4 Local Causes of Oral Pain

Source of Pain	Character	Exacerbating Factors	Associated with	Pain Provoked by
Dentine	Evoked by a stimulus, does not last long	Hot/cold, sweet or sour	Caries, defective restorations, exposed dentine	Hot/cold, probing
Pulp	Severe, intermittent, throbbing	Hot/cold, sometimes biting	Pulpitis	Hot/cold, probing
Periapical area	For hours at same intensity; deep, boring	Biting	Periapical abscess	Percussion, palpation (touch)
Gingiva	Pressing, annoying	Food impaction, toothbrushing	Acute gingivitis	Palpation
Mucosa	Burning, sharp	Sour, sharp food	Erosions or ulcers	Palpation

may be throbbing with an obvious location, the pain of trigeminal neuralgia (see below) is lancinating (stabbing) and unilateral, and **idiopathic** facial pain tends to be dull and may be bilateral.

Trigeminal Neuralgia

This is a severe stabbing pain in the area of the face supplied by the trigeminal nerve (see Figure 4.2.10, p. 126), usually with no evident cause (idiopathic trigeminal neuralgia or simply trigeminal neuralgia). Rarely, it may be secondary to serious disease such as multiple sclerosis or a brain tumour. It is usually treated with an anticonvulsant drug called carbamazepine (Tegretol).

Atypical (Idiopathic) Facial Pain

Some patients have symptoms that seem to have no known organic cause, but rather a psychogenic basis. These patients are said to have persistent idiopathic, or unexplained (or atypical) facial pain. Others may have a burning sensation in the mouth (burning mouth syndrome). Most people with facial pain are or have been under extreme stress, such as concerned about cancer, a few have **hypochondriasis**, neuroses (often depression) or psychoses. Psychological care such as cognitive behavioural therapy (**CBT**) may be needed, and anti-depressants may also be used.

A thorough examination and radiological tests are important in order not to miss detecting organic disease, and thus avoid mislabelling the patient as having psychogenic pain.

HALITOSIS

Halitosis or oral malodour is common on awakening (morning breath). It can be readily rectified by eating, brushing the teeth and rinsing the mouth with fresh water.

Malodour at other times may be due to eating certain food and drinks such as garlic, onion, spices, cabbage, cauliflower or radish. Durian is a fruit with a particular malodour. Habits such as smoking or drinking alcohol also cause malodour.

Individuals who have poor oral hygiene soon develop halitosis, but it is made worse by any form of oral infection, such as:

- Gingivitis
- Periodontitis
- Dental abscess
- Dry (infected) extraction socket

Term to Learn
Idiopathic: a disease that has no evident cause.

Terms to Learn
Hypochondriasis: An excessive worry about being ill or having a disease or deformity despite reassurance by a medical professional that there is no evidence of it.
CBT: A type of talking treatment for mental conditions such as depression, anxiety and panic attacks.

153

- Sinusitis
- Tonsillitis.

Rarer causes of halitosis include more general conditions such as:

- Respiratory disease
- Sinusitis
- Nasal infections
- Lung problems
- Metabolic disease
- Diabetes
- Kidney disease
- Liver disease
- Psychiatric disease (where halitosis may be imagined).

Treatment includes improving oral hygiene and reducing the tongue coating by gentle and regular tongue cleaning. Mouthwashes containing chlorhexidine gluconate, triclosan, cetylpyridinium (essential oils), may help. Toothpastes containing triclosan and a copolymer (e.g. Colgate Total toothpaste) could also be used.

QUICK REVISION AID OF THE MAIN CAUSES OF ORAL SIGNS AND SYMPTOMS

Bleeding:

- Haemangioma (a tumour of the cells that line the blood vessels)
- Trauma
- Bleeding tendency
- Inflammation

Blisters:

- Skin diseases
- Infections
- Burns
- Allergies
- Cysts
- Mucoceles

Discoloured teeth:

- Extrinsic discolorations (brown or black):
  - Poor oral hygiene
  - Smoking
  - Beverages/food (e.g. tea, coffee, red wine)
  - Drugs
  - Betel
- Intrinsic discolorations:
  - Localised: trauma; caries; restorative (filling) materials
  - Generalised: tetracyclines; excessive fluoride; genetic diseases

Dry mouth (xerostomia):

- Drugs
- Dehydration
- Psychogenic cause
- Salivary gland disease

Early tooth loss:

- Trauma
- Dental caries
- Periodontal breakdown
- Tumours

Facial swelling:

- Inflammation (e.g. infections or bites)
- Trauma
- Allergies
- Cysts
- Neoplasms

Halitosis:

- Volatile foodstuffs
- Drugs and tobacco
- Oral disease
- Systemic disease:
  - Respiratory disease
  - Metabolic disease
- Psychogenic cause

Late tooth eruption:

- Impacted teeth
- Cancer treatment

Pain:

- Dental disease
- Migraine and similar vascular disorders
- Trigeminal neuralgia
- Psychogenic pain
- Referred pain (e.g. angina)

Pigmentation:

- Racial
- Food/drugs
- Tobacco
- Betel
- Chlorhexidine
- Minocycline treatment
- Endocrinological (Addison disease)
- Red areas
- Congenital conditions:
  ○ Haemangiomas
- Trauma
- Inflammatory
- Neoplastic and possibly pre-neoplastic

Salivary swelling:

- Inflammatory
- Obstruction
- Neoplasm

Soreness and ulceration:

- Systemic disease
- Malignant disease

- Local causes
- Aphthae (recurrent aphthous stomatitis)
- Drugs

Swellings and lumps:

- Congenital
- Allergic reactions
- Inflammatory lesions
- Neoplasms
- Traumatic

Trismus:

- Infection and inflammation near masticatory muscles
- Temporomandibular joint-dysfunction syndrome (facial arthromyalgia)
- Fractured or dislocated jaw
- Arthritis
- After radiotherapy

White lesions:

- Congenital conditions
- Cheek biting
- Inflammatory:
  ○ Infective (e.g. candidosis)
  ○ Non-infective (e.g. lichen planus)
- Neoplastic and possibly pre-neoplastic:
  ○ Keratoses (leukoplakias)
  ○ Carcinoma

155

FIND OUT MORE

There are several websites that describe oral diseases and conditions for a range of readers. See for example:

- Health Canada (http://www.hc-sc.gc.ca/hl-vs/oral-bucco/disease-maladie/index-eng.php)
- Health Central.com (http://www.healthcentral.com/channel/408/1122.html).

CHAPTER 6

Patient Care and Special Groups

CHAPTER POINTS

- This chapter covers the requirements of the NEBDN syllabus Section 6: patient care and management. The chapter is divided into two subchapters:

  6.1: Patient Care: Diagnosis and Management

  6.2: Special Groups and Minority Issues

6.1 PATIENT CARE: DIAGNOSIS AND MANAGEMENT

- This chapter covers the requirements of the NEBDN syllabus Section 6: patient care and management, part 6.1. This includes the role of a dental nurse in meeting and greeting the patient, and assisting in the dental surgery. You should read this chapter in conjunction with the chapters on legal and ethical issues (Chapter 3), treatment planning (Chapter 7) and communications (Chapter 15).

INTRODUCTION

The dental nurse provides a key link between the dental clinician and patient and partner, family or friends, by supporting the patient as well as assisting clinically. The dental nurse also undertakes several other routines that are more fully explained in Chapters 3, 7 and 15.

CRIMINAL RECORDS BUREAU

The law tries to protect patients from harm, especially serious harm. In the UK, children and vulnerable people are offered formal protection via the Criminal Records Bureau (CRB) checks.

> **KEY POINT** The first rule in health care is 'do no harm'.

The CRB is an executive agency of the Home Office, which vets applications for people who want to work with children and vulnerable people. People working in the UK healthcare sector also require CRB checks. The role of this agency has been enhanced by the Safeguarding Vulnerable People Act (2006) in response to the recommendations of the Bichard Inquiry.

The Foster Review on the regulation of the non-medical healthcare professions, when describing 'good character', referred to objective tests to measure this, such as the absence of criminal convictions and adverse decisions by regulatory bodies, and the information about likely criminal activity contained in a CRB disclosure.

CRB disclosures are either 'standard' or 'enhanced'.

Standard CRB Disclosures

These disclosures reveal details of any convictions, cautions, reprimands and final warnings the applicant has received, regardless of length of time since the incidents. They also reveal details of whether that person is banned from working with children or vulnerable adults (if these details have been requested). The CRB aims to issue Standard Disclosures within 10 days of receipt of the application.

Enhanced CRB Disclosures

These disclosures are for positions involving greater contact with children or vulnerable adults (e.g. most health professionals) and involve an additional check with the police. The police then check if any other information is held on file that may be relevant (for instance, investigations that have not led to a criminal record). The police will decide what (if any) additional information will be added to the Disclosure. The CRB aims to issue enhanced disclosure within 28 days of receiving the application.

FIND OUT MORE

Visit the CRB website (www.crb.gov.uk) to find out more about CRB checks and the Bichard Inquiry.

GENERAL ISSUES REGARDING PATIENT CARE IN THE DENTAL SURGERY

According to the Institute of Healthcare Management: 'customer care fundamentally depends very much on good management and organisation, but individual staff contacts and conducts are crucial to success.'

Customer Service

Patients appreciate good customer care. It makes them feel both welcome and important. The key message is 'goodwill' and never 'bad will'. You can help your workplace achieve this by:

- Always being courteous and helpful to patients
- Knowing them
- Managing their expectations
- Identifying their specific needs
- Treating them fairly
- Giving them control
- Helping them understand the way the practice works.

Behaviour

See also Chapter 15.

Patients have a right to receive attention and to be treated with respect. Remember that like everyone, patients are the experts on their lives, cultures and experiences. If you treat them with respect and sensitivity, they will usually tell you how best to provide care for them. They will usually also tell you if asked, how they wish to be addressed. Many patients are aware of their rights and willing to enforce them if they feel that they are not being cared for appropriately.

KEY POINT Treat patients as you yourself would like to be treated.

Greeting Patients

Communication is discussed in Chapter 15. In addition remember the following good practice points:

- When calling a patient in, walk right into the waiting area and call the patient by their title and surname. (Have you ever waited in a waiting room and heard your name shouted out from afar but could not see the person? How would or did it make you feel?)
- Check that when a patient responds, it is the correct patient; not uncommonly patients get up in expectation that it is their turn to be seen, but are wrong.
- Introduce yourself to the patient with a greeting appropriate to their age and culture.
- Talk to the patient when escorting them into the surgery as this will help them feel at ease.
- All patients' details are confidential and should never be discussed in the waiting or other public areas; this is especially appropriate when a new patient joins the practice. If this is the only place available lower your voice and make sure you are not overheard. (Imagine how you would feel if you were the patient).
- Following the examination or treatment, escort the patient to reception, hand them over to the receptionist and say goodbye.
- As you get to know the patients, remember to follow up a conversation from a previous visit.

Dress Codes

Staff are usually also expected to uphold a dress code which prevents infection, maintains health and safety and keeps a 'professional image'. This is often some type of uniform.

You must wear a name badge that is clearly visible at all times, and which must not be defaced or broken.

Under many codes (Box 6.1.1), clinical staff must tie back long hair, but not with ribbons or combs. Jewellery is limited to simple earrings and one ring, and any clothing that exposes the midriff or cleavage is banned. Nose studs should be covered with a fresh plaster each day. Some codes also cover above-the-knee skirts and high heels. Shoes that are low-heeled, soft-soled, supportive and closed are generally agreed to be best for work. Shoes with holes in the top or side may carry a risk of injury from falling scalpels and needles, or the risk of catching an infection from blood or fluids dropping through the holes.

Whatever is the prescribed code in your workplace, as a healthcare worker, your clothing should clearly conform to health and safety standards. In some organisations, breaching the code could lead to disciplinary action.

Cleanliness and Hygiene

PERSONAL HYGIENE

Hygiene practices are used to reduce the incidence and spread of disease. Poor handwashing for example, is responsible for the spread of many diseases.

Personal hygiene is achieved by using personal hygiene products including: soap, shampoo, toothbrushes, dental floss, toothpaste, deodorants, nail clippers and files, razors, and shaving cream. Things that people might wish to think about are:

- How often to bathe?
- Having fresh breath before working with patients each session?

RECEPTION, WAITING AREA AND TOILETS

The dental team should always ensure that the reception, waiting area, facilities and work environment are clean, safe and user friendly.

Term to Learn
Hygiene: this refers to cleanliness and preventive measures – the practices that are associated with the preservation of health and healthy living.

159

BOX 6.1.1 DRESS CODES IN PRACTICE

Dress codes can be controversial. At least one hospital banned nurses from wearing Croc shoes, suggesting they might be dangerous. But some surgeons use Crocs in the operating theatre, believing they are easier to clean. Even NHS rules can vary. In England and Wales for example, bare-below-the-elbows dress code for clinicians is recommended since it 'helps to support effective hand-washing and may reduce the risk of patients catching infections'. Other codes have caused considerable controversy and even made newspaper headlines. See the *Daily Mail* archive for example, for the article 'Don't forget to wear socks and make sure your shoelaces match' (31 December 2007).

The Scottish code (published on the Scottish Government website, www.scotland.gov.uk/ Publications/2008/08/interimdresscode) is reproduced below:

- 'Staff should dress in a manner which is likely to inspire public confidence:
  - For example: in clean uniform (where uniform is a requirement), with hair tied back off the collar, with nails kept short and clean.
  - Wear clear identifiers, (e.g. badges, epaulets etc).
  - Where changing facilities are available, staff should change into and out of uniform at work. In any case, staff should avoid undertaking activities in public, such as shopping, whilst wearing their uniform, except where such activities form an integral part of their duties.
- Appropriate steps should be taken to minimise the risks of infections and cross contamination for patients and the public:
  - For example: staff should wear short-sleeved shirts/blouses and avoid wearing white coats or neck ties when providing patient care.
  - Staff should not wear false nails or hand or wrist jewellery (other than a plain wedding ring or one other plain band) when providing patient care.
- All appropriate health and safety requirements for staff should be met:
  - For example: Staff should not wear excessive jewellery, such as necklaces, visible piercings and multiple earrings.
  - Staff should wear soft-soled, closed toe shoes.
  - Staff should not carry pens or scissors in outside breast pockets.
- Be sensitive to the social, cultural and diversity and equality needs of staff and patients:
  - For example: tattoos which could be deemed offensive should be covered where this does not compromise good clinical practice.'

FIND OUT MORE

Look around your workplace and answer the following questions:

- Is the waiting area clear and tidy or is there something that could be tripped over?
- Are the facilities in the toilets acceptable?
- Is the reception area tidy or piled high with patient records?
- Can the patient talk to the receptionist, dental nurse or clinician without being overheard?
- Is the route to and in the dental surgery clear and tidy or is there something that could be tripped over?
- Are all cables secured and if possible out of sight?

CLINICAL AREA

In the clinical area, the following points should help you consider how you may increase the comfort and safety of your patients:

- Ensure the patient will not knock their head on the dental light or trip over the foot pedal or cables or pipes.

- Are accompanying children, relatives or friends appropriate in the surgery or will they be a distraction and/or a liability? Where should they sit? Is there enough seating? Are there coat hooks?
- Ask the patient if they will be happy with the chair tilted back (some – especially older people – may have a medical condition that precludes this, or feel anxious when the chair is tilted back).
- Has the dental light been cleaned efficiently or is there dust, or are there finger marks or stains?
- Is the dental surgery tidy?
- Is the spittoon clean with fresh beaker and mouthwash?
- Is there a new clean disposable bib?

Conduct

- Do not interrupt the clinician when they are talking to the patient.
- Ensure any conversation with the clinician includes the patient.
- Do not take personal mobile phone messages in the clinical area.
- Do not discuss other patients or people.
- Do not discuss patients' details outside the surgery as they are confidential.
- Do not eat or drink in a clinical area but rather in another separate designated area for infection control and health and safety reasons.
- Do not chew gum in the workplace.
- Do not wear an iPod or other such device
- Do not carry out personal hygiene measures such as combing hair or blowing your nose in a clinical area.

GOOD PRACTICE POINTS: PATIENT CARE

- Know your patient.
- Act professionally at all times.
- Follow the prescribed dress code.
- Ensure personal hygiene.
- Keep the environment user friendly.
- Minimise hazards in the dental surgery.

161

THE DENTAL APPOINTMENT

Aims of Healthcare

Healthcare aims to improve the health of patients but can itself carry risks.

Hazards of Healthcare

Dentistry is essentially very safe in healthy patients. Thus **morbidity** and **mortality** following dental procedures are even less excusable than when they follow, for example, more invasive surgery.

Drugs, particularly those that act on the central nervous system (CNS; e.g. sedatives and anaesthetic agents) are potentially dangerous and must be carefully administered. Most dental procedures can be carried out under local anaesthesia (LA, sometimes called local analgesia) with minimal morbidity. Conscious sedation (CS) is not as safe as LA alone. CS must be carried out:

- In appropriate facilities
- By adequately trained personnel
- With due consideration of the possible risks.

Terms to Learn
Morbidity: the state of being unwell or having a disease. Here, it means developing a condition or ill health becoming worse after a dental or medical procedure.
Mortality: a term that pertains to death. Here it means a patient dying as a result of a dental procedure.

General anaesthesia (GA) with intravenous or inhalational agents is only permitted in a hospital with appropriate resuscitation facilities. It is not often needed for dental treatment, and then only in a hospital setting: because of its potential dangers it must be carried out by a qualified anaesthetist. CS is considerably safer, and is thus preferred.

Surgical procedures are generally the most hazardous. In the dental environment, operative procedures that involve use of LA and CS, and operative interventions such as drilling teeth and cutting tissues and bone are the main ones that can be hazardous.

Risks mainly happen when staff are overambitious in terms of their skill or knowledge, the patient is not healthy, inadequate time is taken and/or the procedure is invasive (tissues are disrupted).

Thus there is always a need for doing risk assessments and careful **peri-operative** care.

Patient Care during Diagnosis
RISK ASSESSMENT

An adequate risk assessment endeavours to anticipate and to prevent trouble. This topic was covered in the context of a medical emergency in Chapter 2. This chapter explains its relevance in day-to-day practice.

At the start of a patient's visit it is essential to:

1. Assess patient's needs
2. Obtain a careful medical, dental, family, social, (and sometimes developmental) history and make a risk assessment
3. Obtain patient's consent to any investigations required
4. Obtain patient's consent to agreed treatment plan.

A patient's 'fitness' for a procedure depends on several factors (see Chapter 2, Box 2.1 and Table 2.1). Many patients with life-threatening diseases now survive as a result of advances in surgical and medical care. Such diseases can significantly affect the dental management of the patient. A patient attending for dental treatment and apparently 'fit' may actually have a serious **systemic** disease. Or they may be taking drugs (including recreational drugs). Both of these might influence the healthcare that can be delivered to the patient.

The *risk is greatest when surgery is needed*, and when GA or sedation is given. In addition, problems may be compounded if medical support is not at hand.

> **Term to Learn**
> **Peri-operative:** the term that covers the period of time starting from preparation for surgery up to the time the procedure is completed and the patient can go home safely.

162

> **Term to Learn**
> **Systemic:** a condition that affects a system or the whole body as opposed to a distinct local site.

> **KEY POINT** No interventional procedure is entirely free from risk but care can be improved by making an adequate assessment based on history, clinical signs and, where appropriate, investigations, and minimising trauma and stress to the patient.

History Taking
PERSONAL DETAILS

Personal details (first and last names, the name by which the patient wishes to be known, date of birth, gender (sex), religion, occupation, relationship status, address and contact details) are necessary information for administrative purposes. This information may be collected by the dental nurse or receptionist. In fact, obtaining this information provides the patient with the opportunity for a gentle introduction to the dental team, and an opportunity for individual introduction suitable to the particular culture. As stated above, it is usually helpful to ask the patient how they would wish to be addressed.

Having read the previous section, you will appreciate that every effort has to be made to identify the medically compromised patient. For this a medical history is essential.

> ## BOX 6.1.2 ESSENTIALS OF HISTORY TAKING
> - Personal details.
> - The presenting complaint (PC).
> - History of presenting complaint (HPC).
> - Relevant medical history (RMH).
> - Drug history.
> - Social history.
> - Family history.

MEDICAL HISTORY

See also Chapter 2.

When taking a medical history, the dental clinician will usually ask a structured set of questions, such as those shown in Box 6.1.2. Patients are often also given a form for them to supply all the information they can about their health and any medication they are receiving. The history may significantly change with time. Therefore, it is essential to ask about any changes and update the history before each new course of treatment, every sedation session and especially before surgery or GA. For example, a female patient who is not pregnant at one course of treatment could well be at the next. Table 2.2 (p. 47) lists some important medical issues that would affect the dental treatment of a patient.

It is helpful for nurses to have basic knowledge about the essential components of a medical history. Many of the items below may be included on the form that is handed out to the patient to fill in before they see the dental clinician. The completion of such a form provides:

- A useful base for the clinician from which to enquire further about any concerning items on the form
- Useful evidence if the patient makes a complaint or medico-legal claim.

PRESENTING COMPLAINT (PC)

This should be recorded in the patient's own words, e.g. 'I have pain in my face'.

HISTORY OF PRESENTING COMPLAINT (HPC)

The clinician needs to ask about the timing of the complaint and its evolution. For example, if the patient has facial pain, a useful mnemonic is SOCRATES:

S – site
O – onset (gradual/sudden)
C – character
R – radiation
A – associations (other symptoms)
T – timing/duration
E – exacerbating and alleviating factors
S – severity (rate the pain on a visual analogue scale of 1–10).

RELEVANT MEDICAL HISTORY (RMH)

RMH was covered in Chapter 2 in detail. To recapitulate, RMH includes finding out about any past or present medical and surgical problems. Patients are also asked if they carry a medical warning card or device (e.g. Medic-Alert and Talisman). Because patients may not know if they have a condition that may affect their dental treatment, a functional enquiry/review of systems (ROS) can be helpful. This involves asking specifically about certain conditions (see Table 2.2).

SOCIAL HISTORY

The clinician and dental nurse need to tactfully find out about a patient's occupation, marital status, partner's job and health, housing, dependants, mobility, lifestyle habits (alcohol, tobacco, betel and recreational drugs), culture and faith. In addition, it is also worth finding out if the patient has any forthcoming social engagements that are dependent on them being able to carry out their usual activities following a dental treatment (for example, wedding/examination/job interviews). This may require rescheduling of treatment.

FAMILY HISTORY

The medical history of blood relatives may be required as some relevant diseases run in families (e.g. haemophilia).

Clinical Examination

It is important for dental professionals not merely to inspect and examine the mouth and neck, but to look at the patient as a whole. A patient's appearance, behaviour and speech, body language and inspection of the face, neck, arms and hands can reveal many significant conditions. The clinician needs to look for anxiety, movements and tremors, and tiredness, and for facial changes (e.g. expression, pallor, cyanosis or jaundice), dyspnoea or wheezing, or finger clubbing. However, remember that even very ill patients can look remarkably well.

The clinician will examine the neck as swollen lymph nodes are sometimes a sign of disease such as infections or cancer. Hospital in-patients always also have a full physical examination before GA and operation which includes at least the following systems:

- Cardiovascular: Pulse, blood pressure, heart sounds.
- Respiratory: Respiratory rate, lung expansion, tracheal position, lung sounds.
- Gastro-intestinal: Any swelling or tenderness.
- Neurological: Especially the cranial nerves.

Investigations

The history and physical examination often reveal most if not all of the clinically useful information and data. However, in some patients tests (investigations) may be needed.

Before any investigations are initiated, the clinician must obtain the patient's consent.

The Clinical Role of the Dental Nurse: Chaperoning

If you read the introduction to this book and Chapter 3 you will already have an idea of your clinical role (as described by the General Dental Council). When carrying out treatment, the clinician should usually be assisted by a dental nurse, who can also act as a chaperone.

LEGAL IMPORTANCE OF A CHAPERONE

The Council for Healthcare Regulatory Excellence in its 2008 publication *Clear Sexual Boundaries Between Healthcare Professionals and Patients: Responsibilities of Healthcare Professionals* stresses the value of a chaperone: 'Wherever possible patients should be offered the choice of having an impartial observer, or chaperone, present during an examination that the patient considers to be intimate'.

The General Dental Council in its 2009 publication *Principles of Dental Team Working*, does not insist on a chaperone but make it clear that:

(3.7) When treating patients, make sure there is someone else – preferably a registered team member – present in the room, who is trained to deal with medical emergencies.

It also says:

*(3.8) There may be circumstances in which it is not possible for a trained person to be present –
for example, if you are treating a patient in an out-of-hours emergency or on a home visit. If
this is the case, you are responsible for assessing the possible risk to the patient of continuing
with treatment in the absence of a trained person.*

The Scottish Government in its *National Standards for Dental Services* clearly states that the dental
nurse is a 'Person who assists the clinician at the chair-side during dental treatment, *acts as a
chaperone*, often has administrative duties and infection control responsibilities.'

FIND OUT MORE

Visit the following websites to find out more about caring for patients in the most appropriate way:

- NHS National Services Scotland. Patient Details Amendments
  (http://www.psd.scot.nhs.uk/professionals/dental/patient-detail-amendments.html)
- British Dental Health Foundation. Frequently asked questions. Patients' rights
  (http://www.dentalhealth.org.uk/faqs/leafletdetail.php?LeafletID=30)

6.2 SPECIAL GROUPS AND MINORITY ISSUES

- This chapter covers the requirements of the NEBDN syllabus Section 6: patient care
  and management, except for (part 6.1) which was covered in Chapter 6.1.

165

INTRODUCTION

There are people who are disadvantaged for a variety of reasons and in need of special care.
In today's multicultural society, we also must be aware of, and respect, others' points of
view.

PEOPLE WITH SPECIAL NEEDS

People who have special needs is a term used to describe
individuals who require assistance for conditions that
may be medical or psychological. The World Health
Organization's International Classification of Diseases
includes the following definitions:

> **KEY POINT** A dental nurse should
> respect the uniqueness and dignity of each
> individual patient, and respond appropriately to their
> need for care, irrespective of religion, ethnic origin,
> gender, sexual preferences, personal attributes or
> nature of the health problem.

- *Impairment* – a loss or abnormality of structure or
  function including psychological functioning (for
  example problems with vision, diminished hearing capacity, lack of muscular control,
  decreased learning ability, or an inability to concentrate).
- *Disability* – a restriction or lack of ability to perform an activity within the range
  considered normal.
- *Handicap* – a disadvantage resulting from an impairment or disability that limits or
  prevents the fulfilment of a normal role.

FIND OUT MORE

What is the WHO International Classification? Visit the WHO website (http://www.who.int) to find out.

A person has a disability if he or she has a physical or mental impairment which greatly limits one or more major life activities such as:

- Breathing
- Caring for oneself
- Concentrating
- Hearing
- Interacting with other people
- Learning
- Lifting
- Performing manual tasks
- Reaching
- Reading
- Seeing
- Speaking
- Standing
- Thinking
- Walking
- Working.

Table 6.2.1 shows the relationship between disability and impairment. Note that many people do not like the term 'disability' and prefer the term 'difficulties'.

The origin of a disability may be:

- *Developmental* – that is, caused by impairments that occur during development (up to age 18). These include fetal damage from infections, defects of metabolism, alcohol, or hypoxia, chromosomal abnormalities (e.g. Down syndrome), autism, and childhood infections (e.g. meningitis or encephalitis).
- *Acquired* – caused by impairments that are not related to the body's development. For example trauma to the brain or spinal cord, multiple sclerosis, arthritis and Alzheimer disease.

Dental considerations of disability are discussed below.

Oral Health in People with Special Needs

Studies have shown that in the past untreated caries, gingivitis and periodontal disease were more common and rates of extractions were usually higher in people with special needs. The main obstacle or barrier to good oral healthcare in people with special needs in the past was access, either to facilities or because of discrimination. It is crucial to avoid discrimination (Box 6.2.1) on the grounds of:

- Age
- Gender
- Social exclusion
- Disability.

Service providers (an expression which includes all dental staff) have a legal duty not to discriminate against people with special needs. The Disability Discrimination Act 1995 (DDA) states that service providers cannot refuse to provide good facilities or services or provide them at a lower standard or in a worse manner to people with special needs. They also cannot offer a service on worse terms than would be offered to other members of the public.

TABLE 6.2.1 Disability and Impairment

Disabilities	Impairments
Physical	Mobility
	Respiratory
Mental	Emotional
	Social
Sensory	Hearing
	Visual
Cognitive	Learning
	Attention

> ## BOX 6.2.1 REDUCING DISCRIMINATION IN THE DENTAL PRACTICE
>
> - All providers of dentistry need to take reasonable steps to make their dental practices accessible.
> - They should remove, alter or provide means of avoiding physical features that make it impossible or unreasonably difficult for people with disabilities to use their services. This includes possible alterations to the building design or construction, the approach and access to and exit from the building – for example ramp access for wheelchairs, parking bays for those with disabilities, and modifications to fixtures and fittings, furniture and furnishings, and equipment and materials.
> - A 'no dogs' policy needs to have a provision to allow entry to service animals such as guide dogs or hearing dogs into the premises (but not necessarily into the surgery).
> - However, if taking steps to facilitate access to the premises would result in an 'undue burden' or fundamentally alter the nature of the services provided, then exemptions may apply.
> - Dental staff must also treat the person with a disability on the same basis as they treat non-disabled patients. For example, services cannot charge extra from a person with a disability for the cost of auxiliary aids and services.
> - If a person with a disability poses a 'direct threat' (that is a risk that cannot be eliminated using special procedures) to the health or safety of others, a dentist may refuse to admit that person, e.g. an aggressive patient. They may need to be treated in hospital under general anaesthesia.
> - If the person with a disability requires a procedure for which a non-disabled patient would ordinarily be referred, the person with a disability may legally be referred elsewhere for healthcare.

Younger People

- Paediatric dentistry is the speciality that provides primary and comprehensive preventive and therapeutic oral healthcare for infants and children through adolescence, including those with special healthcare needs.
- Dental caries is the most prevalent childhood ailment among children aged 5–16 years.
- When treating children and the adolescents, the dental clinician needs to consider:
- Medical and social history:
  - Medical, physical or psychiatric problems
  - **Patient compliance**
  - Commitment of the parent or guardian to the treatment
- Dental status:
  - Is the tooth (teeth) restorable?
  - Is there an aesthetic problem?
  - Is there a problem with chewing?

Treatment may take longer to plan and carry out and children may need special control of anxiety and pain.

Older People

Geriatric dentistry and special care dentistry are the specialities that provide primary and comprehensive preventive and therapeutic oral healthcare for older people, including those with special healthcare needs. A number of diseases are more common in older people – and many older people have chronic diseases.

People over the age of 65 years are currently regarded as old. By that definition, a growing proportion of the population in many countries, particularly in the developed world, is old. Some older people walk with difficulty or are house-bound or bed-ridden. Based on their capacity to carry out activities of ordinary life (to dress, to eat, to bathe, etc), older people are said to be functionally independent or dependent. This is assessed with specific tests (e.g. Activities of Daily Living Scale (ADLS)).

Oral healthcare may be lacking, and older people generally are more likely to have a drier mouth and a softer, more cariogenic diet than some younger people. For these reasons they may have:

Terms to Learn
Patient compliance: how well a patient correctly follows all the instructions given to them by a healthcare professional about a particular treatment or preventive **regimen.**
Regimen: a systematic plan for therapy (may include diet).

167

- Fewer teeth
- Tooth surface loss – especially due to **gross caries**, root caries and attrition
- Periodontitis.

Independent older people are often reluctant to demand special attention. This is mainly because of fear of loss of their independence and possible consequent hospitalisation, or through apathy. Treatment compliance can be difficult, not least because of forgetfulness or indifference.

The major goals of oral healthcare in older people are:

- Preventive and conservative treatment
- Elimination/avoidance of pain and oral infections.

However, dental staff also have a crucial role in supporting morale and contributing to advice regarding adequate nutrition.

KEY POINT Handling of older patients may require immense patience.

Dependent persons may need **domiciliary dental care** with portable dental equipment. When such patients also have significant medical problems, they may be best seen in a hospital environment. However, this raises issues of adequate transportation and availability of accompanying persons.

Pregnancy

During the first trimester (first three months) of pregnancy, the organs of the fetus are still developing and liable to damage.

KEY POINT Fetal development during the first trimester is especially vulnerable to interference from infections, drugs and irradiation.

Although most developmental defects are of unknown aetiology it is crucial to avoid exposure during dental treatment to:

- Infections (e.g. chickenpox, rubella and HIV)
- Drugs (e.g. tetracyclines – which cause tooth staining) and sedation gases
- Irradiation (dental radiographs must only be taken when clinically necessary).

WHEN TO TREAT IN PREGNANCY

Clinicians advise that non-urgent dental care is best scheduled in the second trimester or during the early part of the third trimester. During the second and third trimester, if the woman lies on her back, the growing uterus will put pressure on the inferior vena cava and decrease the blood circulation to the head. This causes light-headedness and an increase in heart rate (supine hypotensive syndrome). In the last half of the third trimester, the uterus becomes sensitive and stress can lead to a premature delivery.

DENTAL PROBLEMS PECULIAR TO PREGNANCY

Hormonal changes during pregnancy may cause *pregnancy gingivitis* in some women. But this is not severe enough to cause tooth loss. The blood levels of several hormones such as sex hormones, prolactin and thyroid hormones rise in pregnancy. Levels of other hormones fall. All these changes affect the woman's endocrine, cardiovascular and circulatory systems. They can also cause changes in attitude, mood or behaviour. Pregnant women also may have a tendency to diabetes. Pregnant women who have periodontal disease may have a higher chance of a premature delivery.

FIND OUT MORE

Why are some pregnant women prone to getting diabetes?

People with Impaired Vision

People with visual impairments include those who:

- Have never been able to see
- Had normal vision for some years before becoming gradually or suddenly partially or totally blind
- Have other disabilities in addition to the visual loss
- Have selective impairments of parts of the visual field.

In the UK the Blind Persons Act 1920 defines blindness as: 'so blind as to be unable to perform any work for which eyesight is essential'. But in real life, a person is considered blind if:

- They see clearly at 6 m (20 ft) what someone with very good vision can see at 60 m (200 ft)

  and

- Using glasses or contact lenses cannot make them see better.

There is no statutory definition of 'partial sight' although the National Assistance Act 1948 states that a person has partial sight if they are 'substantially and permanently handicapped by defective vision caused by congenital defect, illness or injury'.

You can recognise visual disability if the patient:

- Has difficulty recognising people
- Holds books or reading material close to the face or at arm's length
- Finds lighting always either too bright or too dim
- Squints or tilts the head to see
- Moves about cautiously or bumps into objects
- Acts confusedly or is disoriented.

Totally blind people generally read using Braille or other non-visual media. People with low vision use a combination of vision and other senses (they may require adaptations in lighting or print size) and, sometimes, Braille.

All signs (Figure 6.2.1) and patient information material in dental facilities should use large text. Assistive technology which may help includes:

- *Screen enlargers* (or screen magnifiers) – these work like a magnifying glass.
- *Screen readers* – these are software programs that present graphics and text as speech.
- *Speech recognition systems* (voice recognition programs) – these allow people to give commands and enter data using their voices rather than a mouse or keyboard.
- *Speech synthesisers* (text-to-speech (TTS) systems) – these receive information going to the screen in the form of letters, numbers and punctuation marks, and then 'speak' it out loud.
- *Refreshable Braille displays* – provide tactile output of information on the computer screen. The user reads the Braille letters with their fingers, and then, after a line is read, refreshes the display to read the next line.

169

FIGURE 6.2.1
Example of a sign for people with impaired vision.

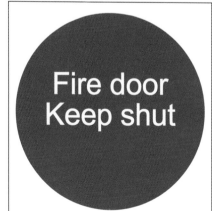

Fire door
Keep shut

- *Braille embossers* – these transfer computer-generated text into embossed Braille output.
- *Talking word processors* – these are software programs that use speech synthesisers to provide auditory feedback of what is typed.
- *Large-print word processors* – these allow the user to view everything in large text without added screen enlargement.
- *Talking PDAs* – these are 'personal digital assistants', e.g. Braille 'n Speak Scholar.

The oral health of people with visual impairment can be compromised since they may not be able to detect and recognise signs of early oral disease.

People with Impaired Hearing

Hearing impairment occurs when there is a problem with one or more parts of the ear, or the main sensory pathway that carries sound signals to the brain. About one in 10 people have hearing impairment. Hearing loss can be sudden or progressive, and it may be congenital or acquired (e.g. chronic infection or trauma). Some people have partial hearing loss, which means that the ear can detect some sounds; others have complete hearing loss, which means that the ear cannot hear at all (they are considered deaf).

The main issue with hearing loss is communication. The higher the frequency of the sound, the louder the sound has to be, in order for the hearing-impaired person to hear it. Thus the patient with a hearing impairment may feel fear or hostility. This is because they may feel they are not going to understand instructions and may pretend to hear just to avoid embarrassment. Hearing loss may be managed with hearing aids (wearable miniature amplifiers which give an amplification of approximately +40 **decibels**) or a cochlear implant.

Communication can be helped by **cued speech**. Communication can be made easier for the hearing-impaired person by:

- Using bright lighting.
- Reducing background noise to a minimum, that is, turning off the high-volume evacuator, saliva ejector, radio or piped-in music. Hearing devices can be adversely affected by the high pitched tone of the handpiece or ultrasonic scaler, which may make the device useless and cause the patient to be less co-operative.
- The speaker facing the patient directly and not wearing a face mask.
- The speaker not moving their head around.
- The speaker speaking slowly, preferably one phrase at a time.
- The speaker at the optimal distance from the person (between 1 and 2 metres).
- Using mirrors, models, drawings and written information to augment communication.
- A sign language interpreter can also be valuable.

Term to Learn
Decibel: a unit that measures sound.
Cued speech: use of hand symbols for each sound; it is used in conjunction with lip reading.

170

FIND OUT MORE

How does your workplace improve communication with hearing-impaired patients?

Hearing induction loops are helpful for the patient with hearing impairment who is wearing a hearing aid. Sometimes it is easier to use a notepad or a keyboard to communicate. Other aids are:

- E-mail
- Blackberry
- i-Pad
- Voice-to-text phone service or text-to-voice phone service or text telephone (TDD/TTY), a special telephone called a Telecommunications Device for the Deaf (TDD) or a TELETYPewriter (TTY)
- Internet relay service
- Voice carry over (VCO)
- Captioned telephones.

People with Medical Problems

People with medical problems (see Subchapter 17.1) require not only safe and appropriate dental care, but also guidance on preventing oral problems occurring. This includes advice on the use of effective preventive measures that they can use to improve their oral health status.

> **KEY POINT** All discussions should be completed and the patient's hearing device turned off before operative dental treatment is begun.

Main objectives when providing oral healthcare to people with medical problems are to:

- Enable the patient to care for their own oral health, with or without assistance
- Keep the patient free from pain and acute disease
- Maintain effective oral function
- Retain aesthetics
- Cause no harm.

The clinician is often the team leader but other dental professionals are essential to successful provision of care in such patients. Such multidisciplinary care may involve the following professional groups:

- Parents/partners/carers
- Social services/social work departments
- Health visitor
- General medical practitioner
- Paediatric consultant/other hospital specialists
- School teacher and assistants
- Colleagues in paediatric dentistry, oral surgery, oral medicine, maxillofacial surgery, periodontics, endodontics, prosthodontics, orthodontics.

ADVANTAGES OF MULTI-DISCIPLINARY WORKING

A multi-disciplinary team (MDT):

- Leads to more effective sharing of resources
- Leads to more creative responses to problems
- Heightens communication skills
- Produces new approaches
- Results in a more practical and appropriate treatment plan
- Ensures other professionals appreciate the importance of oral healthcare, its relationship and general health
- Helps dispel the misconception that oral disease and tooth loss are unavoidable outcomes.

People with Cancer

Oral problems generally become increasingly common in patients with serious illness such as cancer, especially following treatments such as chemotherapy and head and neck radiotherapy. For example, mucositis, dry mouth and oral candidiasis are common in patients on **oncology** wards/hospices. These conditions can impact on the quality of life by causing pain and interfering with:

- Eating and drinking
- Ability to talk comfortably.

Term to Learn
Oncology: The medical specialty concerned with the study, diagnosis and management of cancerous conditions.

171

Regular mouth examination and care reduce the risk of oral problems developing. A typical plan will include:

- Control of sugar intake
- Brushing teeth twice a day with a soft toothbrush and a fluoride-containing toothpaste.
- Removal of visible debris by gently brushing the tongue or mucosal surfaces with a soft toothbrush (after meals and at night, or as often as tolerated). Foam sticks are an alternative if gentle brushing with a soft toothbrush causes pain or bleeding. Alcohol-free chlorhexidine may be helpfully used.
- Rinsing the mouth after meals and at night, with water, aqueous 0.2% chlorhexidine or 0.9% sodium chloride. (Fresh sodium chloride solution can be made for each rinse by dissolving half a teaspoon of domestic salt in 250 ml of fresh water).
- Chewing pineapple may also help to clean the mouth – pineapple contains ananase, an enzyme which may help to break down mouth debris (unsweetened fresh or tinned pineapple can be used).
- Rinsing with a fluoride mouth rinse at night.

Dentures should be removed at night, cleaned with a soft toothbrush and toothpaste, and soaked overnight in chlorhexidine or a denture solution containing sodium hypochlorite, and then rinsed in cool running water before use.

DRY MOUTH

- Dry mouth can be managed by reversing dehydration and with frequent sips or sprays of cold water, sucking ice cubes, or eating partly frozen melon or pineapple chunks.
- Petroleum jelly can help prevent sore, cracked lips.
- Mouth wetting agents (artificial saliva) containing mucin (e.g. AS Saliva Orthana) or lactoperoxidase (e.g. Biotene Oralbalance and BioXtra), or chewing sugar-free gum are also useful.
- Long-term use of acidic products (e.g. Glandosane spray, Salivix pastilles, and SST tablets are slightly acidic) may however, demineralise tooth enamel.
- Dealing with causes of dry mouth including drugs and anxiety.

People with Learning Impairment

People with **learning impairment** may also have physical or neurological impairments (e.g. epilepsy). There has been a move away from people with learning impairment living in institutions to community-based dwellings, which has had implications for education and the provision of medical and dental services.

LEGAL BACKGROUND IN THE UK

The Disability Rights Commission (DRC) which is an independent body established by Act of Parliament, endeavours to stop discrimination and promote equality of opportunity for disabled people.

The Disability Discrimination Act 1995 states that it is unlawful to treat a person with disability less favourably for a reason related to that person's disability (unless it can be justified). This act defines a person with disability as 'A person who has or has had a physical or mental impairment which has a substantial and long-term adverse effect upon his or her ability to carry out normal day-to-day activities.'

> **Term to Learn**
> **Learning disability:**
> 'a significant impairment of intelligence and social functioning acquired before adulthood' (Department of Health, UK).

FIND OUT MORE

Visit the Department for Work and Pensions website (http://www.dwp.gov.uk/employers/dda/) for more facts about the Disability Discrimination Act in relation to your work.

PRINCIPLE OF BEST INTEREST

If a health professional believes a patient lacks the capacity to consent, they cannot give or withhold consent to treatment on behalf of that patient; they may carry out an investigation or treatment judged to be in that patient's **best interest**. In deciding what is in the patient's best interest, the treating clinician will consider:

- The treatment options
- Any evidence of the patient's preferences
- The patient's background
- Views of family members.

THE MENTAL CAPACITY ACT 2005

The Mental Capacity Act 2005 (MCA) applies to everyone involved in the care, treatment or support of people aged 16 years and over in England and Wales and who lack capacity to make all or some decisions for themselves. This Act also applies to situations where a person may lack capacity to make a decision at a particular time due to illness or drugs or alcohol. In Scotland, the equivalent is the Adults with Incapacity (Scotland) Act 2000.

Assessments of capacity should be time and decision specific. The MCA states that a person is unable to make a particular decision if they cannot do one or more of the following:

- Understand information given them
- Retain that information long enough to be able to make the decision
- Weigh up the information available to make the decision
- Communicate their decision.

A new criminal offence of ill-treatment or wilful neglect of people who lack capacity also came into force in 2007. Within the law, 'helping with personal hygiene' (that would include toothbrushing) is protected from liability as long as the person assisting has assessed the disabled person's capacity and is acting in their best interests.

> **Term to Learn**
> **'Best interest' decisions:** decisions made on behalf of people who lack capacity and aimed to be the least restrictive of the disabled person's basic rights and freedoms.

173

CONSENT AND COMPETENCY

For a person 'to be competent' or 'to have the capacity to consent' they must be able to reason and weigh the risks, benefits and consequences of their decision. Some patients with learning disabilities, no matter how well the facts about treatment are explained to them, are incapable of understanding them. Or they may not understand the implications of the treatment decision they are being asked to make. They are then regarded as not competent to give consent.

Under the MCA:

- When a health professional has a significant concern relating to decisions taken under the authority of a Lasting Power of Attorney (**LPA**) about serious medical treatment, the case can be referred for adjudication to the Court of Protection, which is ultimately responsible for the proper functioning of the legislation.
- A 'Public Guardian' has responsibility for the registration and supervision of both LPAs and Court appointed deputies.
- Independent Mental Capacity Advocates (IMCAs) can support particularly vulnerable incapacitated adults – most often those who lack any other forms of external support – in making certain decisions such as consent.

> **Term to Learn**
> **LPA:** When a person authorises another person to act on their behalf in matters concerning the law or business.

Oral Health of People with Learning Disabilities

Rates of untreated caries and extractions are higher in people with learning disabilities compared with the general population. Levels of untreated caries and of gingivitis and periodontal disease are also higher.

The management of patients with learning disabilities depends on the severity of the disability – with some patients requiring examination and treatment under conscious sedation or general anaesthetic. The emphasis should be on preventing disease and promoting good oral health, by:

- Establishing good oral hygiene practices
- Dietary advice
- Use of fissure sealants (see p. 206)
- Topical fluoride application (see p. 197).

Socially Excluded People

Term to Learn
Socially excluded groups: these include institutionalised older people, the homeless, those engaged in substance abuse, refugees and asylum seekers.

Over the years, the inequalities in oral health in, and the use of health services by, **socially excluded groups** have increased. The gap between the deprived (socio-economic classes IV and V) and affluent (I, II and III) social groups has increased.

For example, the homeless often have a greater rate or risk of:

- Missed dental appointments
- Caries
- Periodontal disease
- Oral cancer.

174

FIND OUT MORE

Find out what are the social classes I to V.

People who Abuse Drugs and Alcohol

Trends suggest an increase in the use, particularly by young people, of 'skunk' cannabis/marijuana, amphetamines and Ecstasy, 'crack' cocaine and volatile substances (solvents). There are also many changing vogues of drug use; for example, in the UK, the drug mephedrone ('meow meow', 'plant food' and 'bubbles') has recently been in fashion. People may use drugs occasionally or regularly. Regular use can lead on to tolerance, dependence, and addiction.

Problems for delivery of healthcare to people who abuse drugs relate mainly to:

- Poor oral hygiene
- High rates of smoking – which lead to increased levels of periodontal disease
- Preference for sweet foods – leading to caries
- Facial and dental trauma from violence
- Tooth damage and loss due to convulsions
- Poorly used dental services
- High dental anxiety.

There may also be:

- Anti-social behaviour
- Irregular attendance
- Drug interactions.

In addition, use of certain drugs can cause dehydration. The resultant xerostomia (see Subchapter 6.1) may be relieved by frequent intake of sugary drinks. Some drugs also cause bruxism and tooth attrition (e.g. 'meth mouth' from methylamphetamine, and 'munchies' with Ecstasy).

Alcoholics often have:

- Neglected oral health
- Dental trauma
- Erosion – from frequent acidic drinks and regurgitation due to gastro-oesophageal disorders.

Smoking tobacco or marijuana is also linked to chronic airway limitation and ischaemic heart disease, which may affect dental management. Tobacco and alcohol have a synergistic effect in causing oral cancer; betel and marijuana have also been implicated in cancer.

Withdrawal from drugs can lead to rebound of dental pain that was previously suppressed. Methadone, which is used to manage opioid withdrawal, is cariogenic and erosive, and leads to sugar cravings. It is now available sugar-free.

> **KEY POINT** Intravenous drug abusers have a tendency to have needle phobia. They are at increased risk of infection with blood-borne viruses, such as hepatitis B, C and HIV, as well as of bleeding if there is liver damage.

People in Custodial Care

The prison population:

- Consists primarily of men aged 15-35 years
- Has lower levels of educational attainment
- Has higher levels of mental illness, drug abuse, homosexual activity and previous unemployment.

As a consequence, violence and trauma, sexually transmitted infections and blood-borne viral infections such as hepatitis B, C and HIV, are more common in this population. Oral health may be lacking and the amount of untreated caries is about four times greater than in the general population from similar social backgrounds.

People from Black and Minority Ethnic (BME) Backgrounds

Multicultural societies are increasingly common across the world. Also, increasing numbers of BME groups are seeking access to culturally sensitive oral healthcare provision.

Healthcare professionals as a group have also become much more multicultural, with graduates from different cultures or backgrounds. Most younger clinicians and dental care professionals are more aware of religious and cultural issues (Table 6.2.2) than some older members of the professions.

Culturally sensitive healthcare is a phrase used to describe a healthcare system that is accessible, and respects the:

- Beliefs
- Attitudes
- Cultural lifestyles

of both the professional and the patient.

As a consequence, the care provided is sensitive to issues such as culture, race, gender, sexual orientation, social class and economic situation.

> **KEY POINT** Healthcare should be offered in a way that respects and recognises everyone's religious and cultural needs. For example, at the most simple level, ask people for their 'personal' name rather than their 'Christian' name (as not everyone is a Christian).

175

TABLE 6.2.2 Main Religions and their Relevance

Religion	Main Festival or Religious Occasion(s)	Dietary Points	Main Medical and Other Concerns which Apply to Many
Buddhism	Wesak	Often vegetarian	–
Christianity	Christmas, Easter	–	–
Hinduism	Mahashivaratri, Ram Navami, Janmastami, Diwali, Holi	Often eat no meat (particularly beef), eggs or fish. Some do not drink tea, coffee or alcohol, and others do not eat garlic or onions	Rarely vitamin B12 deficient from veganism
Islam (Muslim)	Ramadan, Mawlid, al-Nabi	Eat only Halal meat, no pork, or alcohol. During Ramadan, between sunrise and sunset, eat and drink nothing (including water), or smoke unless ill, young, old or pregnant	Often cover much of the body and head/face. Handshakes are appropriate only between same gender. Women are usually not permitted to be alone with a man who is not her husband or relative. The right hand is considered clean, and is used for eating, handshaking, etc. In general, Shiites are more strict and restricted in their daily activities than Sunnis, in religious practices, food proscriptions, and especially, treatment of women. May be non-compliant with oral medication during fasts such as Ramadan. It may therefore be best to avoid elective procedures where for example, oral analgesics or antibiotics may be required, or to change to less-frequent oral dose regimens or to parenteral drugs. Alcohol-free oral products should be used.
Jehovah's Witnesses	–	–	Often refuse blood transfusions
Judaism	Rosh Hashanah, Yom Kippur, Pesach	Eat only kosher meat and no pork or shellfish. Fast for 25 hr from eve of Yom Kippur	No work or routine healthcare on Sabbath (Saturday).
Sikhism	Vaisakhi	Eat no fish or eggs, usually no beef or pork. Often vegetarian	Invariably cover head. Rarely, vitamin B12 deficient from veganism

176

Term to Learn
Stereotyping: Making assumptions about a person, based on membership of a certain group, without bothering to learn whether or not the individual fits that assumption.

Never 'stereotype' people.

An understanding of the culture of your practice's patients, and of differences between a healthcare professional and recipient, is vital. Cultures can differ in a number of ways from each other, especially in religion and family values. An important difference between non-Anglo-American and Anglo-American cultures is that the latter emphasise the independence of the individual while the former emphasise the individual's dependence on the family – where the elders act as role models, are in control, and are respected and often the family decides where to seek healthcare. They also may decide whether to comply with appointments, prescribed medication or other treatment.

In terms of health and healthcare, cultures can thus often differ significantly in beliefs about what is regarded as:

- Health
- The cause of illness
- Good healthcare.

Cultures can also differ in attitudes towards:

- How symptoms are perceived
- Traditional medicines and treatments
- Western healing, healthcare professionals and medicines.

These differences have implications for healthcare. Thus it is important for the clinician, dental care professional and other staff to understand and recognise the culture of patients.

People from ethnic minority groups tend to seek dental and related oral healthcare from healthcare professionals within their group. They may have found barriers elsewhere, such as cost, fear, mistrust, the need to travel long distances at inconvenient times, or the absence of dental professionals able and willing to accommodate their cultural and ethnic needs.

The Law

The Race Relations Act, which was passed in 1965 in the UK, outlawed public discrimination, and established the Race Relations Board (RRB).

The Commission for Racial Equality (CRE) later replaced the RRB. The Equality and Human Rights Commission (EHRC) replaced CRE in 2007.

Other Acts forbid direct or indirect racial discrimination in employment, housing and social services. Currently it is illegal in the UK to discriminate by:

- Refusing or omitting to provide services
- Offering services of a lesser quality
- Offering services in different ways or on different terms.

Facilities must also take account of cultural needs. For example, the waiting area should be appropriate for accompanying people such as children or families, and if divided discretely can permit women to sit alone if need be. Toilet facilities should permit perineal washing for those people, such as Muslims, who prefer it. This could be a simple ancillary (bidet) shower, a bidet, or one of the more sophisticated water closets that have perineal washing facility. Separate soap and towels should be provided for use on the upper and lower parts of the body; disposable items are preferred.

177

> **KEY POINTS** Respect others' point of view, culture, background and religion. Treat patients with special needs at least as well as all patients.

CHAPTER 7

Oral Health Needs, Treatment Planning and Appointments

CHAPTER POINTS
- This chapter covers the requirements of the NEBDN syllabus Section 7: Assessing patients' oral health needs and treatment planning.

INTRODUCTION

A dental workplace should have a written protocol for:

- The length of appointments required for different procedures
- What to do if a patient arrives late
- What to do if a patient does not attend
- What to do if emergency treatment is needed
- What to do if families want appointments together.

One way of organising appointments is to leave an 'emergency slot' at the end of each session. This session allows:

- Catch-up time if the clinician is running late
- Seeing an emergency patient
- Seeing a patient who has arrived late for an appointment, as long as:
  - The patient rang to inform the practice of the reason for delay
  - The prescribed treatment for the appointment can still be carried out
  - The treatment of other patients is not delayed.

If it is feasible, another patient could be seen in the late patient's slot and the late patient asked to wait.

PATIENT RECORD CARDS

In NHS practices, clinical records are kept on form FP25. In other dental workplaces other suitable cards can be used.

Patient records should always be:

- Accurate
- Truthful
- Up to date (in correct date order)
- Treated with confidentiality (see Subchapter 3.2).

Records must not be altered after any request for access (see Chapter 3) has been received.

Patient records should include the following:

- Patient details:
  - Last name
  - First name
  - Birth date
  - Address
  - Home, mobile and work telephone number
  - Practice or hospital reference number
  - Occupation
  - General medical practitioner
  - General dental practitioner (if patient is being seen in hospital)
  - Medical history (this should be reviewed at each recall appointment – see Chapters 2 and 6)
  - Initial dental charting.
- Record of:
  - Dental charting
  - Previous dental treatment received
  - Discussions about treatment received and recommendations
  - Laboratory work details and shade nos. if relevant
  - Any requests for private care
  - Charges, payments and method of payment
  - Failed or cancelled appointments
  - Treatments advised but refused by patient
  - Referrals and outcomes
  - Prescriptions
  - Post-operative instructions.
  - Complaints/other letters
  - Consent forms
  - Medical history forms
  - X-rays or other **imaging scans**
  - Referral letters
  - Replies to referral letters
  - Treatment plans.

Term to Learn
Imaging scans:
Besides the more common radiographs (X-rays), some patients may require other scans such as CT (computed tomography) or MRI (magnetic resonance imaging) or ultrasound (US).

TERMINOLOGY

Dental terminology is covered in detail in Chapter 4.2. The following list summarises some key terms:

- Enamel – this is the outer covering of the tooth (it is not sensitive)
- Dentine – this is the next layer (it is sensitive)
- Pulp – the innermost layer of the tooth (it is very sensitive)
- Clinical crown – the part of the tooth visible in the oral cavity.

Surfaces of the Tooth

The various surfaces of a tooth are called by specific names (Box 7.1 and Figure 7.1).

BOX 7.1 SURFACES OF THE TOOTH

- Mesial – surface nearest the midline.
- Distal – surface furthest away from the midline.
- Occlusal – the biting surface of the premolars and molars.
- Incisal – the biting edge of the incisors and canines.
- Palatal – the surface nearest the palate.
- Lingual – the surface nearest the tongue.
- Buccal – the surface of the premolars and molars nearest the cheeks.
- Labial – the surface of the incisors and canines nearest the lips.
- Cervical – the part of any surface nearest the gingival margin.

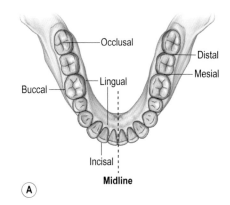

(A)

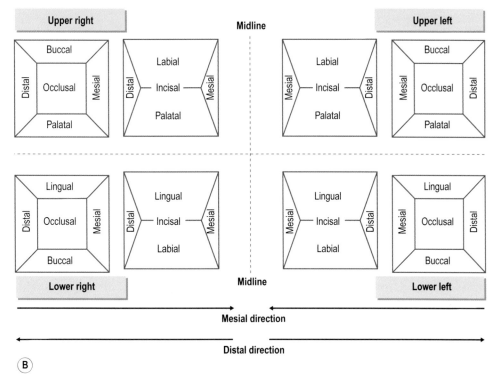

(B)

FIGURE 7.1
(A) The surfaces of the teeth. (B) The surfaces of teeth as appearing on a dental chart.

181

> **BOX 7.2 WHY DO DENTAL CHARTING?**
>
> A record of the condition of the patient's teeth and surrounding tissues provides:
>
> - Basic information for dental treatment planning
> - Evidence in medico-legal cases
> - Evidence in cases of identification of a dead person.
>
> It is vital therefore that dental charting is accurate.

DENTAL CHARTING

Dental and periodontal charting is the 'recording of clinical details of a patient's dentition and surrounding tissues'. As a part of the dental clinical team, you will be required to know how to complete a dental chart. Box 7.2 lists the main reasons for doing dental charting.

Dental charting includes:

- State of the dentition:
  - Caries
  - Restorations
  - Missing or malpositioned teeth
  - Implants
  - Teeth to be extracted.
- Periodontal problems:
  - Pocket depth
  - Bleeding sites
  - Clinical attachment levels (see below)
  - **Furcation** (root) involvement
  - Mobile teeth.
- Other dental conditions:
  - Erosion
  - Abrasion
  - Attrition
  - Developmental anomalies
  - Prostheses.

Term to Learn
Furcation: the area where the root of multi-rooted teeth divides into two or more roots.

182

KEY POINT Charting provides a pictorial description of the health of a patient's mouth.

How to Chart

KEY POINT Remember while charting, the dental chart is opposite to *your* left and right.

The teeth present in each quadrant of the mouth and their condition is recorded. You need to record these in relation to the patient's left or right side. That is, with the patient sitting in the dental chair, a tooth on the patient's left side (your right side) is recorded as on the 'left' on the chart.

Most dental charts consist of a diagrammatic representation of all the teeth with surfaces shown as flat (Figure 7.2). Imagine the face is divided into four equal parts (quadrants):

- A line straight down the middle of the eyes, nose and chin (called the midline)
- A line straight across the middle between the maxilla and mandible
- The two upper quadrants include the maxilla
- The two lower quadrants include the mandible.

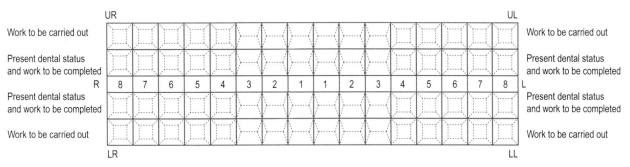

FIGURE 7.2
Blank dental chart. The inner grid is for present dental status and work already present in the mouth. The outer grid is for work to be carried out.

Charting begins with noting the names and numbers of the teeth. Charting by hand is most efficient with the clinician performing the examination and the dental nurse recording the findings on the chart (Figure 7.3) or computer (Figure 7.4). Some clinicians use a headset microphone and voice-activated charting software for ease and convenience.

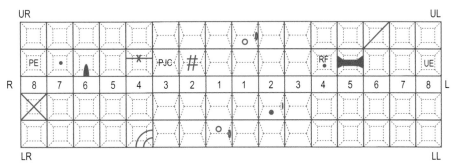

FIGURE 7.3
Completed dental chart.

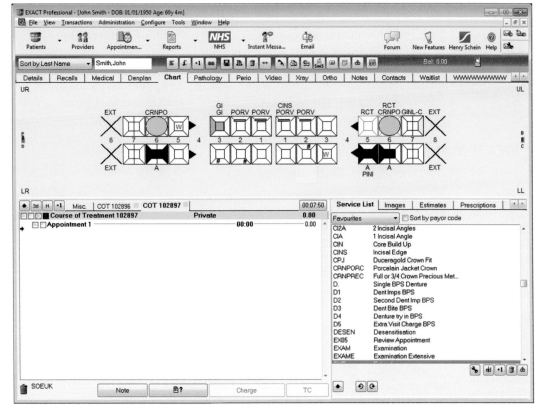

FIGURE 7.4
Computerised dental chart.

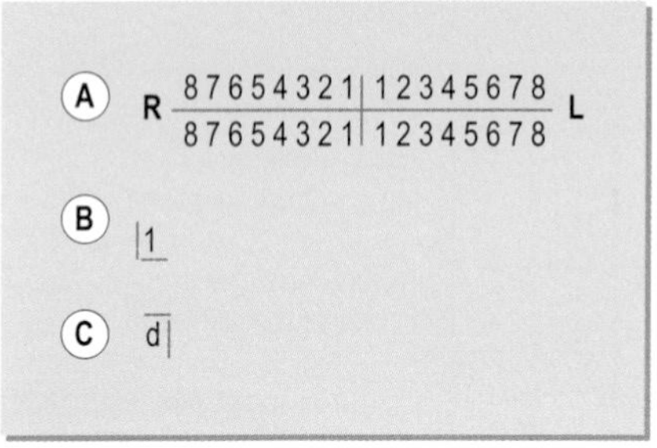

FIGURE 7.5
Examples of Zsigmondy-Palmer system notation. (A) The full permanent dentition. (B) The upper left permanent central incisor. (C) The lower right deciduous first molar.

Permanent dentition
1 for upper right
2 for upper left
3 for lower left
4 for lower right

18 17 16 15 14 13 12 11	21 22 23 24 25 26 27 28
48 47 46 45 44 43 42 41	31 32 33 34 35 36 37 38

Deciduous dentition
5 for upper right
6 for upper left
7 for lower left
8 for lower right

55 54 53 52 51	61 62 63 64 65
85 84 83 82 81	71 72 73 74 75

FIGURE 7.6
The FDI notation two-digit charting system. In this system, the quadrant name is replaced by a number and this is the first of the two digit code while the second number identifies the individual tooth.

Charting Systems

There are two systems of dental charting commonly used:

- Zsigmondy-Palmer (Figure 7.5)
- FDI (Fédération Dentale Internationale) (Figure 7.6).

THE ZSIGMONDY–PALMER SYSTEM

This system is commonly used in the UK but only rarely in other countries.

In this system, in each quadrant, the permanent teeth are represented by the numbers 1 to 8, beginning from the midline. So the permanent maxillary lateral incisors, for instance, are referred to as 'upper right 2' (UR2) and 'upper left 2' (UL2). Similarly, the deciduous teeth are represented by the letters A to E, beginning at the midline (Table 7.1). So the primary mandibular first molars are referred to as 'lower right D' (LRD) and 'lower left D' (LLD). When written down, two lines are drawn at right angles to denote the quadrants and the numbers or letters are placed in the quadrant in which they belong. If only one tooth is written in the patient records, the lines are shortened as shown in Figure 7.5.

IDENTIFY AND LEARN

Identify the following teeth: e⎤e, 2⎤1 6, 8⎤8, 5⎤, ⎣3

THE FDI TWO-DIGIT CHARTING SYSTEM

The FDI system is widely used in many countries. It is easy to understand, to teach, to pronounce and to write/type. Each tooth is represented by a two-digit number. The first number represents the quadrant and the second number is the tooth number. The quadrants are numbered in a clockwise direction commencing with the upper right quadrant (see Figure 7.6).

Thus the permanent teeth quadrants are numbered from upper right (1) to upper left (2), lower left (3) and lower right (4). The teeth are numbered starting from the central incisor (1) to the third molar (8). The primary teeth quadrants are numbered from upper right (5), to upper left (6), lower left (7) and lower right (8). The teeth are numbered starting from the central incisor (1) to the second molar (5).

IDENTIFY AND LEARN

Name the following teeth: 21, 44, 55, 73 (see Appendix 7.1, p. 192, for the answers).

TABLE 7.1 The Zsigmondy-Palmer System of Dental Charting

Permanent Dentition		Deciduous Dentition	
Tooth	Denoted as	Tooth	Denoted as
Central incisor	1	Central incisor	A
Lateral incisor	2	Lateral incisor	B
Canine	3	Canine	C
First premolar	4	First molar	D
Second premolar	5	Second molar	E
First molar	6		
Second molar	7		
Third molar	8		

184

Tooth decay or cavities can involve more than one surface of a tooth. When this happens the cavity is referred to by the names of the surfaces that are involved:

- Mesio-occlusal
- Disto-occlusal
- Mesio-occluso-distal
- Mesio-incisal
- Disto-incisal.

If the decay or cavity has just entered a surface from another surface, this is called an extension, for example:

- Mesio-occlusal with a palatal extension
- Mesio-occlusal-distal with lingual and buccal extensions.

Symbols, Signs and Abbreviations used in Dental Charting

A cavity (on the surface of a tooth) is represented by a symbol (an empty shape, e.g. ◯).

A restoration or filling on the surface of a tooth is represented by the same symbol but is shaded in (e.g. ●).

Figures 7.7 and 7.8 illustrate the accepted symbols for use in incisors, premolars and molars. Box 7.3 shows the abbreviations and signs used in dental charting.

IDENTIFY AND LEARN

Ask your supervisor to show you examples of an F/S, BP, BA, FRC, PJC, PBC, IMP, PV, GI, PI, RCT, TEMP material. How many of these did you already know?

185

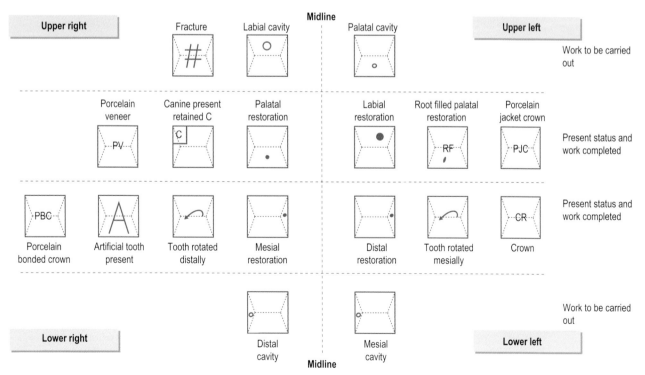

FIGURE 7.7
Accepted notations – incisor teeth.

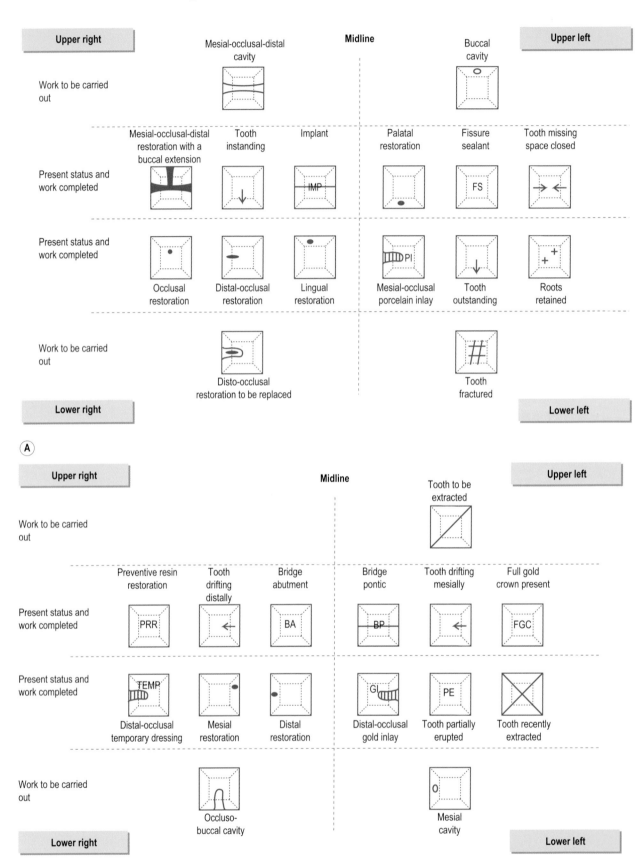

FIGURE 7.8
(A, B) Accepted notations – premolar and molar teeth.

186

BOX 7.3 ABBREVIATIONS AND SIGNS USED IN CHARTING

C	Canine present	PV	Porcelain veneer
PE	Partially erupted tooth	GI	Gold inlay
A	Artificial tooth present	PI	Porcelain inlay
F/S	Fissure sealant	RCT	Root canal treated
BP	Bridge pontic	TEMP	Temporary dressing
BA	Bridge abutment	++	Roots retained
CR	Crown	#	Tooth fractured
FGC	Full gold crown	-	Space
PJC	Porcelain jacket crown	/	Tooth to be extracted
PBC	Porcelain bonded crown	X	Tooth extracted
IMP	Implant		

Periodontal Charting

In a healthy mouth, each tooth is surrounded by a collar of marginal gingiva, 0–3 mm deep. Below this, the gingiva is attached to the cementum, the surface layer of the tooth root. The 0–3 mm space within the free collar is called the *gingival crevice* or sulcus. In patients with periodontal disease the point of attachment of the gingiva to tooth moves deeper down the tooth surface or is fully lost and the deepened crevice is called a *periodontal pocket*.

- Periodontal charting is when the clinician measures and records the depths of these pockets and bleeding that is caused by inflammation. The measurements are done by hand with a calibrated periodontal probe, which is inserted into the sulcus parallel to the tooth long axis.
- The *basic periodontal examination* (BPE) is the accepted standard procedure of periodontal charting in the UK. In this method, the clinician examines the periodontal tissues using light pressure with a standardised periodontal BPE probe (Figure 7.9).

The BPE probe (Figure 7.9) is ball-tipped and coded with a single coloured marking from 3.5 mm to 5.5 mm. The probe is also known as the WHO 621 or CPITN probe. This is because the BPE is based on the Community Periodontal Index of Treatment Needs (CPITN) system. In this system, the mouth is divided into sextants: maxillary right, anterior and left; and mandibular right, anterior and left. The clinician records the worst score for each sextant (Table 7.2), that is the deepest probing depth found in that sextant. The scores are recorded in a table like the one shown in Table 7.3. Electronic probes are also available that record pocket depths automatically on a computerised chart.

For a *full periodontal charting*, readings are taken at six points on each tooth and recorded in boxes above and below the teeth on the chart. This includes looking for four features:

- Bleeding
- Plaque and calculus
- Pocket formation
- Furcation involvement.

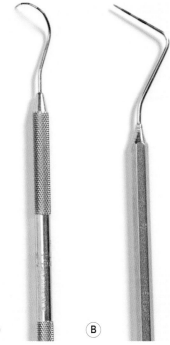

FIGURE 7.9
(A) Naber's and (B) BPE probes.

Ⓐ   Ⓑ

TABLE 7.2 BPE Examination Codes

Code	
0	No bleeding or pockets detected
1	Bleeding on probing – no pockets >3.5 mm
2	Plaque retentive factors present – no pockets >3.5 mm
3	Pockets >3.5 mm but <5.5 mm in depth
4	Pockets >5.5 mm in depth
*	Furcation involvement, or total attachment loss

TABLE 7.3 Grid to Record the BPE Scores

Root furcation involvement is measured with Naber's probe (Figure 7.9). It is graded as:

- 1 = probe enters furcation to one-third of its length
- 2 = probe enters furcation between one-third and two-thirds of its length.
- 3 = probe completely penetrates the furcation.

NATIONAL HEALTH SERVICE (NHS) TREATMENT
NHS or Other Welfare Entitlement

The NHS is the UK's state health service which provides treatment for UK residents. Some services are free, others have to be paid for and some people are exempt from payment.

The regulations that govern who can and cannot receive (free) treatment and payments, are complex and may change with time. A person who is regarded as ordinarily resident in the UK is eligible for free treatment under certain circumstances. A person is 'ordinarily resident' for this purpose if lawfully living in the UK for a settled purpose as part of the regular order of his or her life for the time being. Anyone coming to live in this country would qualify as ordinarily resident. Overseas visitors to the UK are not regarded as ordinarily resident if they do not meet this description.

The following NHS treatment is available to all people:

- Treatment in an emergency (but not follow-up treatment)
- Treatment of certain **communicable diseases**
- Compulsory psychiatric treatment.

A patient will often enquire as to whether they are entitled to free or help towards the cost of dental treatment. Remember that the NHS Leaflet HC11, 'Help with health costs', is a useful guide. To qualify for other NHS treatments, patients must meet certain conditions (Box 7.4).

> **Term to Learn**
> **Communicable disease:** a disease that can be passed on from one person to another, e.g. tuberculosis.

FIND OUT MORE

Find an H2 and H3 form in your workplace office. Who is responsible for filling them?

If patients need information on dentists who may be prepared to register them under the NHS, they should telephone NHS Direct. If there is a dental emergency, they should contact the dentist they are registered with. If a person is not registered with a dentist they can obtain advice from NHS Direct.

188

> **BOX 7.4 FREE DENTAL CARE**
>
> 1. Entitlements to free dental care in UK
>
>   Patients are entitled to free dental care if they are:
>
>   - Under 18 years
>   - 18 or over and in full time education
>   - Pregnant or had a baby in the previous 12 months before treatment commences
>   - In hospital
>   - Treated in a dental hospital or dental department in a general hospital (there may be a charge for dentures and bridges)
>   - Receiving income support
>   - Receiving income-based Jobseeker's Allowance
>   - Receiving income-related Employment and Support Allowance
>   - Receiving Pension Credit/Guarantee Credit
>   - Named on a valid HC2 certificate.
>
>   People with an NHS tax credit exemption certificate are also entitled to free treatment.
>
> 2. Entitlements to partial help
>
>   Patients are entitled to partial help with dental care payments if they are:
>
>   - Named on a valid HC3 Certificate
>
>   For each course of treatment the patient will be asked to pay whichever is less:
>
>   - The actual cost
>   - The maximum patient's charge.

NHS Direct contact details:

- Tel: 0845 4647
- Website: http://www.nhsdirect.nhs.uk

NHS Travel Costs

A patient may get help travelling to and from hospital to receive NHS treatment under the care of a consultant. If a patient requires an escort for medical reasons, the escort's travel costs are dealt with the patient's costs.

Claim Forms

There are a range of NHS and Department of Health forms that you should be familiar with (Table 7.4). Other important points to note are:

- The NHS form for treatment cost estimates is FP17DC.
- NHS payment for orthodontic examination, assessment and treatment is claimed on NHS form FP170.
- The NHS claim forms for treatment must be submitted for payment within six months from the end of treatment.

OVERSEAS PATIENTS

European Union (EU) Nationals

There are reciprocal arrangements for foreign nationals from EU member states for both dental and medical healthcare. So they can access the full range of NHS services.

TABLE 7.4 NHS and Department of Health Forms

Form	Purpose
NHS	
FP 10 D	Dental prescription pads
FP 17	Dental payment claim
FP 17 B	Dental Practice Board addressed envelopes
FP 17 DC	NHS Acceptance form
FP 17 DCO	NHS Orthodontic Acceptance form
FP 17(PL)	General Dental Services (GDS) Dental Department, Dental Practice Board addressed envelope
FP 17(PM)	Dental Payments Department, Dental Practice Board addressed envelope
FP17RN	Referral Notice form
FP 18	Withdrawal notice from a capitation/continuing care arrangement
FP 25	NHS Dental Record Card
FP 25 A	NHS Dental Record Envelope
FP 25 C	NHS Dental Record Card – Continuation
FP 25 P	NHS Dental Record – Periodontal
FP 30D	Dental Stationery Requisition Forms
FP 64	Receipt for Clinician's Charges
FP 170	Dental Payments Form – Orthodontic
Plain	Hospital Referral Letter
PR	Practice Record Patient Declaration
Department of Health (low income scheme)	
HC 1	Claims for Help with NHS Costs (form/pre-paid envelope)
HC 5 (D)	Refund Claim form
HC 11QG	Help with NHS costs
HC 12	NHS Charges (leaflet)
HC 10	Help with Health Cost poster
HC 20	Paying NHS Prescription Charges poster

Non-EU Nationals

Foreign nationals from non-EU countries have no automatic right to NHS healthcare (other than those outlined on p. 188). These include visitors and students who are going to stay in the UK for less than six months. These individuals would have to be seen as private patients and would have to pay for their treatment.

Patients entitled to NHS treatment should receive the following services free of charge:

- Consulting a general practitioner (GP) and most other GP services
- Treatment in hospital (both emergency and non-emergency treatment).

They will need to pay for:

- Medicines prescribed by the GP (there are some exceptions to this)
- Some GP services
- Dental treatment
- Optical treatment.

In January 2005 the Department of Health issued guidance on healthcare provision for refugees and asylum seekers. There has been tightening of controls on welfare entitlements in the Nationality, Immigration and Asylum Act 2002, which declares that, although refugees and those granted asylum in the UK will retain their entitlement to the full range of NHS services both in primary and secondary care, failed asylum seekers will no longer be eligible for treatment in secondary care.

REFERRAL PROCEDURES

On occasion, treatment may be indicated at another location or the treatment may not be covered by the primary care trust (PCT) service agreement. The request for funding of such treatment may come from the patient themselves, from the patient's dentist, or from another provider unit. The principles of most PCT commissioning teams are as follows:

- The general dental practitioner (GDP) should continue to play a major role in the appropriate use of resources.
- GDPs should apply the criteria as they would if managing the budget at a practice level, that is:
  - Is there an appropriate service available within the contract portfolio?
  - Does the service provide value for money?
  - Is it of proven clinical effectiveness
  - Does it fit with current clinical priorities?
- Tertiary referrals (referrals from hospital clinicians) to non-contracted providers will require the support of a patient's GDP.
- Referrals should take into account the countywide purchasing policies that are endorsed by the PCT.
- A PCT Complex Case Panel is often used to consider complex funding requests.
- There will also be instances where providers wish to pursue new treatments or developments: PCTs usually wish to be involved in deciding whether to support the funding of these developments.
- If the GDP wishes to continue with the referral, they should submit a request to the PCT for consideration, giving the following information:
  - Patient details (within Caldicott and confidentiality guidelines): date of birth; initials of patient; gender; daytime telephone number; NHS number
  - Practice address
  - Condition
  - Date of onset of condition
  - Treatment
  - Prognosis
  - Provider organisation and consultant providing care
  - Provider organisation where care is requested
  - Reason for referral outside of existing portfolio
  - Any evidence base known of the intervention
  - Relevant clinical information and indication of urgency
  - Information on any relevant pathology tests or X-rays carried out
  - Whether the patient needs an interpreter.

Delivery of a two-week cancer outpatient waiting time standard is a priority in the National Priorities Guidance 2000/01 to 2002/3.

191

APPENDIX 7.1
The FDI System of Dental Charting

Permanent				Deciduous			
Upper Right (1)		**Upper Left (2)**		**Upper Right (5)**		**Upper Left (6)**	
Central incisor	11	Central incisor	21	Central incisor	51	Central incisor	61
Lateral incisor	12	Lateral incisor	22	Lateral incisor	52	Lateral incisor	62
Canine	13	Canine	23	Canine	53	Canine	63
First premolar	14	First premolar	24	First molar	54	First molar	64
Second premolar	15	Second premolar	25	Second molar	55	Second molar	65
First molar	16	First molar	26				
Second molar	17	Second molar	27				
Third molar	18	Third molar	28				
Lower Right (4)		**Lower Left (3)**		**Lower Right (8)**		**Lower Left (7)**	
Central incisor	41	Central incisor	31	Central incisor	81	Central incisor	71
Lateral incisor	42	Lateral incisor	32	Lateral incisor	82	Lateral incisor	72
Canine	43	Canine	33	Canine	83	Canine	73
First premolar	44	First premolar	34	First molar	84	First molar	74
Second premolar	45	Second premolar	35	Second molar	85	Second molar	75
First molar	46	First molar	36				
Second molar	47	Second molar	37				
Third molar	48	Third molar	38				

Oral Health Promotion

INTRODUCTION

Oral health promotion involves educating people about how to achieve and maintain good oral health. A dental nurse should be able to provide competent and complete oral health promotion. This includes:

● Instructions in toothbrushing, flossing, use of disclosing tablets and other dental aids
● Dietary advice
● Advice on how often a dental examination (check-up or recall) is required
● Advice to mothers on preventing **nursing bottle caries**.

This chapter presents an overview of the oral health messages that you should know and should be able to educate patients about. It will describe the measures and oral health devices (dental care accessories) and materials and techniques that patients can use to achieve and maintain oral health.

DENTAL RECALL GUIDELINES

Guidelines from the National Institute for Health and Clinical Excellence (NICE) and the National Collaborating Centre for Acute Care (**NCAC**) recommend the following general intervals between check-ups:

● Under-18s: between 3 and 12 months
● Adults: between 3 and 24 months.

However, the interval between check-ups needs to be decided on a patient-by-patient basis. Each patient's check-up routine should be based on their needs, their disease levels and their risk of developing dental disease. The guideline also recommends that during a check-up, the dental team should ensure that:

● A comprehensive history is taken (see Chapters 2 and 6)
● A thorough examination is conducted
● Preventive advice is reinforced.

The following issues need to be discussed or reinforced with the patient where relevant:

● Maintaining oral health by practising oral hygiene, dietary precautions, fluoride use
● Any factors that may influence the patient's oral health, e.g. tobacco and alcohol use, and their implications for deciding the appropriate recall interval

Term to Learn
Nursing bottle caries: the decay of the upper incisors related to drinking milk through a bottle just before sleeping. The milk remains on the teeth and acts as a substrate for dental caries.

193

Term to Learn
NCAC: There are four national collaborating centres that help NICE to develop the clinical guidelines.

- The outcome of previous treatments and visits and the suitability of previously recommended intervals
- The patient's ability or desire to visit the dentist at the recommended interval
- The costs involved in having regular check-ups and any further treatments.

THE ORAL HEALTH MESSAGE

Most oral diseases, including not only the more common problems (such as tooth surface loss due to caries, trauma, abrasion, erosion and periodontal disease) but also potentially fatal diseases (such as cancer), are largely related to people's lifestyle and habits (Table 8.1). Thus these diseases are often preventable by careful attention to lifestyle. For example, oral health can be improved by:

- Reducing frequency and amount of sugar and acidic drinks in the diet
- Using fluoride toothpaste/mouthwash regularly
- Using amorphous calcium phosphate (ACP) topically
- Practising oral hygiene at least twice daily
- Using mouth protection against trauma
- Avoiding alcohol, tobacco and betel habits
- Attending for dental professional attention as required for:
  - Scaling and polishing
  - Fissure sealing
  - Fluoride applications
- Using other oral hygiene measures, e.g. chewing gum.

194

FIND OUT MORE

This chapter is based on the toolkit 'Delivering better oral health: An evidence-based toolkit for prevention' by the Department of Health and British Association for the Study of Community Dentistry. See the Department of Health website for the full toolkit (http://www.dh.gov.uk/en/Publicationsandstatistics/Publications/PublicationsPolicyAndGuidance/DH_078742)

Diet

GENERAL ADVICE

Refined carbohydrates and sugars, particularly non-milk extrinsic sugars in items other than fresh fruits and vegetables, are the major causes of dental caries (Chapter 5). The frequency of intake is more important than the amount. Thus to lessen the chances of accumulating dental plaque, and developing caries, it is important to limit and reduce the frequency of consumption of sugary foods, such as restricting them to meal times.

TABLE 8.1 Oral Diseases Related to Lifestyle Habits

Disease	Risk Factor
Abrasion	Incorrect toothbrushing
Cancer	Tobacco, alcohol, betel nut use
Candidosis	Dry mouth, antibiotic use, HIV and other immunity problems
Caries	High sugar diet, low fluoride
Erosion	Soft drinks, fruit juices, alcohol
Gingivitis	Plaque accumulation
Halitosis	Plaque accumulation, tobacco use, alcohol use
Periodontitis	Plaque and calculus accumulation, tobacco use
Trauma	Alcohol use; some contact sports

BABIES

Breast-feeding is best for babies, and they should be weaned onto sugar-free foods. From 6 months of age infants should be introduced to drinking from a cup and from 1 year of age bottle-feeding should be discouraged. Drinks other than milk and water should not be given to pre-school children in feeding bottles, and should be given only at main meals. Foods should be free of or very low in sugars other than those in fresh milk and raw fruits or vegetables.

OLDER CHILDREN AND ADULTS

- Foods and drinks for snacking should be free of sugars. Because of the risk of erosion, as well as of caries, discourage frequent consumption of carbonated, cola-type drinks and fruit juices such as grapefruit, apple, or orange. Children should preferably drink water and milk. Wine and some other alcohol-containing drinks can also cause erosion.
- Chewing sugar-free gum or cheese after meals can help by increasing salivary flow, as this helps wash off the acids in the plaque and on tooth surfaces.
- Most sugars in the diet come from consuming processed foods and drinks.
- Consumption of sugary foods and drinks should be restricted to meal times and to a maximum of four times a day.
- Sugars (excluding those naturally present in whole fruit) should provide less than 10% of total energy in the diet or less than 60 g per person per day. Note that for young children this will be around 33 g per day.
- Potentially cariogenic foods and drinks include:

> **KEY POINT** Remember that honey, fresh fruit juice and dried fruit all contain cariogenic sugars.

- Sugar and chocolate confectionery
- Cakes and biscuits
- Buns, pastries, fruit pies
- Sponge puddings and other puddings
- Table sugar
- Sugared breakfast cereals
- Jams, preserves, honey
- Ice cream
- Fruit in syrup
- Fresh fruit juices
- Sugared soft drinks
- Sugared, milk-based beverages
- Sugar-containing alcoholic drinks
- Dried fruits
- Syrups and sweet sauces.

195

SUGAR-FREE MEDICINES

The National Pharmacy Association leaflet 'sugar in medicines', and the Delivering better oral health' toolkit contain information about the sugar (fructose/glucose/sucrose) content of branded oral liquid medicines, both over-the-counter and prescription-only medicines. Products that do not contain these sugars are listed as being sugar-free. Preparations containing hydrogenated glucose syrup (Lycasin), maltitol, sorbitol or xylitol are also listed as sugar-free, since there is evidence that they are non-cariogenic.

Fluoride

Fluoride can protect teeth against caries by:

- Strengthening the enamel
- Inhibiting acid production by oral cariogenic bacteria
- Helping tooth remineralisation.

WATER FLUORIDATION

- Water fluoridation has consistently been shown to be the most effective, safe means of preventing caries, resulting in a decrease of approximately 50%.
- Information about the fluoride status of the water supplies can be obtained from the water supplier in your area by quoting the residential postcode.
- The West Midlands is the most extensively fluoridated area in the UK, followed by parts of the North East of England.
- In 2003 the UK law was changed to enable strategic health authorities to require water companies to fluoridate water supplies as long as there was support from the local population.
- The use of bottled *non-fluoridated* water in contrast may be linked with increased dental caries.

FIND OUT MORE

What is the level of fluoride in the drinking water supply in your area?

Term to Learn
ppm: Short for 'parts per million'; 0.7 ppm is equivalent to 700 micrograms per litre of fluoride.

196

FLUORIDE SUPPLEMENTS

- No fluoride supplements are required if the water supply contains more than 0.7 **ppm** of fluoride. Where the water supply contains less than 0.3 ppm of fluoride, children over the age of 6 months may benefit from taking fluoride supplements daily (see Table 8.2).
- While it is safe for pregnant women to take fluoride supplements, this has little impact on the future dental health of the child.
- Fluoride supplements should be stored out of reach of children.

KEY POINT Excess fluoride may cause tooth discoloration (fluorosis); the risk of this is higher from the use of fluoride supplements or topical fluorides in water-fluoridated areas.

FLUORIDE TOOTHPASTES

- Fluoride toothpastes have probably been largely responsible for most of the decline in caries over the past decades.
- Fluoride toothpastes are usually available over the counter in one of three strengths (Table 8.3). Toothpastes with 2800 ppm (Figure 8.1) and over 5000 ppm are considered prescription-only medicines.

TABLE 8.2 Sodium Fluoride Supplement Doses (Tablets) to Reduce Caries in Children in Relation to Water Fluoride Content

Fluoride in Water Supply* (ppm)	Infant up to 6 Months	6 Months to 3 Years	3 to 6 Years	Over 6 Years
Less than 0.3	Not advised	250 micrograms fluoride daily	500 micrograms fluoride daily	1 gram fluoride daily
0.3–0.7	Not advised	Not advised	250 micrograms fluoride daily	500 micrograms fluoride daily
Over 0.7	Not advised	Not advised	Not advised	Not advised

*Your local District Dental Officer or equivalent or your water company should be able to help with this information.

TABLE 8.3 Fluoride Toothpastes

Availability	Content of Fluoride in Toothpaste	Fluoride Content (ppm)	Comments
Over the counter	*Low*	<500	Give little protection against caries. Useful mainly in children with low risk of caries who live in areas with fluoridated water or receive fluoride supplements
	Medium	1000–1300	Useful for all children over 6 years of age
	High	1350–1500	Useful for people with increased caries risk
Prescription only	Sodium fluoride toothpaste 0.619% (**DPF**)	2800	For patients aged 10 years and over with high caries risk (e.g. root caries, dry mouth, orthodontic appliances, overdentures, those consuming a highly cariogenic diet or medication)
	Sodium fluoride toothpaste 1.1% (*DPF*)	5000	For patients aged 16 years and over with high caries risk (e.g. root caries, dry mouth, orthodontic appliances, overdentures, consuming a highly cariogenic diet or medication)

Term to Learn
DPF: This is the abbreviation for the *Dental Practitioners' Formulary.* (The BNF is the *British National Formulary*, which contains the DPF).

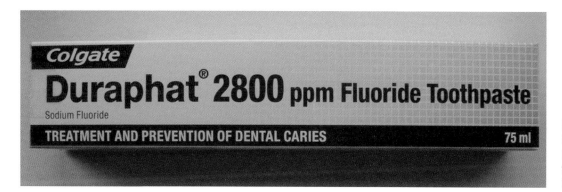

FIGURE 8.1
Duraphat by Colgate is a prescription-only toothpaste because of its high fluoride content.

FLUORIDE VARNISHES

Fluoride varnish is one of the best options for the application of topical fluoride to teeth. Fluoride varnish can also arrest existing caries (stop it spreading) on the smooth surfaces of deciduous teeth and roots of permanent teeth.

WELL-KNOWN BRANDS OF FLUORIDE VARNISH

- Fluorprotector – 8000 ppm (0.8% F)
- Lawefluor – 22 600 ppm (2.2% F)
- Duraphat – 22 600 ppm (2.2% F)
- Bifluorid – 56 300 ppm (5.6% F)

Sodium fluoride varnish is well accepted and considered safe. The application process is simple and requires minimal training:

1. Remove gross plaque (thorough **prophylaxis** is not essential)
2. Dry teeth with cotton rolls or a 3-in-1 syringe.
3. Use a microbrush to apply a small quantity of fluoride varnish to pits, fissures and proximal surfaces of primary and permanent teeth.
4. Advise the patient to avoid eating, drinking or toothbrushing for 30 minutes after application.

Term to Learn
Prophylaxis: In the dental context prophylaxis refers to cleaning the surface of teeth with a rotary brush (see Figure 8.8 below) to remove all plaque and fine deposits before treatment.

IDENTIFY AND LEARN

Identify a microbrush in your workplace.

There is a small risk of allergy to the colophony component of Duraphat. Therefore varnish application is contraindicated for children who have a history of allergies, including asthma. Duraphat is also contraindicated in patients with ulcerative gingivitis and stomatitis (see Chapter 5).

FLUORIDE MOUTHWASHES AND GELS

Fluoride mouthwashes or rinses can be prescribed for patients aged 8 years and above, for daily or weekly use, in addition to twice-daily brushing with toothpaste containing at least 1350 ppm fluoride. They should be used at a different time to toothbrushing to maximise the topical effect. Fluoride mouthwashes and gels are particularly recommended for people with a dry mouth (hyposalivation; see Chapter 5), who are otherwise particularly at risk of caries.

> **KEY POINT** Use of mouthwashes is reliant on patient compliance.

Amorphous Calcium Phosphate

Amorphous calcium phosphate (ACP) is derived from the milk protein casein and is the active ingredient of Tooth Mousse, which is found in certain crèmes and chewing gums. ACP works by neutralising acids and remineralising early enamel caries lesions. However, it is still not known for how long it remains effective.

Oral Hygiene

Oral hygiene measures that remove plaque can prevent gingivitis, periodontitis, and halitosis (malodour), and may help reduce caries, if teeth are brushed at least twice each day.

> **KEY POINT** Plaque on the tongue and other tissues is also stained when using disclosing tablets. Thus they are best used at night, so the patient does not go to work or school with a red/blue tongue.

DISCLOSING TABLETS OR RINSES

Disclosing tablets or rinses are harmless dyes which stain the plaque red or blue. When used after tooth cleaning the dye shows where plaque has been left behind on the teeth.

TOOTHBRUSHES AND TOOTHBRUSHING

Toothbrushes are the most important oral hygiene devices. However, they do not reach all areas of the teeth (for example the interdental areas) so other devices can help (Table 8.4; Figures 8.2 and 8.3). Toothbrushes can be *manual* or *powered*.

IDENTIFY AND LEARN

In your local supermarket or pharmacy, look at the various oral hygiene devices available and see which category they fit into in Table 8.4.

Manual Brushes

- Manual brushes should ideally have synthetic bristles of medium hardness (0.15–0.2 mm diameter bristles) and of an even length.
- The head should be small enough to be easily placed in the mouth, yet suitably designed to effectively remove all the dental plaque. For children, a brush head of 2 cm length by 1 cm width is suitable. For adults, a brush head of about 2–3 cm length and 1 cm width is usually sufficient.
- Altered bristle length brushes, with the middle row of bristles shorter than the outer rows, clean above and below the gingiva without causing over-brushing and are excellent for patients with generally healthy mouths.

198

TABLE 8.4 Tooth Cleaning Devices

Devices	Types
Floss	Monofilament (single-stranded)
	Braided
	Waxed
	Unwaxed
	With or without fluoride
	With or without chlorhexidine
	Power flosser (e.g. Hummingbird; Oral-B)
Interdental brushes	Tapered (e.g. Proxa)
	Uni-tufted
	Bottle type (e.g. TePe brushes, see p. 200)
Interdental sticks	Plastic
	Wood
	Hybrid with floss (e.g. Flixsticks)
Miswak or chewing sticks	A wooden stick with the end frayed to clean the teeth
Dental tape	With or without fluoride
Toothbrushes	Manual
	Powered
Waterpik	Pulsating water

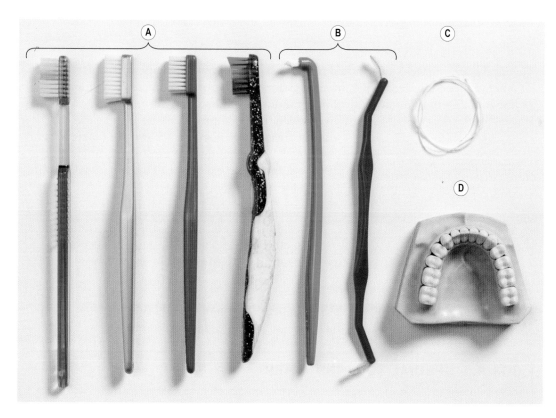

FIGURE 8.2
(A) A selection of toothbrushes;
(B) interdental aids;
(C) dental floss; and
(D) a model of the teeth that can be used to demonstrate brushing to patients.

- Hard brushes are not advisable as they can cause wearing of the teeth and gingiva and may lead to tooth hypersensitivity.
- Brushes that are too soft will not effectively remove plaque and debris, and are only recommended for patients who have extreme tooth hypersensitivity.

KEY POINT Replace toothbrushes at least every three to four months: bristles fray with use and cleaning effectiveness decreases.

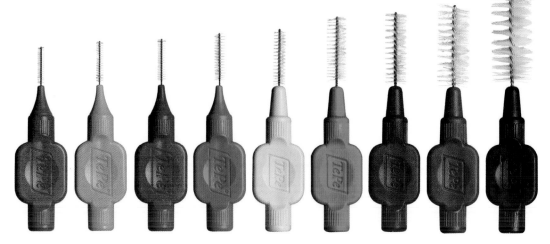

FIGURE 8.3
TePe interdental brushes. Pink = 0.4 mm; orange = 0.45 mm; red = 0.5 mm; blue = 0.6 mm; yellow = 0.7 mm; green = 0.8 mm; purple = 1.1 mm; grey = 1.3 mm.

A variety of toothbrushes are available on the market. Manufacturers are ingenious in how they almost annually produce a new model and introduce gadgets or gimmicks such as lights or music. Some toothbrushes also claim to have therapeutic advantages, but there is not much good evidence for this.

Special toothbrushes are also available for certain patients or situations such as for cleaning difficult areas including implants, braces, crowns and bridges (Box 8.1).

Toothbrushing Techniques

The ideal brushing technique should remove plaque without damaging the teeth, gingiva or other tissues. Many techniques have been developed, involving different combinations of horizontal, vertical, rotary and vibratory motions: all can clean the occlusal, facial and lingual tooth surfaces, but few effectively clean interproximally, and none can clean the contact areas – only floss can achieve this (Table 8.4 and Figure 8.2). Recommended brushing techniques are those that achieve a degree of interproximal cleaning (Table 8.5):

> **KEY POINTS** Patients should try to have a routine brushing pattern to avoid forgetting any areas.
>
> A three-minute brushing time is ideal.

- Roll technique
- Modified Bass technique –the only technique that at all effectively cleans the gingival sulcus
- Modified Charters technique – useful for cleaning fixed orthodontic appliances.

Powered (Electric) Toothbrushes

- Powered toothbrushes are consistently superior to manual toothbrushes for removing plaque, reducing staining and gingivitis, and avoiding gingival abrasions.

BOX 8.1 SPECIAL TOOTHBRUSHES

- Angled brushes – access areas of the mouth that are difficult to reach (Figure 8.2).
- Easy-grip brushes – useful for people whose grip is weak (e.g. people with arthritis). The toothbrush can be enlarged, for example by fixing a ball of sponge rubber, or bicycle handlebar grip to the brush handle (Figure 8.4).
- Extended-handle brushes – effective for patients who cannot lift their arms.
- Interspace and interdental brushes (e.g. TePe brushes, Figure 8.3) – these are helpful for cleaning between teeth and underneath bridges. They consist of a plastic-covered metal wire (to prevent scratching) and come in eight sizes with colour-coded handles, ranging from pink for narrow interdental spaces to grey for larger spaces.
- Proximal brushes – these have a much longer, detachable handle than conventional interdental brushes and are thus easier to use towards the back of the mouth (Figure 8.2B).

TABLE 8.5 Toothbrushing Techniques

Technique	Initial Position of the Bristles	Bristle Movements	Comments
Bass (modified Bass)	45° to the tooth	Vibrated backwards and forwards with a horizontal scrubbing movement	Cleans gingival sulcus but can be time consuming, difficult to master and may cause mild trauma if not done properly with the correct brush. Useful for patients with gingival disease
Charters (modified Charters)	90° to the tooth	Sweep occlusally, vibrate circularly	Fairly good interproximal cleaning
Roll	Apically on attached gingiva	Pressed onto the gingiva to make them spread out, then swept onto the tooth surface. Behind the anterior teeth, the brush is held vertically and pulled upwards or downwards	Particularly useful for people with healthy gingiva
Scrub	90° to tooth	Horizontal brushing	May cause abrasion
Fones	90° to tooth	Circular brushing	May cause abrasion
Leonard	90° to tooth	Vertical brushing	

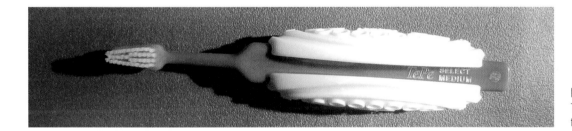

201

FIGURE 8.4
TePe Extra Grip toothbrush.

- They are often light and easy to hold, and are ideal for people with limited manual dexterity.
- Some have timers and displays to guide brushing.
- Some are designed for interspace use.
- Cost is a factor but they are increasingly popular.

Powered brushes with an oscillating/rotating action remove plaque more effectively than do manual brushes and studies show they reduce gingivitis when used for over 3 months. Other powered brushes have not been shown to be as consistently superior to manual brushes.

IDENTIFY AND LEARN
In your local supermarket or pharmacy, look at the various powered toothbrushes available. How much more costly are they than the average manual toothbrush?

Toothbrushing in Children
Brushing should start as soon as the first deciduous tooth erupts. The teeth should be brushed at least twice daily – last thing at night before bed and one other time each day. Few children develop sufficient manual dexterity to clean teeth effectively before about 6 years of age, so either a powered brush should be used or parents should manually brush the teeth. This is best achieved by standing behind the child, and tilting the child's head back so that teeth can be brushed.

Children under about 6 years of age may swallow toothpaste, so only a pea-sized amount of a toothpaste with less than 1000 ppm of fluoride should be used – and brushing should be supervised.

Toothbrushing Damage

Gingival recession and tooth abrasion can be caused by:

- A horizontal scrubbing technique
- Excessive pressure
- Abrasive toothpaste
- Vigorous pressure technique (e.g. Fones and Leonard).

The roll technique can traumatise the mucogingival junction and alveolar mucosa.

Toothbrush Care

Various microorganisms can grow on toothbrushes. There is little evidence that this could lead to adverse oral or systemic health effects. However, some dental associations recommend:

- Do not share toothbrushes (micro-organisms could be transmitted)
- Thoroughly rinse toothbrushes with tap water after brushing to remove any remaining toothpaste and debris
- Store the brush in an upright position if possible and allow the toothbrush to air-dry until used again
- Do not routinely cover toothbrushes or store them in closed containers.

FLOSS AND OTHER TOOTH CLEANING AIDS

As mentioned above, toothbrushes can only remove plaque from smooth surfaces and not from the depths of pits and fissures of teeth, or interproximally. Removal of plaque from between teeth requires regular interdental cleaning (dental floss and dental tape, Figure 8.2).

Most dental associations advise flossing once or more per day after brushing teeth.

- Whether to use regular floss or tape, Teflon or polyethylene, waxed or unwaxed, mint flavour or unflavoured, depends on personal preference and convenience.
- The aid should be threaded between the teeth and gently curled around the side of the tooth, slid down to the gingiva and gently brought back up to the top of the tooth.
- Floss can be difficult to use and can damage the gingiva, so it may be best to use a dental floss holder, such as a Flossette.

TOOTHPASTES (DENTIFRICES)

Toothpastes typically:

- Help remove plaque by their detergent and abrasive activity
- Deliver active ingredients
- Provide a pleasant-tasting mouth and fresh breath.

Toothpastes should not be used by very young children, or anyone else who is likely to swallow a large amount – though small amounts appear not to cause harm. Toothpastes contain:

- Abrasives (to remove plaque and stain) – silica, dicalcium phosphate, calcium carbonate, aluminium oxide (alumina)
- Detergents – sodium lauryl sulphate
- Binders – gums or alginates

- Humectants (to conserve moisture)
- Preservatives – parabens or sodium benzoate
- Sweeteners such as sorbitol
- Flavourings
- Active ingredients – designed for a particular oral health purpose (Box 8.2 and Table 8.6).
  - *Caries protection* – fluorides harden enamel and protect against caries.
  - *Periodontal disease protection* – triclosan (e.g. Total) and chlorhexidine (e.g. Curaprox) have significant anti-plaque activity and protect against periodontitis without harmful reactions.
  - *Anti-calculus activity* – phosphates and phosphonates help prevent calculus but may produce unfavourable mucosal reactions.
  - *Anti-sensitivity action*: strontium fluoride (e.g. Sensodyne), potassium nitrate and potassium oxalate (Protect), potassium nitrate (Emoform), and potassium chloride help reduce tooth sensitivity.
  - *Anti-breath odour* action: triclosan and a copolymer (Colgate Total Toothpaste).
  - *Whitening*: toothpastes often contain carbamide peroxide and can marginally lighten teeth, but the effect is not great and few have reliable supporting evidence for claims.

MOUTHWASHES (MOUTH RINSES)

- *Mouthwashes used by children* may be accidentally swallowed, so they should only be used under adult supervision.
- *Mouthwashes containing alcohol* may cause dryness, burning and, at least theoretically might predispose to cancer. They can be swallowed and cause intoxication, so they should be avoided.
- *Cosmetic mouthwashes* are commercial over-the-counter (OTC) products that:
  - Help remove oral debris before or after brushing
  - Decrease bacterial counts in the mouth
  - Temporarily suppress halitosis
  - Refresh the mouth with a pleasant taste.
- *Therapeutic mouthwashes* have the benefits of the cosmetic counterparts, plus an added active ingredient intended to help protect against some oral condition, usually caries, periodontal disease, and/or halitosis. Therapeutic mouthwashes include those with:
  - Fluoride – these are effective in caries prevention (Figure 8.5): most contain sodium fluoride. If taken excessively or swallowed they can lead over time to fluoride toxicity.
  - Chlorhexidine (e.g. Corsodyl, Figure 8.6) – significantly controls plaque and periodontal disease, and also has some anti-fungal activity. The 0.12% solution is as active in plaque control as is the 0.2% solution. Chlorhexidine can affect taste briefly and it binds tannins and thereby can cause superficial staining if a person drinks coffee, tea, or red wine – but the staining can be cleaned by a dental professional.
  - Triclosan (e.g. Plax) – significantly controls plaque and does not cause tooth-staining.

TABLE 8.6 Examples of Active Principles in Toothpastes

Anti-caries	Antibacterials	Anti-Hypersensitivity	Anti-tartar	Whiteners	Anti-malodour	Others
Calcium phosphate	Chlorhexidine	Potassium citrate	Gantrez acid	Benzalkonium chloride	Chlorhexidine	Essential oils:
Potassium fluoride	Fluorides	Potassium chloride	Potassium pyrophosphate	Calcium phosphates	Zinc citrate	Permethol
Sodium fluoride (NaF) 1450–1500 ppm (<600 ppm in children's toothpaste)	Hexetidine	Sodium citrate	Zinc chloride		Triclosan	Provitamin B5
Sodium monofluorophosphate	Hydrogen peroxide	Sodium fluoride	Zinc citrate	Sodium bicarbonate	Zinc chloride	Tocopherol
Stannous fluoride	Plant extracts	Stannous fluoride		Sodium tripolyphosphate		Vitamin E
Xylitol	Triclosan Urea peroxide Xylitol Zinc citrate	Strontium chloride Strontium fluoride		Calcium carbonate		Keratin Panthenol

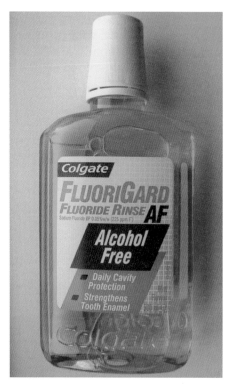

FIGURE 8.5
A fluoridated mouthwash.

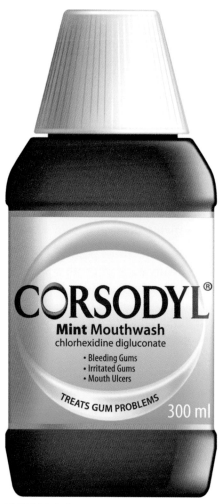

FIGURE 8.6
A chlorhexidine-containing mouthwash.

○ Essential oils – Listerine contains thymol, menthol and eucalyptus oils, helps control plaque and also has some anti-fungal activity. It does not cause tooth staining.

○ Cetylpyridinium chloride (CPC) – possibly helps control plaque and also has some anti-fungal activity. It does not cause tooth staining.

> **KEY POINT** Most of the therapeutic mouthwashes can be safely used for up to one month (but alcohol-free preparations are preferred).

CHEWING GUM

Chewing gum is traditionally made of a natural latex product called chicle, but many modern gums use rubber (polyisobutylene) instead. Chewing gum is available in flavours such as mint, spearmint, wintergreen, cinnamon and various fruits. Sugar-free chewing gum may help contribute to:

- Oral hygiene improvement
- Fresher breath
- Remineralisation of tooth surfaces (those containing calcium phosphate in particular)
- Relief of dry mouth

KEY POINT There are no proven health hazards from chewing gum use but it must always be disposed of carefully. It is banned in Singapore!

- And reduction of:
  - Plaque
  - Calculus
  - Gingivitis
  - Caries.

FISSURE SEALING

Tooth pits and fissures are virtually impossible to clean thoroughly, even with vigorous toothbrushing. Thus these areas can accumulate plaque and are sites prone to caries. Dental sealants are plastic resin coatings placed by the clinician, in the pits and fissures of permanent teeth, designed to reduce caries.

To apply sealants, the dental team involved will:

- Clean the tooth, using pumice
- Wash and dry the tooth with a 3-in-1 syringe
- Apply **acid etchant** solution for 30–60 seconds
- Wash and dry again with a 3-in-1 syringe
- Paint the sealant over pits and fissures
- Cure the sealant with a special blue halogen light (some brands self-cure chemically).

Fissure sealants are especially indicated for people at high risk for caries, such as:

- High caries rate in the deciduous dentition
- Caries in first permanent molars
- Teeth at high risk of caries (e.g. dens in dente (a tooth within a tooth)).

Sealants wear and degrade naturally over time but may last for five or more years and can then be replaced.

Preventive resin restorations are similar, but require some tooth preparation (drilling) first.

> **Term to Learn**
> **Acid etchant:** an acid solution that dissolves away bits of the enamel surface to create 'pores' into which the resin then flows to attach to the tooth. An etched tooth surface appears frosted and dull.

FIND OUT MORE

Use Google image search to look for images of 'dens in dente'.

SCALING, POLISHING AND ROOT PLANING

- Clinicians often achieve good periodontal health by using non-surgical treatments such as scaling and root planing.
- Scaling aims to remove the calculus deposits on the teeth that act an irritant for the gingiva.
- Root planing is the careful cleaning of root surfaces to remove plaque and calculus (tartar) from deep periodontal pockets with scalers (Figure 8.7) and to smooth the tooth root and remove necrotic (dead) cementum.
- The teeth are then polished using a mildly abrasive, flavoured and often fluoride-containing paste (also called prophylaxis paste or 'prophy paste'), which is used with rotating bristle brush or rubber cup (Figure 8.8) in a dental handpiece.
- Instruments that may be used are listed in Table 8.7. Sometimes a local anaesthetic is used topically or by injection to prevent discomfort from scaling.
- Scaling may be followed by adjunctive therapy such as antimicrobials delivered locally.
- Most patients with chronic periodontitis require ongoing maintenance therapy for sustained good oral health.

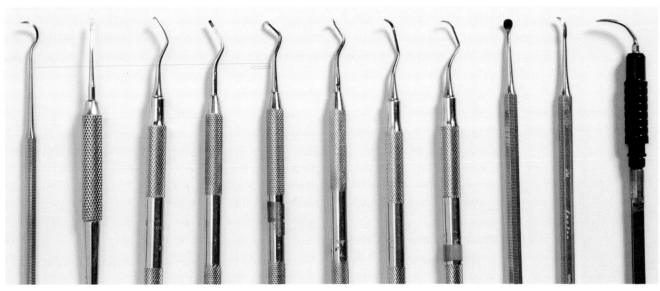

FIGURE 8.7
A selection of scaling instruments. How many can you recognise?

ORAL HEALTH PROCEDURES FOR CHILDREN
Children under 3 Years

- As soon as teeth erupt in the mouth brush them twice daily.
- Brushing should occur twice daily – clean teeth last thing at night before bed and at least one other time each day.
- Children need to be helped or supervised by an adult when brushing.
- Use no more than a smear of toothpaste (a thin film of paste covering less than three-quarters of the brush).
- Children must not be permitted to eat or lick toothpaste from the tube.
- Use a toothpaste containing no less than 1000 ppm fluoride. Family fluoride toothpaste (1350–1500 ppm fluoride) is indicated for maximum caries control for all children except those who cannot be prevented from eating toothpaste.
- Rinsing with lots of water after brushing should be discouraged – spitting out excess toothpaste is preferable.
- Fluoride varnish should be applied to teeth twice yearly.

207

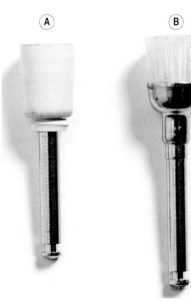

Ⓐ   Ⓑ

FIGURE 8.8
(A) Latch grip rubber cup and (B) bristle brush.

TABLE 8.7 **Instruments Used during Scaling and Polishing**

Function	Instrument*
Pocket depth measurement	BPE probe (Figure 7.9)
Supra-gingival scaling only	Sickle scaler
	Cumine scaler
	Jaquette scaler
	Watchspring scaler (push)
Sub-gingival scaling also	Gracey curette
	Ultrasonic scaler

*To avoid damage, Teflon-coated or plastic scalers, and no ultrasonics are used when working around dental implants.

Terms to Learn
Supra-gingival: the part of the tooth outside the gingival cuff.
Sub-gingival: part of the tooth covered by the gingiva.

Children between 3 and 6 Years

- Children need to be helped or supervised by an adult when brushing until at least 7 years of age and must not be permitted to eat or lick toothpaste from the tube.
- Use no more than a pea-sized amount of toothpaste.
- Rinsing with lots of water after brushing should be discouraged – spitting out excess toothpaste is preferable.
- Disclosing tablets can help to indicate areas that are being missed.
- Brushing is more effective with a small-headed toothbrush with soft (ISO 8627:1987 standard 1–3), round-ended filaments, a compact, angled arrangement of long and short filaments, and a handle which is comfortable.
- Powered brushes with an oscillating/rotating action can be helpful.
- Parents should help with toothbrushing.

Children 7 Years and Older

- Use a pea-sized amount or smear of fluoridated toothpaste – 1450 ppm (unless the child cannot be prevented from eating toothpaste).
- Encourage spitting out toothpaste after brushing rather than rinsing.
- Fluoride varnish should be applied by the clinician three to four times yearly (2.2% NaF = 22 600 ppm fluoride).
- The permanent molars should be fissure sealed with resin sealant.
- Encourage use of toothpastes containing triclosan with copolymer to improve levels of plaque control or use toothpastes containing triclosan with zinc citrate. Chlorhexidine varnish can help.
- These children should clean interdentally using interdental brushes or floss.
- For those with active caries:
    - 8+ years – the clinician will prescribe daily fluoride rinse
    - 10+ years – the clinician will prescribe 2800 ppm fluoride toothpaste
    - 18+ years – the clinician will consider prescription of 5000 ppm fluoride toothpaste.

FIND OUT MORE

The ISO is the International Organization for Standardization. Visit the ISO website (http://www.iso.org/iso/home.htm) to find out more about its work.

PREVENTION OF OTHER ORAL DISEASE
Tooth Erosion

Drinks, foods and medication with tooth erosive potential include:

- Drinks containing citric acid, e.g. orange, grapefruit, lemon, blackcurrant
- Carbonated drinks
- Alcopops and designer drinks
- Cider
- White wine
- Fruit teas (but not camomile)
- Some sports drinks which contain acid
- Acidic fresh fruit (lemons, oranges, grapefruit) that are consumed with high frequency
- Pickles
- Chewable vitamin C tablets, aspirin, some iron preparations.

Erosion prevention includes:

- Reducing the amount and frequency of intake of the above foods and drinks
- Avoiding gastric regurgitation and exposure to other erosive acids.

ADVICE TO PREVENT EROSION PROGRESSING

- Avoid frequent intake of acidic foods or drinks – keep them to meal times, and use a straw for acidic drinks.
- Do not brush immediately after eating or drinking acidic food or drinks.
- Do not brush immediately after vomiting.
- Use toothpaste containing 1450 ppm fluoride twice daily.
- Professional action that may be taken:
  - Sensitive investigation of diet to identify the source of acid
  - Investigation of habits which exacerbate effects of erosion
  - Tailored, specific advice for each individual patient.

Tooth Hypersensitivity

Hypersensitivity prevention includes avoiding tooth surface loss, which exposes the sensitive dentine at the neck of the tooth. The treatment includes:

- Modification of toothbrushing technique to ensure the gingiva are not damaged by excessive or inappropriate toothbrushing
- Application of desensitising agents, e.g. fluoride varnish
- Daily use of a fluoride mouthwash
- Regular daily use of a desensitising toothpaste.

Mouth Trauma

Damage to the mouth can be avoided by:

- Careful behaviour
- Avoiding dangerous activities, violence and assaults
- Wearing protective wear such as a mouth guard or a splint for:
  - Contact sports
  - Tooth grinding (bruxism)
  - Acid erosion
  - Radiotherapy.

Cancer

Given that lifestyle factors are the main risk factors for oral cancer, the clinician will take history of tobacco, betel and alcohol use. The patients will require advice and some contact details for services that will help them stop using these. Take a history of the diet and encourage them to adopt good dietary practices.

Patients should:

- Not smoke
- Not use smokeless tobacco (e.g. betel, chewing tobacco, gutkha)
- Reduce alcohol consumption to moderate (recommended) levels
- Maintain good dietary practices and increase fruit and vegetable intake to at least five portions per day.

FIND OUT MORE

Find out more about oral cancer prevention at:
http://www.cancer.gov/cancertopics/pdq/prevention/oral/Patient

209

SUMMARY

Box 8.3 summarises the key oral health messages you have learnt in this chapter.

BOX 8.3 MAIN WAYS TO MAINTAIN ORAL HEALTH

Diet
- Reduce the consumption and especially the frequency of intake of sugar-containing food and drink.
- Sugar-containing food and drink should be consumed as part of a meal
- Snacks and drinks should be free of sugars
- Avoid the frequent consumption of acidic drinks.

Tooth Cleansing
- Brush and floss the teeth thoroughly twice every day and use a fluoride toothpaste.
- Toothbrushing alone cannot prevent dental decay but fluoride toothpastes offer major benefits.
- Effective plaque removal is essential to prevent periodontal disease.

Fluoridation
- Request the local water company to supply water with the optimum fluoride level.
- Consider use of fluoride supplements for children at high risk and those living in areas without water fluoridation.

Regular Visits to the Dentist
- Have an oral examination every year.
- Children or other people at special risk from oral disease (e.g. people with hyposalivation), and those for whom oral disease can be a particular risk to their health (e.g. people with heart problems) may need to be examined more frequently.

CHAPTER 9

Restorative Procedures and Materials

> **CHAPTER POINTS**
> - This chapter covers the requirements of the NEBDN syllabus Section 9: Restorative dentistry.

WHAT IS RESTORATIVE DENTISTRY?

Restorative dentistry forms a major part of the workload of general dentistry, being the branch of dentistry involved in treatment of the common dental diseases – dental caries and periodontal disease, and their sequelae, including loss of teeth. Thus the specialty of restorative dentistry includes **endodontics**, **periodontics** and **prosthodontics**. Prosthodontists are also sometimes called 'conservative clinicians'.

A dental *restoration* (filling) is used to restore the tooth shape (morphology) and function. Restorations have to be custom-made for every patient, because each patient presents with a unique colour, shape and size of their teeth and relationship of their upper and lower jaws. Each patient also has their own unique aesthetics, depending on the colour, size and shape of their teeth, face and jaws and tone of their facial muscles.

OVERVIEW OF THE ROLE OF THE DENTAL NURSE IN RESTORATIVE PROCEDURES

Before Restorative Treatment

- Retrieve case notes, radiographs, consent forms and check medical history.
- Prepare the dental environment, ensuring effective infection control.
- Prepare trolley or tray using aseptic technique.
- Greet and reassure the patient in the waiting area and be their advocate.
- Ensure pre-operative advice has been followed.
- Inform the clinician of any changes/comment from the patient.
- Assist the patient to the dental chair and make comfortable.
- Provide the patient with protective equipment (bib and glasses, Figure 9.1).
- Provide a bowl with water for dentures (if required).

During Restorative Treatment

- Reassure patient.
- Assist with topical and local anaesthetic administration if required (see Chapter 13).
- Assist with rubber dam placement if required.

> **Terms to Learn**
> **Endodontics:** the dental specialty concerned with the management of the diseases of the pulp.
> **Periodontics:** the specialty of dentistry concerned with the study and management of gingival and periodontal diseases.
> **Prosthodontics:** the specialty of dentistry concerned with the replacement of missing teeth or other oral structures.

211

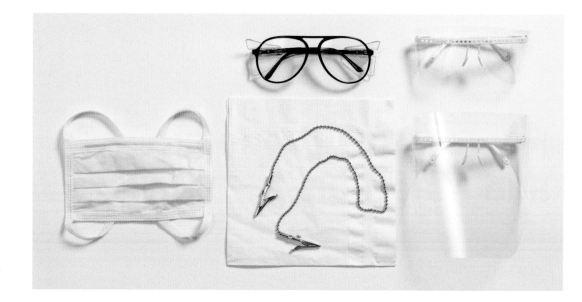

FIGURE 9.1
Protective wear for patients and dental care professionals.

212

Term to Learn
Impression material: a viscous mouldable material that sets to a firm consistency in the mouth to make an 'impression' of the teeth and surrounding structures.

- Aspirate to ensure a clear field and patient comfort if required.
- Anticipate and pass instruments/items as required.
- Mix materials as appropriate and pass as required.
- Develop and label radiographs as required.

After Restorative Treatment

- Provide a mirror and tissues for the patient to wipe their face and assist if necessary.
- Assist patient to the recovery room or waiting area.
- Ensure the patient has a post-operative instruction sheet if required.
- Make a follow up appointment as required.
- Decontaminate the environment and sterilise instruments.
- Dispose of local anaesthetic needle in the correct sharps container.
- Dispose of clinical waste in yellow bags.
- Disinfect and label impressions ready for laboratory with clinician's prescription as required.

DENTAL IMPRESSIONS

A dental impression is an accurate representation of part or all of a person's dentition and adjacent tissue of the mouth. A dental impression is usually made by placing an **impression material** into the mouth, usually in an impression tray (Figure 9.2). The impression material then sets or hardens so that, when removed from the mouth, it retains the shape of the teeth and/or mouth. It forms a 'negative' of a person's teeth and adjacent soft tissues, which is then used to make a cast or model (Figure 9.3) of the dentition, usually from *dental plaster*. The model may be used either as a record of the person's dentition (called a *study model*) or by the dental technician to make:

- Special impression trays which more closely fit the individual patient, in preparation for making dentures
- Indirect restorations: e.g. **inlays**, **onlays**, **crowns** (these are all discussed later in the chapter)
- Other dental prostheses or appliances.

There are several different kinds of impression materials and their properties are described in detail below and in Chapter 12. Impressions are increasingly being made using computers, the basis of **CAD-CAM dentistry**.

Terms to Learn
Inlay: a restoration (such as gold or porcelain) fitted into a cavity and cemented into place.
Onlay: a restoration (such as gold or porcelain) fitted over the occlusal surface of a tooth and cemented into place.
Crown: a crown is like a cap that completely or partially covers a tooth's natural crown.
CAD-CAM dentistry: computer-aided design and computer-aided manufacturing in dentistry.

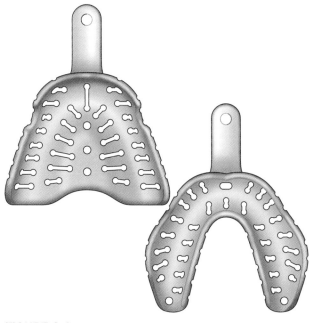

FIGURE 9.2
Upper and lower impression trays.

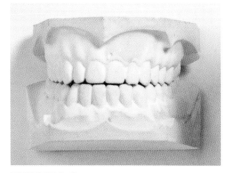

FIGURE 9.3
Upper and lower dental models.

PRIMARY AND SECONDARY IMPRESSIONS

Primary impressions, which are the initial impressions, are often taken using alginates (p. 214) in a *stock impression tray* (see Figure 9.4). The resulting cast is then used by the dental technician to make a *special tray*. Then a *secondary impression* is made – using a more accurate impression material such as an elastomer (p. 215) – in the special tray.

213

The Dental Nurse's Role in Impression Taking

You will need to offer a range of impression trays of different sizes for the clinician to select for use. Differently shaped trays are available for people with or without natural teeth (Figure 9.4). In order that the impression material once set remains firmly in position in the tray, the trays may be perforated, rim locked and/or you may need to apply a special adhesive to the tray before use. You then mix the impression material and place it in the impression tray chosen. With suitable training, dental nurses can also take certain impressions.

You must wash and disinfect the impressions once they are removed from the mouth and label them before despatching to the laboratory with a prescription:

1. Rinse under running cold tap water to remove blood/saliva.
2. Disinfect as appropriate (see Box 9.1).
3. Seal in plastic biological hazard bag with label (name, date of return and prescription).

BOX 9.1 POINTS TO REMEMBER WHEN DISINFECTING IMPRESSION MATERIALS

- No single disinfectant is ideal or compatible with all items: iodophors, sodium hypochlorite (1:10 concentration), chlorine dioxide, phenols are examples of acceptable disinfectants.
- The exposure time should be that recommended by the manufacturer of the disinfectant for tuberculocidal disinfection.
- The **dimensional stability** of impressions is rarely much affected by immersion techniques; however, polyether materials cannot be immersed for long periods in disinfectants due to potential for absorption and distortion.

Term to Learn
Dimensional stability: impressions can distort when taken out of the mouth or shrink if they dry out. They can also expand if left in liquids too long due to absorption (imbibition).

Alginate Impression Material ('Alginate')

Alginate is one of the most commonly used impression materials. It is supplied as a powder, which is mixed with tap water to make a gelatinous mass. This mass then sets (hardens) rapidly. Alginate powder must be stored in a cool dry place in a tightly closed container to protect it from absorbing moisture from the air and from contamination. Shake the container before use to loosen the powder and then leave it for a few minutes before opening to let the dust settle. Powder and water measuring cups are provided by the manufacturer. Measure out the powder into the mixing bowl (Figure 9.4) and add a measured amount of tap water at room temperature (21 °C). Alginates set fairly quickly; the best method of controlling the setting time is to slightly alter the temperature of the water used in the mix. The higher the water temperature, the faster the material will set.

ADVANTAGES

- Alginates are relatively cheap.
- They are flexible once set.
- They are sufficiently elastic to return to their original shape after the slight distortion during their removal from the mouth once set.

DISADVANTAGES

- Alginates are weak materials and may tear on removal from deep undercuts (e.g. when teeth are tilted and the material gets under them).
- They can also distort with time, especially if they dry out, so they must always be kept moist.

To keep moist, wrap the impression in damp gauze or, if the impression must be stored for a short period of time, place it in a humidor in which the relative humidity is 100%. The cast should be poured soon after the impression is removed from the mouth.

USES

Alginates are satisfactory for taking primary impressions and for many of the impressions required in prosthetic work. But they can also distort due to syneresis (separation of liquid

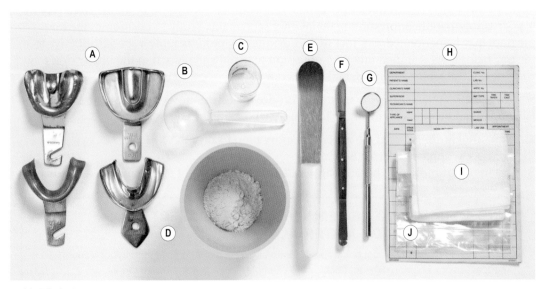

FIGURE 9.4
Items required for an alginate impression: (A) stock impression trays; (B) scoop for measuring out alginate powder; (C) water measure; (D) plastic mixing bowl with alginate powder; (E) plaster spatula; (F) wax knife; (G) mouth mirror; (H) laboratory prescription (instruction) sheet and label; (I) gauze for keeping the impressions moist; and (J) plastic bag to put the impressions in for sending to the laboratory.

214

from the gel), imbibition etc. So for the more accurate impressions, as are required for crowns and bridges (see later), other impression materials such as elastomers are used.

Elastomeric Impression Materials (Elastomers, 'Rubber Base')

Elastomers give better impressions (more accurate and stable) than do alginates. There are three main types of elastomers:

- *Silicone-based*: The silicone base is a paste that comes packaged in tubes. The paste reacts with another material (the chemical reactor), which may be either a paste or a bottled liquid that must be stored in a cool place. This is because it deteriorates after about six months. Varying the amount of chemical reactor changes the setting time of the elastomer. There are two types of silicone impression material depending on the chemical reactor: addition cured (the accuracy of these is very good) and condensation cured.
- *Polysulphide*: The polysulphide base and its chemical reactor are both provided as pastes packaged in separate tubes. Polysulphide impressions do not require special storage and can be stored indefinitely. Increased relative humidity and temperature shorten both setting and mixing time. The accuracy of polysulphides is good but they have an unpleasant smell (bad eggs) and are messy to use.
- *Polyethers*: Polyethers have good accuracy but are rather stiff, and this can cause problems, particularly where the **preparations** are small and narrow or the undercuts deep or multiple. The lower central and lateral incisors are good examples of this. There is a risk of damage to the plaster teeth on the model as the impression is removed from it. For this reason, some technicians are not enthusiastic about the use of polyethers.

> **Term to Learn**
> **Preparation:** a tooth that has been carefully shaped with a dental drill for receiving a crown or filling.

The bases and the chemical reactors of elastomers are usually of different colours. Some products are provided in special mixing syringes. For others, you will need to lay out equal lengths of both the base material and the chemical reactor (*catalyst*) separately but side by side onto a special polymer paper or parchment pad. The reactor should not touch the base material until everything is ready to mix: then you mix the two pastes with a spatula in the prescribed time, until no streaks remain. A thin uniform layer of elastomer impression material is required to give the most accurate impression, so the materials are used in individually designed (*custom* or *special tray*) acrylic trays. You will need to apply a tray adhesive to prevent the impression from pulling away from the tray and distorting. Most elastomer impressions are dimensionally stable if stored dry, and thus they may be sent to the technician without a major risk of dimensional change.

215

> **KEY POINT** Polyether elastomeric impressions will distort if sharing a bag with a damp alginate impression.

ADVANTAGES

- Elastomers are flexible and rubber-like once they set, and sufficiently elastic to return to their original shape after slight distortion.
- They do not significantly distort after setting.
- They do not tend to dry out but the cast is still best poured within 30 minutes after an impression is made. This is because some elastomers undergo shrinkage on setting that continues for some time after the impression is made, particularly the condensation silicone type. However, these materials are not subject to syneresis and imbibition because they are hydrophobic (water-hating).

DISADVANTAGES

- Elastomers are expensive compared with alginates.
- They are more liable than alginates to produce allergic reactions, so should be handled carefully and sparingly.

USES

Elastomers are used for making impressions of areas containing undercuts, especially for crowns, inlays, bridges, **dental implants** and removable and fixed partial dentures (see p. 215).

IMPRESSION TRAY SET-UP (Figure 9.4)

Impression trays	To carry impression materials
Impression adhesive	For aiding adhesion of material to tray
Straight handpiece and acrylic trimmer (Figure 9.5)	For adjustment of tray if needed
Impression material	
Mixing bowl or pad	
Spatula	
Shade guide	
Laboratory prescription (instruction) sheet and label	For custom instruction to technician
Gauze swabs	For damping and placing over alginate impression
Self-seal plastic bag	For transporting to the laboratory
Mirror	For patient to view their appearance for shade selection and ensuring face is clean

TREATMENT OF CARIES

Caries prevention is discussed in Chapter 8, both the measures that the patient can take and the measures that the clinician can take (applying dental fissure sealants). Here we discuss the restoration of teeth which have been damaged by caries.

REPAIRING DAMAGED OR DISEASED TEETH – MAKING A RESTORATION

The Dental Nurse's Role

REMOVING THE CARIES

You will need to assist the clinician, mainly by controlling moisture and debris; they remove the caries and prepare the tooth for a restoration (this can be a filling, inlay, crown or bridge).

MOISTURE CONTROL AND RUBBER DAM

Moisture control is very important for two reasons:

- To allow the clinician to be able to see clearly what they are doing in the mouth
- Moisture can damage the restoration or its adherence to the tooth (Table 9.1).

Moisture control is also crucial in endodontics to prevent spread of infection.

When preparing and placing fillings there are several ways to control moisture (Box 9.2). Use of rubber dam (or dental dam, Figure 9.6) is the most effective.

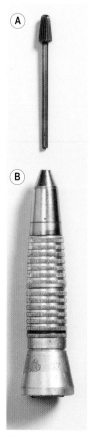

FIGURE 9.5
(A) Acrylic trimmer
(B) Straight handpiece.

TABLE 9.1 Damaging Effects of Moisture on the Setting of Restorations

Materials	Effects of Moisture
Amalgam	Expansion of material
Cement	Fails to adhere to tooth structure; setting time altered
Composite	Fails to adhere to tooth structure
Glass ionomer	Fails to set properly

216

The rubber dam is a thin square of latex rubber (also available in silicone for latex-sensitive patients). To accommodate the teeth being treated, holes are made in the sheet with a rubber dam punch, and the dam is held in place on the teeth by rubber dam clamps or dental floss (Figure 9.6).

> **KEY POINT** The rubber dam isolates the tooth being treated from its environment, retracts and protects the lips and cheeks, and avoids inhalation of small instruments or debris.

You will need to prepare the rubber dam, assist the clinician with placement and use the suction during cavity preparation or endodontics to remove debris, saliva and water. Figure 9.7 shows a selection of suction tips that can be attached to the suction machine and are placed inside mouth.

FIND OUT MORE

Not all suction tips are suitable for all procedures. Try to match the tips shown in Figure 9.7 with the procedures they are best suited for.

BOX 9.2 METHODS OF MOISTURE CONTROL

- Rubber dam placed on the teeth being treated.
- Aspiration by the dental nurse.
- Saliva ejector in the floor of the mouth.
- Cotton wool rolls placed near the openings of the major salivary gland ducts inside the cheeks, and in the floor of the mouth.
- 'Dry guards' placed in the buccal and lingual sulci.

217

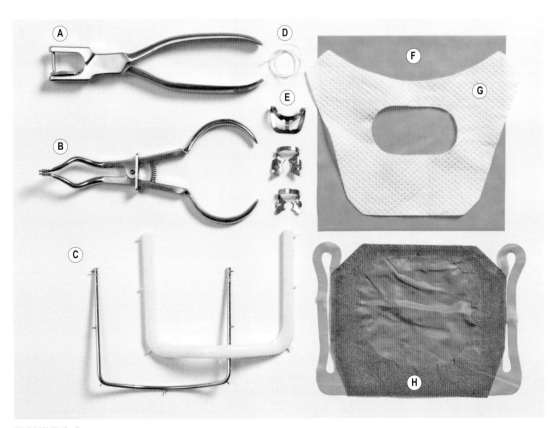

FIGURE 9.6
Rubber dam equipment: (A) rubber dam punch; (B) rubber dam clamp; (C) rubber dam frames; (D) dental floss; (E) a selection of rubber dam clamps; (F) rubber dam sheet; (G) rubber dam napkin; and (H) dry dam.

CAVITY PREPARATION

Teeth are prepared for the restoration using:

- Burs (Figure 9.8): either in an air-rotor (fast speed) or contra-angle (slow speed) handpiece (Figure 9.9)

and/or

- Hand instruments such as excavators (Figure 9.10).

The main aim is to remove all of the decayed parts of the tooth but at the same time avoid damage to the underlying dental pulp. Once the clinician has prepared the cavity, the pulp is protected by applying a lining cement with an instrument called a 'plastic' (labelled H in Figure 9.10).

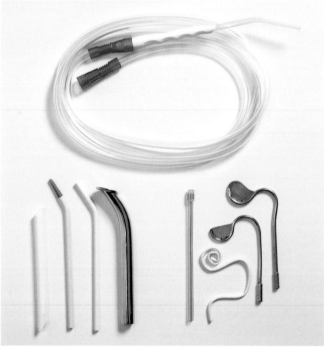

FIGURE 9.7
A selection of suction tips.

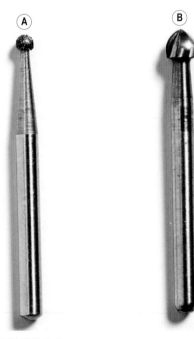

FIGURE 9.8
(A) A diamond bur and (B) a steel bur.

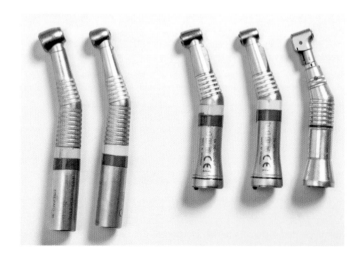

FIGURE 9.9
A selection of air-rotor and latch-grip, contra-angle handpieces.

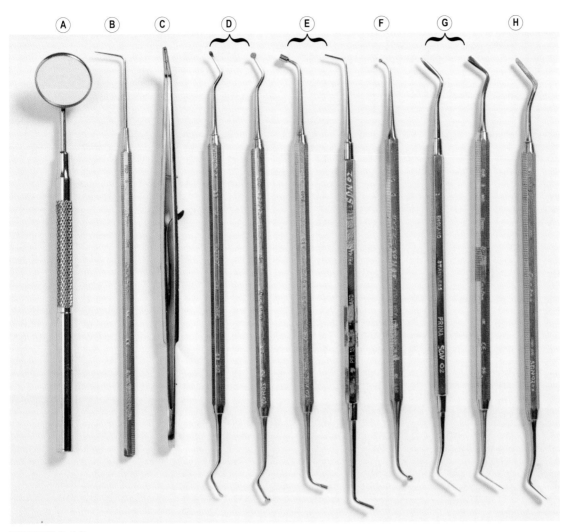

FIGURE 9.10
Instruments used for cavity preparation and amalgam restorations: (A) mouth mirror; (B) straight probe; (C) tweezers; (D) excavators; (E) amalgam condensers (pluggers); (F) amalgam burnisher; (G) amalgam carvers; and (H) flat plastic instrument.

DENTAL CEMENTS

Dental cements are used to:

- Line deep cavities to protect the pulp from thermal and other types of irritation.
- Secure indirect restorations (crowns, inlays, bridges) into or on the teeth (often called luting cement).

Cements are described in Chapter 12. They are usually prepared by the dental nurse. Several cements are supplied in capsules containing pre-proportioned powder and liquid. These are not only convenient but ensure consistent powder/liquid ratios and thus predictable setting times and ultimately the lining strength.

If cement is supplied in bottle form:

- Follow the manufacturer's instructions both for storage and mixing of the material.
- Ask the clinician whether they want you to cool the glass mixing slab (Figure 9.11) in the refrigerator prior to mixing, to slow down the reaction rate and increase the working time.

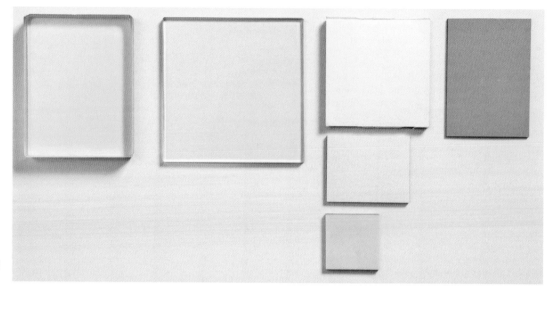

FIGURE 9.11
Selection of glass slabs and paper pads for mixing dental cements.

- Dispense the powder before the liquid, to minimise the loss of water due to evaporation. Fluff up the powder in the bottle before using the dispensing measuring scoop – this will help distribute particles evenly and will assist in providing an even mix.
- Hold the bottle or vial upright to ensure consistent sized drops when dispensing the liquid.
- Use the correct powder/liquid ratio since this influences:
  - The working and setting time
  - The consistency and flow
  - The degree of solubility
  - Erosion
  - Strength.

Mix the powder and liquid using the cement spatula (Figure 9.12).

FACTORS THAT INFLUENCE THE PERFORMANCE OF CEMENTS

- Incorporating too much or too little powder.
- Room or mixing slab temperature too high.
- Premature exposure of cement to moisture.
- Delay between completion of the mix and seating in restoration.
- Surface contamination of the crown or tooth preparation.
- Whether the cement is adhesive and the tooth surface has been etched.

DENTAL RESTORATIONS

These can be divided into:

- Direct restorations (made in the clinic)
- Indirect restorations (made in the laboratory).

They can be further classified by their location and size, or type of material used as discussed below and in Chapter 12.

Direct dental restorations are usually made by the clinician in the clinic, by filling the cavity with a material such as amalgam or a plastic resin, which then sets hard. Indirect restorations are made by the technician in the laboratory. Then the clinician must usually first take an

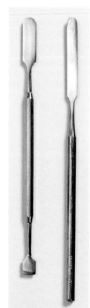

FIGURE 9.12
Cement spatulas.

impression of the tooth cavity so that the technician can make a **die** on which to produce the restoration. This is then cemented by the clinician into the cavity, using cement as above. Occasionally, a clinician will make a wax restoration in the mouth which is then sent to the laboratory for the technician to cast in gold.

The main advantages of the indirect method of tooth restoration are that the materials used in these restorations have better mechanical properties (such as strength) than do those used for direct restorations. Also much of the work is done away from the dental chairside by the technician, on a die created from an impression of the teeth.

Direct Restorations

PROVISIONAL OR TEMPORARY RESTORATIONS

These are made as a temporary measure during the course of complex treatments or when diagnosing pain. For these restorations, the materials used are relatively soft and easy to remove, such as zinc oxide eugenol (see Chapter 12).

PERMANENT RESTORATIONS

Common materials used for permanent direct restorations are: dental amalgam, glass ionomer cement and composite resins. The properties of all these materials are described in Chapter 12. Here we describe the role of the dental nurse in handling of these materials in the clinic.

AMALGAM RESTORATIONS

The cavity preparation for an amalgam filling is fairly destructive. This means some sound tooth structure must be removed to ensure the cavity will mechanically retain the filling when set. This is because amalgam does not adhere to tooth structure.

Steps in Placing an Amalgam Filling

1. The rubber dam is placed and the cavity prepared.
2. In teeth with loss of marginal tooth structure the cavity may lack a wall on one or more sides. In such cases offer the clinician a matrix band (Figure 9.13) and wedges (Figure 9.14).

> **Term to Learn**
> **Die:** this is a positive likeness of the teeth that is usually composed of a special kind of plaster called dental stone which is much harder than plaster of Paris.

221

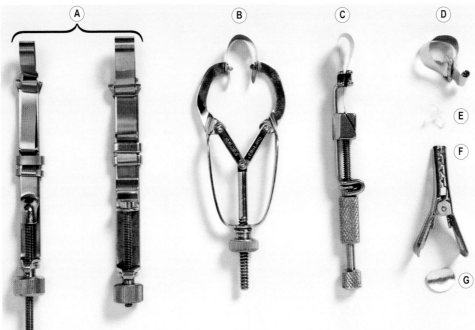
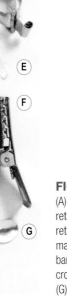

FIGURE 9.13
(A) Siqveland matrix retainers; (B) Ivory matrix retainer; (C) Tofflemire matrix retainer; (D) matrix band; (E) temporary acrylic crown; (F) butterfly clip; (G) cervical matrix.

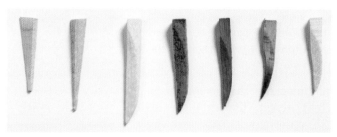

FIGURE 9.14

A selection of wedges.

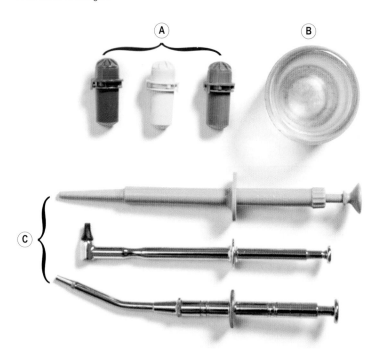

FIGURE 9.15

(A) Amalgam capsules; (B) glass amalgam pot; (C) straight and right-angled amalgam carriers.

The clinician will use these to form a temporary wall when packing the filling.

3. Mix the amalgam in an amalgamator by placing a capsule (Figure 9.15) in it.

Fill the amalgam carrier (Figure 9.15) with the mixed amalgam and give it to the clinician.

- The clinician places the amalgam in the cavity.
- Amalgam remains plastic for a short time so it can be packed (condensed) to fill the cavity with the amalgam plugger (Figure 9.10, E) or automatic vibrator.
- Before it hardens to a strong filling, the clinician carves it to a tooth shape using amalgam carvers (Figure 9.10, G) and may smooth the surface with cotton pledgets or a burnisher (Figure 9.10, F).
- At a later appointment, the amalgam is polished.
- Amalgam waste must be disposed of safely (see Subchapter 1.2).

IDENTIFY AND LEARN

Identify an amalgamator in your workplace and learn how it works.

Try fitting a metal matrix band in its holder.

FIND OUT MORE

What is used for polishing amalgam?

THE AMALGAM TRAY

Amalgam carrier (Figure 9.15)	Used to deliver amalgam to cavity
Amalgam plugger (Figure 9.10)	Used to compact amalgam
Carver (e.g. Ward's) (Figure 9.10)	Used to carve the amalgam surface to the original anatomical shape
Burnisher (Figure 9.10)	Used to smooth the amalgam
Cotton wool pellets/pledgets (Figure 9.16) and tweezers (Figure 9.17)	Used to smooth the surface of the filling
Enamel chisel (Figure 9.18)	Used to remove unsupported enamel
Excavator (Figure 9.10)	Used to remove carious dentine
Flat plastic (Figure 9.10)	Used to carry and adapt restorative materials to cavity
Gauze swabs (Figure 9.16)	
Gingival margin trimmer (Figure 9.19)	Used to remove unsupported enamel
Matrix bands (Figure 9.13) and wedges (Figure 9.14)	Used to produce a correctly shaped filling
Mouth mirror (Figure 9.17)	Aids direct vision
Straight probe (Figure 9.17)	

COMPOSITE RESINS

The cavity preparation for a resin filling is fairly conservative. The bare minimum of tooth structure is removed since resins adhere to tooth structure. Composite resin fillings (also called white or tooth-coloured fillings) *bond* (adhere) to the tooth surface after the enamel has been first *etched* with a special weak acid (phosphoric acid). Composite resin fillings require a clean dry surface to bond with the tooth. *Dentine-bonding agents* are resin materials used to make a composite filling material adhere to both dentine and enamel.

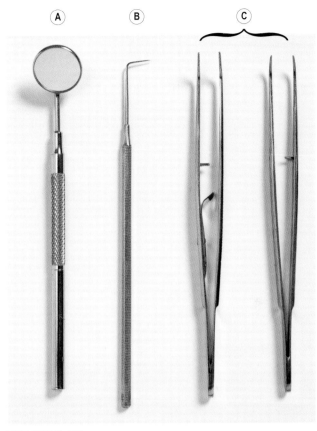

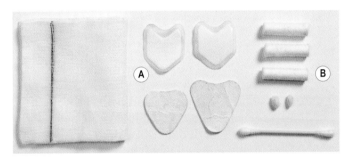

FIGURE 9.16
A selection of (A) gauze swabs; (B) cotton rolls and pledgets.

FIGURE 9.17
(A) Mouth mirror; (B) straight probe; (C) tweezers.

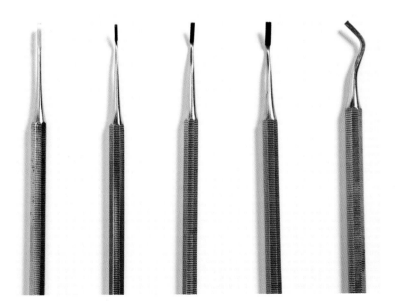

FIGURE 9.18
A selection of enamel chisels.

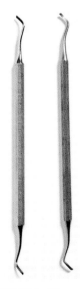

FIGURE 9.19
Gingival margin trimmers.

Term to Learn
Polymerisation:
The process by which thousands of small molecules of a substance (called monomers) combine together to form three-dimensional networks of long-chain molecules. The substance is then called a polymer.

Steps in Placing a Composite Filling

1. Acid-etch enamel conditioning: a 37% solution of phosphoric acid is placed on the enamel (check manufacturer's instructions for amount of time: usually between 15 and 60 seconds), then washed off with water from the 3-in-1 syringe, and dried with air to leave a chalky, or frosted, etched surface to which the resin will bond mechanically.
2. Dentine bonding: if this is required, an aqueous solution of 2-hydroxyethyl methacrylate (HEMA) – a plastic material – is applied to the conditioned dentine. This flows into the dentine tubules and bonds with the collagen inside and around each tubule.

Then mix the two parts of the composite and give it to the clinician using a plastic instrument rather than a metal one as that can stain the material.

The composite is placed in the cavity by the clinician. A clear matrix band may sometimes be used to achieve the correct shape. Composite resin remains soft until cured.

The resin may be cured (**polymerised**) by:

- *Chemical reaction* – between the two parts when they are mixed together.
- *Action of light* – a special hand-held curing light source (Figure 9.20) is used that emits light of a specific wavelength onto the resin. This sets off a reaction in the material and it hardens. The curing light should be held as close to the resin surface as possible, and a shield must be placed between the light tip and the eyes (operator's and dental nurse's) to protect their eyes from damage.
- *Both chemical and light action* – these are called dual-cure resins.

IDENTIFY AND LEARN

Identify in your workplace a clear matrix band and plastic wedge.

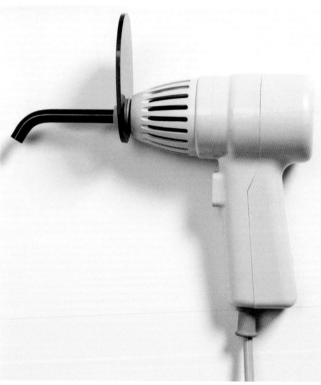

FIGURE 9.20
Blue halogen light source.

THE COMPOSITE TRAY

Rubber dam (Figure 9.6)	Isolation of field
Excavator (Figure 9.10)	To remove carious dentine
Clear matrix bands and plastic wedges (Figures 9.13 and 9.14)	To produce a correctly shaped filling
Etchant and brush	
Flat plastic (not metal) (Figure 9.10)	To carry and adapt restorative materials to cavity
Mouth mirror (Figure 9.17)	
Straight probe (Figure 9.17)	
Tweezers (Figure 9.17)	

GLASS IONOMER CEMENTS (GICS) AND RESIN-MODIFIED GICS

The cavity preparation for a GIC filling is the same as for a composite resin; it is fairly conservative and a bare minimum of tooth structure should be removed. When GIC is applied directly to enamel and dentine that has not been conditioned with acid etch or dentine conditioner it dissolves some **hydroxyapatite**. The metallic polyalkenoate salts in the GIC combine with the hydroxyapatite helping the GIC to chemically adhere to the tooth.

Term to Learn
Hydroxyapatite: the main inorganic material that forms the tooth's hard tissues.

Indirect Restorations

Materials for indirect restorations are also described in Chapter 12. All of these are retained in the tooth with cements. Indirect restorations can be inlays or onlays. Common indirect restorative materials are gold, porcelain and zirconia. Indirect restorations can also be fabricated from composites. These are used for full crowns (Figure 9.21) and even for bridges (Figures 9.21 and 9.22).

FIND OUT MORE

Computers are increasingly becoming a part of crown and bridge fabrication, such as in CAD/CAM technology. Does your workplace laboratory use CAD/CAM?

GOLD

Advantages of gold fillings (inlays or onlays):

- Excellent durability
- Wear well
- Do not cause excessive wear of the opposing teeth.

Disadvantages:

- Unaesthetic
- Expensive
- Conduct heat and cold.

PORCELAIN (CERAMIC)

Porcelain crowns usually have a ceramic coping of either alumina porcelain or zirconia, called the 'core'. The porcelain crown covers the core. Porcelain is also used for veneers.

Advantages of porcelain restorations:

- Excellent aesthetics

Disadvantages:

- Brittle and hard and can break
- Can cause wear on opposing teeth because they are harder than enamel.

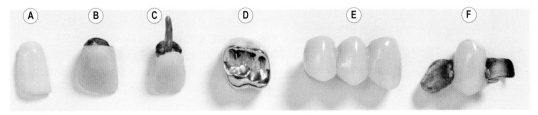

FIGURE 9.21
A selection of restorations: (A) porcelain veneer; (B) porcelain bonded jacket crown; (C) post crown; (D) full gold crown; (E) conventional bridge; (F) resin-retained bridge.

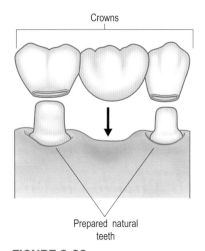

FIGURE 9.22
A bridge with abutment teeth.

CROWNS

Temporary Crowns (Figure 9.23)

Temporary crowns are used to cover the tooth while the laboratory is making the permanent gold or porcelain crowns.

Full Gold Crowns

Full gold crowns (FGCs; Figure 9.21) are cast from gold alloy in the laboratory, using the *lost-wax technique*:

1. After the clinician prepares the tooth for a crown, he or she will take an impression.
2. This is sent to a dental laboratory where a die is made.
3. The dental laboratory technician will then build up on the die the pattern of the crown restoration in wax.
4. This wax pattern is then invested in a special investment material, and placed in a furnace to burn off the wax to leave a space within the investment material.
5. This investment pattern is then placed in a centrifuge where gold alloy is melted down and rapidly shot through into the investment to make the gold crown.

Porcelain-fused-to-metal Crowns

- Porcelain-fused-to-metal (PFM; Figure 9.21BC) crowns consist of a metal shell or *coping*, which is covered with feldspathic porcelain.
  - The alloy used is different from that used in conventional gold crowns.
  - This alloy is able to withstand the intense temperatures of the ceramic furnace, which are necessary to bake the porcelain.

Porcelain Crowns

- Porcelain crowns (Figure 9.21A) are aesthetic but they are less durable than PFM crowns.
- In-ceram is an 'all-ceramic crown' with glass.
- Procera AllCeram is a CAD/CAM based method that produces a crown by overlaying a very durable ceramic coping.
- The coping or core is made of either alumina or zirconium.
- The Empress system is similar to a lost-wax technique in that a hollow investment pattern is made. A specially designed pressure-injected leucite-reinforced ceramic is then pressed into the mould.

CEREC is a CAD/CAM all-ceramic restoration made by electronically capturing and storing a photographic image of the prepared tooth. Using computer technology, a three-dimensional restoration design is made that conforms to all the necessary specifications of the proposed inlay; there is no need for an impression.

Other Crowns

Crowns may also be made of zirconia or yttria-stabilised zirconia (see Chapter 12).

226

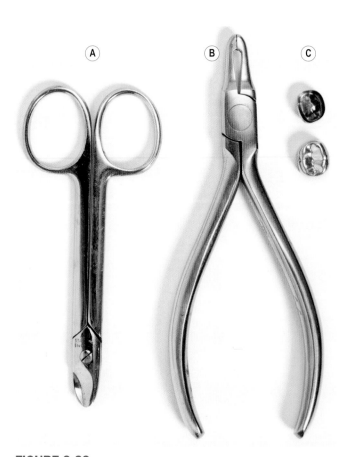

FIGURE 9.23
(A) Crown-cutting Bee bee scissors; (B) contouring pliers; (C) stainless steel temporary crowns.

Bridges

A dental bridge (sometimes called a fixed partial denture; Figures 9.21 and 9.22) is used to replace missing teeth. However, unlike a denture (Figure 9.21) it cannot be removed by the patient. The materials used to make bridges are composite resins, gold, PFM or occasionally, porcelain or zirconia.

A *conventional bridge* is made by preparing the teeth on either side of a missing tooth or teeth. These are called the abutment teeth. The preparation helps accommodate the material to be used to restore the size and shape of the original teeth in a correct alignment and contact with the opposing teeth. Thus a disadvantage of a bridge is the damage to the adjacent abutment teeth. The artificial teeth between abutments are called 'pontics'.

For anterior bridges, where aesthetics are usually more important than strength, *resin-retained bridges* are often used (Figure 9.21). These require little or no preparation to the abutment teeth as they rely on a composite resin for retention. They are a good treatment option for many single missing anterior teeth as they can be good aesthetically, relatively cheap and well tolerated by most patients. They can also readily be replaced if they fail.

DENTAL IMPLANTS (Figure 9.24)

The most widely accepted and successful type of dental implant is the osseointegrated (endosseous) implant, based on the discovery by Professor Per-Ingvar Brånemark that the inert metal titanium can successfully fuse to bone (Box 9.3). Implants are now also available in stable metal compounds such as stainless steel, titanium alloy (e.g. 6% aluminium and 4% vanadium), and zirconium. Some cheaper metal implants on the market may leach components. Ceramic implants are also available.

The implant procedure is sophisticated and expensive. It involves drilling a precision hole in the jaw bone often guided by cone-beam computed tomography, while cooling the drill tip. Then the implant is placed in the drilled hole. Healing and integration of the implant(s) with the jawbone occurs over months (osseointegration; see Box 9.3). As the implant is integrated it becomes biomechanically stable and strong. After a few months the implant is uncovered in another surgical procedure, and a healing abutment or sometimes a temporary crown placed onto the exposed implant. Later, a permanent crown, bridge, or denture or other restoration will be made using the implant for retention and support.

For implants to be successful, there must be enough jaw bone to hold and support the implants. *Bone grafting* is used in cases where there is inadequate bone. A wide range of grafting materials and substances may be used:

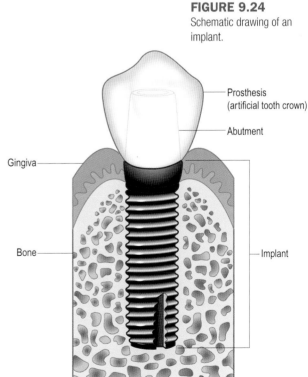

FIGURE 9.24
Schematic drawing of an implant.

- From the patient's own bone (*autograft*):
  ○ From the hip (iliac crest)
  ○ From spare jawbone
- From processed cadaver bone (*allograft*)
- Using bovine bone
- Using coral (*xenograft*) or artificially produced bone-like substances (calcium sulphate or hydroxyapatite).

Sinus lifting is a common surgical procedure to thicken the resorbed part of a maxilla (atrophic maxilla) under the sinus by transplanting bone.

> ## BOX 9.3 OSSEOINTEGRATED IMPLANTS
> - These implants are embedded in the maxillary or mandibular bone and projected through the ridge mucosa.
> - This is often a two-stage procedure.
> - The cylindrical, threaded, endosteal osseointegrated titanium implant is the most successful version (Brånemark; Nobel Biocare). There are many other variations in design also available.

The success rate of dental implants is about 90–95% at 5 years. The success of an implant depends largely on the operator's skill and experience, but other factors are discussed below.

FIND OUT MORE

Cone-beam computed tomography is a special, advanced radiological technique. Find out what role it has in dentistry.

Patient factors, such as oral and general health or smoking (smokers have poorer success rates because smoking impairs the healing process), can reduce implant success, but a crucial factor is the quality and quantity of the available jaw bone.

Term to Learn
Dentures (prostheses): removable prosthetic devices used to replace missing teeth; they are supported by the surrounding soft (the alveolar ridge) and/or hard tissues (usually the teeth).

228

Advantages of Implants
- Independent of, and no need to prepare, adjacent teeth.
- Feel like they belong and not foreign.
- The **prosthesis** is well retained.
- Improved chewing function.
- Low risk of side effects.
- Immune to caries.

Disadvantages of Implants
- Invasive procedure: surgery is required.
- Costly procedure.
- Time-consuming procedure.
- An adequate amount of bone must be present.
- Must be precisely positioned.

DENTURES

Complete Dentures

Complete (or full) dentures are meant for patients who have no teeth in the upper or lower arch (Figure 9.25).

Partial Dentures

Removable partial dentures are used for patients who are missing some of their teeth in a particular arch (Figure 9.26).

Conventional dentures are removable. Some types have better stability and retention through clasping (clipping) onto teeth or dental implants. (In some countries a bridge is called a fixed partial denture.)

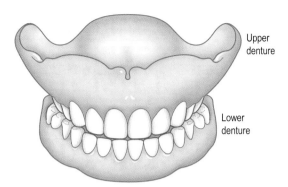

FIGURE 9.25
Full dentures.

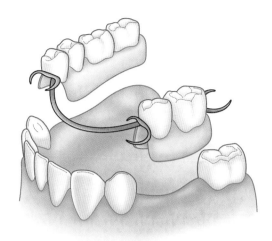

Dentures are made of acrylic resin but sometimes contain chrome
cobalt or even gold metal parts such as bars and clasps.

FIGURE 9.26
Removable partial denture.

STEPS IN MAKING A DENTURE

1. The clinician will do an assessment and take an initial (primary) impression. This is made using a stock tray and usually alginate impression material (Figure 9.4).
2. A secondary, highly accurate impression is taken using a custom-made (special) impression tray.
3. Next is occlusal registration. This is recorded on wax rims on plastic bases called occlusal rims or bite blocks (Figure 9.27). The wax rim is warmed and altered to establish the correct occlusion (bite), lip support, and orientation of the denture teeth for the laboratory.
4. The shape, size, and shade of teeth are selected.
5. Try-in: (At this point the laboratory has set the pre-made plastic or porcelain teeth into the wax rim according to the prescription from the clinician.) Using the wax rims again, the occlusion and orientation are checked and the aesthetics of the teeth checked by the clinician *and* the patient.

229

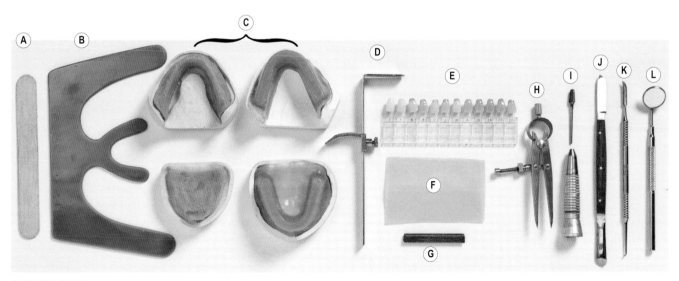

FIGURE 9.27
Dental instruments and materials required for bite registration: (A) wooden spatula; (B) Fox bite plane; (C) bite rims on models; (D) Willis bite gauge; (E) shade guide; (F) sheet of wax; (G) green stick compound; (H) dividers; (I) straight handpiece and acrylic trimmer; (J) wax knife; (K) LeCron carver; (L) mouth mirror.

6. Fitting stage: (The technician has now processed the pre-made teeth onto a hard, tissue coloured acrylic base.) Adjustments are made to the fit and bite using articulation strips (Figure 9.28).
7. Review: The patient is given another appointment after 24–48 hours to check the denture and adjust any sore spots. They may need to be seen again after another seven days.

THE DENTURE TRAY (Figure 9.29)

Laboratory work	
Straight handpiece	
Straight carbon steel acrylic trimmers	For denture /tray adjustment
Occlusal registration paste	For occlusal registration
Articulating paper and Miller's forceps, or occlusal indicator wax	To indicate occlusal problems
Pressure-indicating cream and applicator brush	To highlight high spots beneath a denture
Wax	
Willis bite gauge	
Wax knife and heat source	
Shade and mould guide	
Gauze swabs (Figure 9.16)	
Cotton wool rolls (Figure 9.16)	
Mirror	For patient to view their appearance

Reassuring the Patient about their New Dentures

It may take some time for the patient to get used to a new denture, particularly if it is their first. Some may initially have difficulty speaking but most quickly adapt with practice. Eating also takes practice: the important thing to tell the patient is to remember to cut food into small pieces and use a *side to side* motion to mash down food.

All patients improve with practice, time, and a lot of patience. Upper dentures usually fit snugly and are retained well with suction. However, lower dentures cannot develop this suction due to the considerable movement of the tongue, lips and cheeks. They may tend to 'float', though most patients learn with time to control them. All dentures loosen over time because the alveolar bone which supported the natural teeth gradually shrinks away once the teeth have been lost. Denture adhesives or relining or rebasing can help but, for some patients, implants may be the only real solution.

Immediate Dentures

Immediate dentures are inserted immediately after the extraction of the natural teeth that they are replacing. From the patient's perspective this is excellent in terms of aesthetics. However, immediate dentures will loosen over the following three to six months as the alveolar bone resorbs, so that adjustments are then required, such as relining, rebasing and possibly even a new denture.

Relining Dentures

Relining is the resurfacing of the denture's fitting surface with a new material. This is done in one of two ways, direct (chairside) or indirect (laboratory). It is usually carried out when the fit of the denture has deteriorated but is not necessary otherwise to construct a new denture (e.g. an immediate replacement denture).

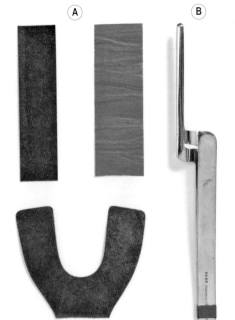

FIGURE 9.28
(A) Articulation strips
(B) Willis bite gauge.

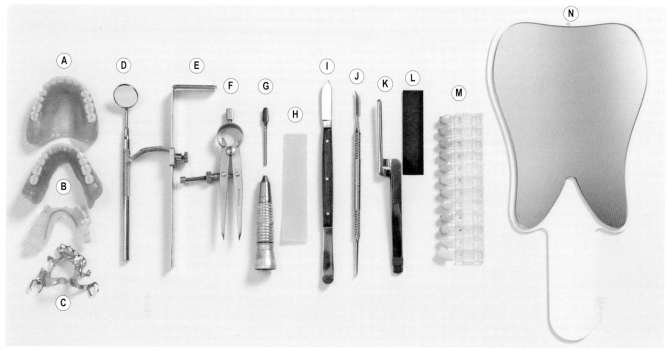

FIGURE 9.29
Dental instruments and materials required for fitting of dentures: (A) upper and lower full dentures; (B) acrylic removable partial denture; (C) chrome-cobalt removable partial denture; (D) mouth mirror; (E) Willis bite gauge; (F) dividers; (G) straight handpiece and acrylic trimmer; (H) strip of wax; (I) wax knife; (J) LeCron's carver; (K) Willis bite gauge; (L) articulation strip; (M) shade guide; and (N) mirror.

231

STEPS IN RELINING OF DENTURES

1. At the chairside, for a direct reline, cold-cured (self-cure) acrylic is used.
2. The clinician will clean, roughen and slightly reduce the denture's fitting surface.
3. The flanges are trimmed (to reduce danger of over-extension) and the undercuts are removed.
4. Mix the new relining material and give it to the clinician to apply to the fitting surface.
5. The denture is inserted and the patient asked to close gently on the denture to ensure that the occlusion is not altered by the procedure.
6. The clinician may then carry out **border moulding**.
7. The denture is kept in situ for about five minutes after which it is removed and carefully examined.
8. If cold-cured acrylic (see Chapter 12) was used, place the denture in a hydroflask to complete the curing and to reduce the possibility of porosity.
9. The result is a better fitting denture due to its new and well-adapted fitting surface, but the new plastic tends to discolour over time.

If a laboratory (indirect) reline is to be carried out, the fitting surface is cleaned, the undercuts removed and the flanges shortened. Minor defects and extensions can be corrected with self-cured acrylic such as Total or tracing compound. A **wash impression** is then taken on the fitting surface of the denture with impression paste, with the patient in light occlusal contact. In the laboratory, the technician replaces the impression paste with heat-cured acrylic (see Chapter 12) which is more durable than the materials used for direct relines.

Term to Learn
Border moulding:
shaping the borders of the dentures so that they form a good seal with the mucosa and thus aid retention of the dentures.

Term to Learn
Wash impression:
putting a thin layer of an accurate impression material inside a cruder impression and then taking an impression again.

KEY POINT Tissue conditioner may also be used as a reline material, but is not very durable and is only a short term solution.

KEY POINT Relines lead to an increase in palate thickness. When a number of relines have been carried out a rebase can be carried out to reduce the palatal thickness.

Rebasing Dentures

Rebase technique is the same as for reline except that, in the laboratory, the palate and fit surface is removed and a new one waxed in before processing.

CARE OF REMOVABLE DENTAL APPLIANCES

- Remove during contact sports.
- Avoid chewing gum and sweets.
- After every meal, remove appliance and rinse in cold running water, over a bowl of water lest the appliance falls and breaks, and brush natural teeth.
- During sleep dentures should be removed and stored in denture soak or similar provided there are no metal parts, then rinsed in water before re-inserting on waking.
- Do not let the appliance dry out; always store in water or another liquid such as denture cleaner, provided there are no metal parts.

MANAGEMENT OF PULP DISEASE (ENDODONTICS)

If damaged by caries or trauma such as tooth fracture, heat or chemical irritation from a filling, the dental pulp becomes inflamed (pulpitis) and infected and eventually dies. The infection is caused by micro-organisms from the mouth flora or blood stream entering into the tooth. Pulpitis is usually painful. Infected pulp tissue will continue to be a problem unless it is removed by:

- Endodontic therapy ('root canal' treatment)
- Tooth extraction.

Pulpotomy/Pulpectomy/Pulp Capping

In a primary tooth the clinician may also remove just part of the dental pulp and leave the healthy pulp in the root canals (*pulpotomy*). The tooth can be temporarily filled with calcium hydroxide paste for a week or more to disinfect and reduce inflammation. If the problematic tooth is not fully developed (as in a child), the initial treatment may be a *pulpectomy*. This involves the removal of all the infected pulp and applying a dressing and temporary filling. If a pulp is only slightly damaged and lightly infected, such as may occur accidentally during cavity preparation, *pulp capping* with calcium hydroxide paste may suffice. This means just applying the material to the top of the pulp without disturbing it.

If all this is not indicated as the pulp is beyond repair, the clinician will suggest endodontic therapy.

Endodontic Therapy

Endodontic therapy is a sequence of treatments aimed at eliminating infection and then protecting the decontaminated tooth from future microbial invasion. It is usually carried out under local anaesthesia. Rubber dam (Figure 9.6) is needed to isolate the tooth from its environment, to retract and protect the soft tissues, and to avoid inhalation of instruments or debris.

Once the rubber dam is placed, the clinician drills into the tooth to access the pulp chamber and remove the diseased pulp. Then the lengths of the canals are measured by taking an X-ray with an endodontic file (Figure 9.30) in the canal or by using an electronic

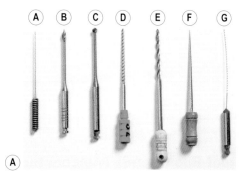

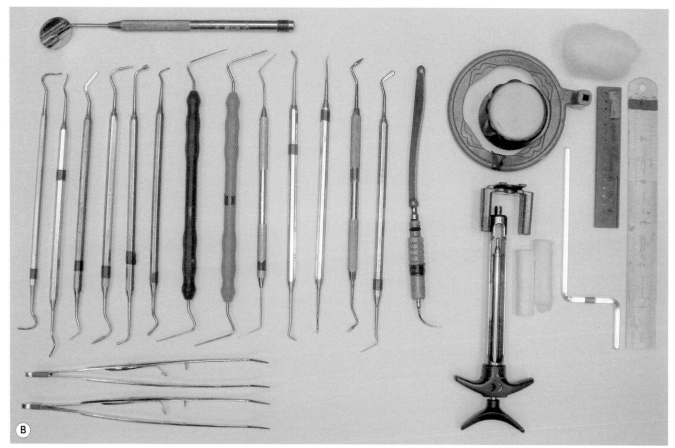

FIGURE 9.30
(A): (A) Barbed broach (B) Gates Glidden bur; (C) goose (long) neck bur (D) endodontic hand file; (E) hand reamer (F) finger spreader; and (G) spiral root filler.
(B): A selection of instruments and items used in endodontic treatment. Do you use them in your workplace? Try to identify as many as you can.

233

device (an apex locator). The clinician may use a microscope to visualise the tooth and canals more clearly. On removal of the pulp the canals are cleaned using reamers and files; an antiseptic solution (often sodium hypochlorite), is used to irrigate the canal to help combat infection.

IDENTIFY AND LEARN

Identify an apex locator in your workplace and find out how it works.

Once the canals have been thoroughly cleaned and disinfected they are filled (*obturated*) with an inert filling, often gutta-percha (Figure 9.31) along with a eugenol-based cement (see Chapter 12). The tooth crown is restored with a temporary and later a permanent filling or crown.

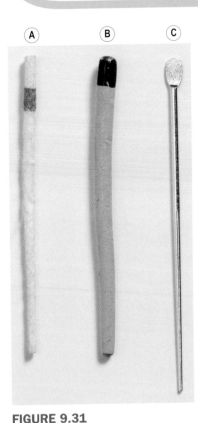

FIGURE 9.31
(A) Paper point;
(B) gutta-percha point;
(C) silver point.

234

Root canals are very complex, with many small branches coming off the main canal. Occasionally even after very good root canal treatment, infected debris can remain in these branches. This can possibly prevent healing or cause re-infection later.

If infection recurs and if it spreads beyond the root apex it can cause pain. Then re-treatment, or root end surgery (apicectomy or apicoectomy; see below) may be needed.

Root End Surgery (Apicoectomy, Apicectomy or Endodontic Microsurgery)

In root end surgery:

- The root tip, or apex, is exposed by raising a gingival flap and removing bone over the root tip.
- The root tip is cut.
- A filling is placed, usually of amalgam, glass ionomer or MTA (mineral trioxide aggregate) in the canal at the root end to seal it (retrograde root filling).
- The gingival flap is then sutured back in place.

Being a surgical operation, the usual pre- and post-operative care is indicated; complications can also be similar.

IDENTIFY AND LEARN

Identify irrigation solution and syringes and a file holder in your workplace.

Root Amputation

Root amputation or resection is the removal of an entire root of a multirooted tooth.

Hemisection

Hemisection is the removal of one-half of a tooth. The remaining half will be restored as a one-rooted tooth.

ENDODONTIC TRAY

Broaches – smooth and barbed (Figure 9.30)	For removing pulp tissue
Gates Glidden bur (Figure 9.30)	For cleaning and shaping the canals
Endodontic files (Flexofile, Hedstroem) (hand or handpiece driven) (Figure 9.30)	For cleaning and shaping the canals
Paper points (Figure 9.31)	For drying the canal
Irrigation syringes	Monojet syringe 27G
Irrigation solutions	
Hypochlorite – sterile water	
Antiseptic dressings	Calcium hydroxide, Ledermix
Gutta-percha (Figure 9.30) (silver points rarely used now) and cement	For occluding canal
File holder	
Apex locator	
Gauze swabs (Figure 9.16)	
Cotton wool rolls (Figure 9.16)	
Temporary dressing (provisional restoration)	

FIND OUT MORE
Which antiseptic and temporary dressings are used in your workplace?

GINGIVAL AND PERIODONTAL DISEASE TREATMENT (PERIODONTAL TREATMENT)

Prevention of disease is crucial for maintaining oral health: tooth brushing at least twice a day and cleaning between the teeth with floss or other interdental oral hygiene aids (see Chapter 8) helps prevent dental plaque accumulation.

Chronic Gingivitis

Chronic gingivitis is reversible: once dental plaque and calculus are removed and prevented from returning (by regular tooth brushing and inter-dental cleaning), gingivitis should resolve.

Scaling and polishing are carried out by the clinician.

Chronic Periodontitis

Chronic periodontitis is not reversible but it can be halted or slowed by:

- Practising good oral hygiene
- Scaling, polishing and root planing (which removes subgingival calculus, plaque and dead cementum)
- Patients with more advanced disease may require appropriate treatment (periodontal surgery) by a periodontist. This is usually aimed at facilitating easier cleaning for the patient.

Periodontal Surgery

Periodontal surgery may be needed to:

- Remove calculus from deep pockets
- Reduce the pocket depths
- Smooth root surfaces
- Arrange gingival tissue into a shape that will enable easier access and facilitate oral hygiene practices.

It is also carried out to correct gingival recession and elongation of the clinical crown of a tooth.

Periodontal surgical procedures include the following.

GINGIVECTOMY

In gingivectomy, the clinician removes and reshapes loose, diseased gingival tissue to eliminate pockets. Under local anaesthesia, the tissue is cut with laser or scalpel. The wound is dressed with a periodontal dressing, for example Coepak.

FLAP OPERATIONS

Flap operations also allow the removal and reshaping of loose, diseased gingival tissue as well as providing access to clean deep (infrabony) pockets. The flap is replaced so as to remove pockets. Under local anaesthesia, the flap is raised and tissue is removed with curettes and the flap sutured and dressed with, for example, Coepak.

PERIODONTAL REGENERATIVE THERAPY

Periodontal regenerative therapy uses a bone graft material or bone regenerative material (e.g. Emdogain) to restore bony defects deep within the pockets in a technique similar to a flap

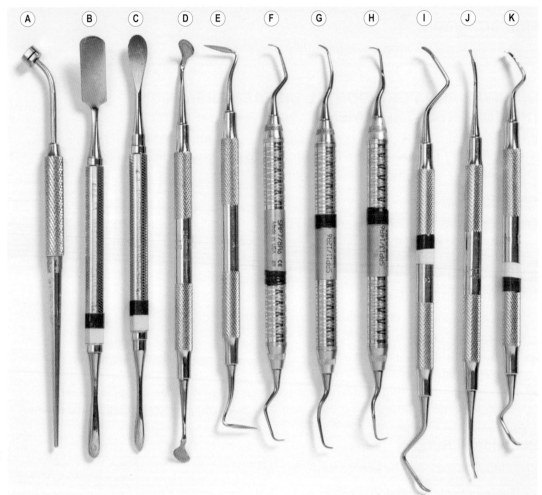

FIGURE 9.32
A selection of periodontal surgical instruments. (A) Blakes gingivectomy knife; (B) shortened Pritchard periosteal elevator; (C) Molt no. 9 periosteal elevator; (D) Goldman Fox no. 7 heavy periodontal knife; (E) Buck 5/6 periodontal knife; (F) Gracey curette 7/8; (G) Gracey curette 11/12; (H) Gracey curette 13/14; (I) Pritchard surgical curette; (J) Fedi 2 bone chisel; (K) Rhodes back action bone chisel.

operation. It may also be necessary to place a special membrane such as Gore-Tex over the graft to protect the material and to help it regenerate the tissues (guided tissue regeneration; GTR).

Figure 9.32 shows a selection of periodontal surgical instruments. Being surgical operations, the usual pre- and post-operative care is indicated and complications can be similar.

COSMETIC (AESTHETIC) DENTAL TREATMENTS

Common cosmetic treatments comprise: cleaning and whitening the teeth; realignment of teeth (orthodontics); and restorative dental procedures (see Table 9.2).

Veneers

A veneer is a thin layer of restorative material (composite resin or porcelain) placed over a tooth facial surface, either to improve the aesthetics (Figure 9.33), or to protect a damaged tooth surface. Veneers typically last 10–15 years.

A composite veneer may be:

- Directly placed (built up in the mouth)
- Indirectly fabricated by a dental technician in a laboratory, and later bonded to the tooth, typically using a resin cement (Figure 9.34).

A porcelain veneer can only be indirectly fabricated but has overall better aesthetics in the long-term.

TABLE 9.2 Cosmetic Procedures

Procedure	Comments
Bonding	Composite material is applied to the tooth, shaped, cured, and polished: an option for chipped or cracked teeth
Enamel shaping	Re-shaping the enamel to improve the shape of the tooth appearance
Gingival repositioning	Restoring the gingival contour especially where there has been *recession*
Gingival lift	Raising and contouring the gingival line
Micro-abrasion	Thoroughly cleaning the teeth using pumice and weak acid; it tends to slightly darken teeth but removes white spots
Orthodontics	Aligning misplaced teeth (see Chapter 11)
Scaling and polishing ('prophylaxis')	Common and least invasive procedure to remove stain and deposits
Veneers	Applying a new tooth facing (Figure 9.34)
Whitening ('tooth bleaching')	Commonest procedure for lightening discoloured teeth

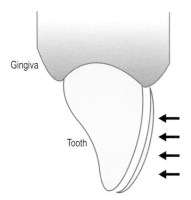

FIGURE 9.33
Illustration of the principle underlying veneers.

Procedures such as body art, piercings, dental 'grillz', tattooing, lip augmentation and use of Botox which might be said to be more at the boundaries of 'healthcare' are not included here. However, they are likely to be more regulated by the government in the near future.

REFERRAL

Referral of patients with restorative problems, to either specialist practitioners or hospital consultants, depends on several factors:

- The GDP's knowledge and ability to treat patients.
- The patient's desire to see a specialist or undergo specialist treatment.
- The age and general health status of the patient.
- The complexity of treatment required.

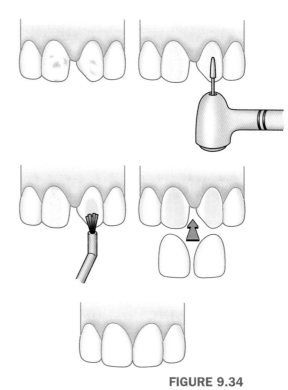

FIGURE 9.34
Cosmetic treatment with veneers: the process.

237

FIND OUT MORE

To read more about:

- How porcelain crowns are made, visit: http://www.qualitydentistry.com/dental/restorative/candb.html
- Impression materials, visit: http://www.dentistry.bham.ac.uk/cal/impress/intromat.html

CHAPTER 10

Surgical Procedures

INTRODUCTION

Oral surgery deals with the treatment and ongoing management of irregularities and pathology of the jaw and mouth that require surgical intervention. In the UK, oral surgery is a specialty regulated by the General Dental Council and includes the specialty previously called surgical dentistry. Oral surgery procedures are sometimes termed dento-alveolar surgery (or minor oral surgery) and are commonly undertaken in the dental surgery.

Oral and maxillofacial surgery deals with mouth, jaws, face and neck surgery. In the UK, this specialty is regulated by the General Medical Council. Oral and maxillofacial surgery is sometimes termed major oral surgery, and is undertaken mainly in a hospital. Oral and maxillofacial surgeons can also undertake oral surgery.

As a dental nurse, you must have the knowledge and understanding of the procedures required to:

- Assist effectively at the chairside
- Provide the patient with advice both before (pre-operative) and after (post-operative) the procedure.

The dental nurse may assist the clinician undertaking dento-alveolar surgery, which may involve:

- Extraction of teeth or roots
- Treatment of complications arising from diseases affecting the teeth, periodontium or alveolar bone (such as infections and cysts)
- Root end surgery (*apicectomy*) for recurrent periapical infections
- Periodontal surgery to facilitate oral hygiene in areas affected by chronic periodontitis
- Implant surgery, that is, placement of endosseous implants and associated procedures such as bone grafting and sinus lifts.

Dental nurses in a hospital may also assist in major oral and maxillofacial surgery, which deals with:

- Effects of trauma
- Effects of oral cancer
- Severe orofacial deformities or malocclusions (*orthognathic surgery*).

239

> **KEY POINT** Informed consent means that the patient must be made fully aware of the procedure, and its intended benefits and possible risks.

CONSENT

Informed consent is required before any operative procedure, especially before surgery. *Written informed consent* must be obtained from all patients having any surgical procedure. The possible benefits of treatment must be weighed against the risks and always discussed by the person carrying out the procedure. If for some good reason this is not possible, a delegated person with the appropriate expertise should do so.

'Informed' consent means that the patient must be fully aware of the procedure, its intended benefits, its possible risks, and the level of these. In particular, patients must be warned carefully and clearly about:

- Pre-operative preparation that may be required
- Possible adverse effects or outcomes (e.g. deformity)
- Post-operative sequelae (e.g. pain, swelling, bruising)
- Where the patient will be during their recovery.

> **KEY POINT** Warnings about surgical procedures must be properly recorded in the case notes and signed by operator and patient.

An example of a patient information sheet is given in Box 10.1. To read more about patient consent, see Subchapter 3.2.

BOX 10.1 PATIENT INFORMATION SHEET: REMOVAL OF WISDOM TEETH

Dear Patient,

As you know we feel that your wisdom teeth should be removed. Here is some information that we hope will answer some of your questions.

Wisdom teeth removal is often necessary because of infection (which causes pain and swelling), decay, serious gingiva (gum) disease, the development of a cyst or because teeth are overcrowded. Wisdom teeth are removed under local anaesthetic (injection in the mouth), sedation or general anaesthetic in hospital, depending on your preference, the number of teeth to be removed and the difficulty of removal.

It is often necessary to make a small incision in the gingiva, which is stitched afterwards. After removal of the teeth, your mouth will be sore and swollen and mouth movements will usually be stiff. Slight bleeding is also very common. These symptoms are quite normal, but can be expected to improve rapidly during the first week. It is quite normal for some stiffness and slight soreness to persist for two to three weeks. Pain and discomfort can be controlled with ordinary painkillers, such as paracetamol, and you might be prescribed antibiotic tablets. A clinician will be available to see you afterwards if you are worried, and will want to check that healing is satisfactory.

Complications are rare, but occasionally wisdom tooth sockets become infected, when pain, swelling and stiffness will last longer than normal. Occasionally patients have tingling or numbness of the lower lip or tongue after lower wisdom teeth removal. This is because nerves to these areas pass very close to the wisdom teeth and may get bruised or damaged. The numbness nearly always disappears after about one month, but very occasionally lasts for a year or more. Jaw fracture is very rare.

Please let us know if we can give you any more information.

SURGICAL PROCEDURES

Soft Tissue Surgery

A range of instruments are used for soft tissue surgery.

The disposable surgical scalpel blades used are:

- No. 11 – for incising abscesses
- No. 12 – for periodontal surgery
- No. 15 – for intraoral and small skin incisions, incising the **mucoperiosteum**, and excision of soft tissue lesions
- No. 10 – for larger skin incisions.

IDENTIFY AND LEARN
Try to find the various scalpels listed above in your workplace and learn the differences and similarities between them.

CUTTING DIATHERMY AND ELECTROSURGERY
These procedures use an electric current to cut or cut and coagulate the tissue. They may be used for extensive oral incisions, or removal of soft tissue, because bleeding from wound edges is reduced.

These procedures should be avoided in patients with **artificial cardiac pacemakers**.

CRYOSURGERY
This procedure uses freezing to destroy tissue.

Advantages
- It can sometimes be used without analgesia.
- There is no haemorrhage.
- There is little post-operative infection.

Disadvantages
- No biopsy specimen can be taken.
- Depth and extent of tissue damage is difficult to predict.
- There is substantial post-operative swelling (**oedema**).

Indications
Cryosurgery is useful for:

- Controlling intractable facial pain (cryoanalgesia to the peripheral nerve)
- Removal of:
  - Leukoplakias (also called keratoses; see Chapter 5). The diagnosis should be confirmed by taking a biopsy and sending it for histological examination prior to cryosurgery, in case it is a malignancy
  - Warts and papillomas
  - Mucus extravasation cysts (mucoceles)
  - Haemangiomas (see Chapter 5).
- Palliation (producing some relief) of:
  - Severe ulcers
  - Cancerous lesions.

Procedure
Liquid nitrogen (N_2) or nitrous oxide (N_2O) is applied to the diseased area. This is done either by spraying it directly or circulating it through a probe called a cryoprobe. The very low temperatures –about $-70°C$ – achieved with liquid N_2 make this particularly useful in the

Term to Learn
Mucoperiosteum: the combined term for the mucous membrane and the periosteum that covers the bone (see Subchapter 4.1).

Term to Learn
Artificial cardiac pacemaker: this is a medical device that regulates the heart beat. It is placed in people whose natural heart beat is not fast enough or in those who have a problem with the system that conducts the heart beat from the atria to the ventricles (see Subchapter 4.1). The pacemaker consists of electrodes that are placed in contact with the heart muscles and which send out electrical signals to the heart.

241

Term to Learn
Oedema: the medical term for swelling that results from excessive accumulation of watery fluid in a particular part of the body.

Mosby's Textbook of Dental Nursing

management of intractable lesions. Liquid N_2 probes and sprays can cause full-thickness skin necrosis, and therefore must be handled very carefully.

- Local analgesia is given if required.
- The clinician ensures good contact of the cryoprobe with the lesion by coating it with a jelly such as KY jelly.
- The clinician freezes the lesion.
- The freezing is turned off. The cryoprobe is left on the lesion until it thaws and de-frosts.
- Multiple freezes, with thawing between each freeze, maximise the effect. The ice crystals formed in the tissue spaces between the cells kill the cells.

LASER SURGERY

Lasers can be used for surgery but can also damage normal tissues, especially the eyes. The hard laser, especially the carbon dioxide laser, is the most useful (see Subchapter 1.1).

Advantages

Laser surgery usually:

- Causes little bleeding. Haemostasis occurs during vaporisation to coagulate small vessels in the wound bed
- Is followed by less pain and swelling than that which follows surgical excision or cryotherapy
- Results in little post-operative scarring
- Is particularly helpful for surgery close to important anatomical structures, e.g. lesions affecting the floor of the mouth.

Disadvantages

Laser surgery usually:

- Is best conducted under general anaesthesia (GA)
- Requires expensive equipment
- Can damage the eyes, skin, mucosae and teeth.

Also, because laser light travels in straight lines, access to some lesions can be difficult.

POTENTIAL HAZARDS

- Damage to the eyes and other tissues from reflection of the laser beam from retractors, mouth props or anaesthetic tube couplings.
- Vaporisation of anaesthetic tubes, leading to ignition of inflammable anaesthetic agents or oxygen.

Indications

- Leukoplakias.
- Early tumours.
- Haemangiomas.

Procedure

The carbon dioxide laser is a cutting laser, which can be used to: excise, much as does a scalpel; or to fulgurate (destroy) the lesion. It is important to:

- Follow laser safety recommendations (see Subchapter 1.1)
- Use non-inflammable general anaesthetic agents
- Avoid reflections from instruments or other metal objects.

Surgery Involving Hard Tissues (Bone and Teeth)

Bone and teeth are usually cut with rotating instruments (burs) in a surgical handpiece. This involves the production of heat, so simultaneous cooling by constant running sterile water or sterile saline (irrigation) is important. Air-rotors are less commonly used as they can contaminate wounds unless using a sterile coolant, and occasionally cause surgical emphysema (see Chapter 16). Laser and ultrasonic cutting are uncommonly used. Piezosurgery is a new but expensive technique that cuts only hard tissues, increasingly used in apical and implant surgery as the danger of damage to nerves or arteries or the sinus membrane is less. However, this kind of surgery can generate significant heat, and cutting is slower than with many high-speed drills.

▎IDENTIFY AND LEARN

Identify two surgical handpieces in your workplace. Note the fitted tube for irrigation.

Wound Closure

Incisions are usually an integral part of surgery. The wound thus created needs to be closed so that it **heals by primary intention**. The would is closed usually with cyanoacrylate tissue adhesive or tapes (e.g. Steri-Strip), or sutures (stitches) (Box 10.2). This results in a small line of scar tissue, which is the goal whenever a wound is closed. In some circumstances, an open wound is left to **heal by secondary intention**. In the mouth it is then protected by a dressing such as Coepak. Wounds in bone are sometimes protected by BIPP (bismuth iodoform paraffin paste), or Whitehead's varnish (compound iodoform paint).

> **Terms to Learn**
> **Healing by primary intention:** when the wound edges heal directly touching each other.
> **Healing by secondary intention:** when the wound is left open to fill with granulation tissue, which will subsequently turn into scar tissue.

BOX 10.2 CLOSING A WOUND

Skin Tapes
- Closure of skin wounds by adhesive tapes is convenient.
- It produces a strong wound with little infection and with good cosmetic results.
- The skin and wound should be thoroughly cleaned as above, and all bleeding within the wound must cease before tapes are applied.
- The tapes are left in place for seven to 10 days and then gently removed by traction.

Sutures
- Atraumatic needles are generally preferred.
- Monofilament materials are associated with a lower rate of wound infection compared with multifilament sutures.
- Sutures (stitches) are used for most:
  - ❍ Oral wounds – 3.0 Vicryl (resorbable) or black silk (non-resorbable but pliable and easily seen)
  - ❍ Facial wounds – 5.0 or 6.0 polypropylene or nylon
  - ❍ Other skin wounds – 3.0 nylon or Prolene (polypropylene).

Technique
The simple interrupted stitch is most commonly used because it allows good approximation of the wound edges, and is easy to place. Various other suturing techniques can be used. The surgeon will often ask the dental nurse to cut the stitch once placed.
1. Care of sutures
   - Clean wounds twice daily with chlorhexidine 0.1% aqueous solution.
   - Apply Polyfax ointment (antibiotics – polymyxin and bacitracin) twice daily to prevent scab formation, facilitate suture removal and reduce scarring.
2. Suture removal
   - Facial sutures should be removed within three to five days, to keep scarring to a minimum.
   - Mucosal sutures are usually resorbable, but otherwise are removed at five to seven days.

Continued...

> ## BOX 10.2 CLOSING A WOUND—continued
> - Many patients are apprehensive and need reassurance.
> - Clean the wound and surrounding mucosa or skin with aqueous 0.2% chlorhexidine.
> - Lift the suture with sterile forceps and cut the stitch on one side, as close to the skin or mucosa as possible (this avoids pulling contaminated suture material through the wound).
> - Pull the suture out using traction on the long end, across the wound so as to avoid pulling apart the edges.
> - Clean the area again with an antiseptic solution.
> - Remove alternate sutures first to see if wound has healed adequately. If yes, remove the remaining sutures a day later.
> - If wounds tend to gape a little, use tapes (but not in the mouth).

KEY POINT The suture (stitch) should be cut about 5 mm away from the knot.

FIND OUT MORE

Look at some wound closure materials in your workplace and try to think of a situation each of them could be used in.

SURGICAL OPERATIONS: SAFEGUARDS
Operating on the Wrong Patient
CAUSES

- Tiredness or lack of care.
- Notes attached to the wrong patient following emergency admission.
- Last-minute changes in operating lists.

PREVENTION

- Taking general care.
- Patients should have one identifying number, which should always be quoted on every paper.
- All patients should have a wristband.
- The wristband should bear the patient's surname, forenames and accident or in-patient number.
- Providing the patient with a wristband should be the responsibility of the sister or their deputy, or, at night, by the nurse in charge or their deputy.
- All unconscious patients admitted through the accident department should be given a wristband before being taken to the ward.
- The surgeon or accident officer should see that unconscious patients are escorted by a nurse to the ward or theatre.
- The dental surgeon who is to operate should check the patient before operation; check that the medical or dental record relates to the patient; and *ask the patient their name and the operation they are to have.*
- The anaesthetist should check that the medical record relates to the patient.
- The operations list should carry the patient's surname in full, forenames, hospital number, and the operation planned.
- The list should be displayed in the surgery or theatre, in the anaesthetic room, and in every ward which has a patient on the list or is to receive a patient from the list.
- When sending from theatre for a patient, the theatre porter should bring a slip bearing the surname, forenames and number of the patient.

- The ward sister or deputy should be responsible for seeing that:
  - ○ The correct patient is sent to theatre
  - ○ The patient has signed a consent form
  - ○ The patient has received the prescribed pre-medications
  - ○ Where appropriate, the side of the operation has been marked
  - ○ The correct records and radiographs accompany the patient.
- In theatre, the theatre superintendent or deputy should be responsible for sending for patients.
- Day patients who are undergoing minor operations, and out-patients undergoing any operation under GA should be labelled in the same way as in-patients.

Operating on the Wrong Side or Area
CAUSES

- Tiredness or lack of care.
- Wrong information on case papers.
- Illegible case papers.
- Abbreviation of the words 'right' and 'left'.
- Mistakes in dental charting.
- Failure to check the entry on the operating lists against the notes in theatre, together with the wrong case papers or the preparation of the wrong side or area.
- Wrong radiographs provided.
- No routine procedure for marking operation side.

PREVENTION

- It is the responsibility of the surgeon who explains the operation to the patient to witness the patient signing the correct consent form.
- The surgeon should mark the side or area with an indelible skin pencil before the patient is sent to theatre.
- Nurses should inform the operating surgeon if they find that a patient due to be sent to theatre has not been so marked, but they should not undertake the marking themselves.
- The words LEFT and RIGHT should always be written in full and in block letters, at least on operating theatre lists.
- When extracting teeth, especially for orthodontic reasons (where the teeth may not be carious), the clinician should count the teeth carefully, and double-check/confirm with a colleague. This elementary exercise can prevent the patient losing a tooth unnecessarily (which can become a medico-legal problem).

THE ROLE OF A DENTAL NURSE IN ORAL SURGERY
Before the Procedure

- Retrieve patient notes, radiographs, consent form.
- Prepare the dental environmental ensuring infection control.
- Prepare the surgical tray or trolley using an aseptic technique.
- Greet and reassure the patient in the waiting area.
- Ensure pre-operative advice has been followed.
- Inform the clinician of any changes/comment from the patient.
- Assist the patient to the dental chair.
- Provide the patient with protective equipment (bib and glasses).
- Provide a bowl with water for dentures.

> ### BASIC SURGICAL TRAY (Figure 10.4)
>
> | Instrument | Purpose |
> |---|---|
> | Scalpel blade (Nos 11,12,15) | To cut the flap |
> | Scalpel handle (e.g. Swann Morton) | |
> | Mitchell's trimmer | To raise the flap |
> | Periosteal elevator (e.g. Howarth's) | To raise the flap and protect soft tissues |
> | Surgical handpiece | To remove bone or cut tooth |
> | Surgical selection of burs | |
> | Retractors: flap; cheek; tongue | To retract flap for visibility to operative site, and protect tissues |
> | Surgical aspirator | To remove saliva, blood, water and debris |
> | Irrigation syringe | To irrigate the site with sterile saline or water |
> | Suture | To reposition and fix mucoperiosteal flap |
> | Needle holders | To hold the suture needle |
> | Rat-toothed tissue dissecting forceps | To hold the flap while suturing |
> | Suture scissors | To cut sutures |
> | Gauze swabs | |
> | Cotton wool rolls | |

During the Procedure

- Reassure patient.
- Assist with giving topical and local anaesthetic.
- Retract the soft tissues, lips, cheek and /or tongue as required.
- Aspirate to ensure a clear field and patient comfort.
- Anticipate and pass instruments/items as required.
- Mix materials as appropriate and pass as required.
- Develop radiographs if another appropriately qualified dental nurse is not available.
- Cut sutures as required.
- Wipe patient's face.

After the Procedure

- Provide a mirror and tissues for the patient to wipe their face and assist if necessary.
- Assist patient to the recovery room or waiting area.
- Ensure the patient has another appointment and has the post-operative instruction sheet.
- Make a follow-up appointment as required.
- Decontaminate the environment and sterilise instruments.
- Dispose of the local anaesthetic needle in the correct sharps container.
- Dispose of the clinical waste in the yellow bags.

EXTRACTION OF TEETH (EXODONTIA)

Instruments Used

Figures 10.1–10.3 show a selection of forceps and elevators used for extraction of teeth, both straightforward and impacted teeth. Figure 10.4 shows a selection of other surgical instruments.

| IDENTIFY AND LEARN

Write down the names of all the items shown in Figure 10.4 and get it checked by your supervisor.

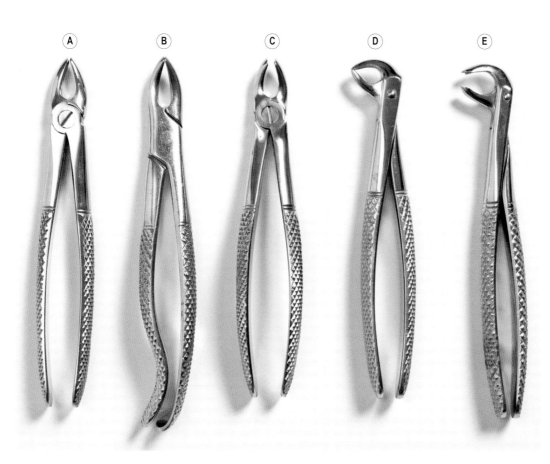

FIGURE 10.1
Forceps for extracting deciduous teeth: (A) upper straight; (B) upper root; (C) upper molar; (D) lower root; (E) lower molar.

247

Extraction of Deciduous Teeth

There is seldom a case for the removal of only one deciduous tooth, unless it:

- Is close to being shed naturally
- Has been retained so long that it impedes the eruption of its successor
- Is **infra-occluded**.

Enforced extractions of deciduous canines or molars are usually balanced by extraction of a contralateral tooth in the same arch. This is to prevent a centre-line shift. Radiographs are usually taken to ensure that there are no other problems (e.g. a midline supernumerary tooth), which may also require attention.

Extraction of Permanent Teeth

Many orthodontic treatments require the extraction of premolars. However, in some patients there may be indications for the removal of a different tooth.

> **Term to Learn**
> **Infra-occluded:** a tooth whose incisal edge or occlusal surface appears 'sunken' in comparison with the rest of the teeth in the arch. So for an upper tooth this would mean the incisal edge or occlusal surface is 'higher' than the rest of the teeth, and in the lower teeth it would appear to be lower down. Conversely, teeth can also supra-occlude (over-erupt) in comparison with the rest.

CHECKS REQUIRED BEFORE EXTRACTION OF A TOOTH

- Check that the name of the correct tooth to be removed is written down clearly in the notes.
- Check that the patient (or in the case of a child, both patient and parent) understands that a permanent tooth is being removed – and the reason for removal.
- Check that any orthodontic appliance (see Chapter 11) that is meant to be worn is being worn satisfactorily before orthodontic extractions are performed.

248

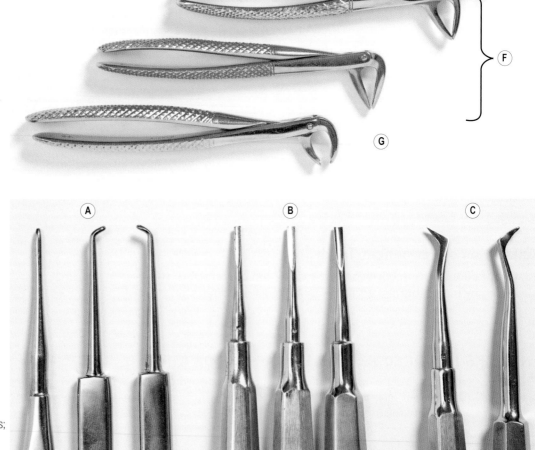

FIGURE 10.2
Forceps for extracting
permanent teeth: (A) upper
straight; (B) upper root;
(C) upper right molar;
(D) upper left molar;
(E) bayonet; (F) lower root;
(G) lower molar.

FIGURE 10.3
(A) Warwick James elevators;
(B) Coupland chisels;
(C) Cryer elevators.

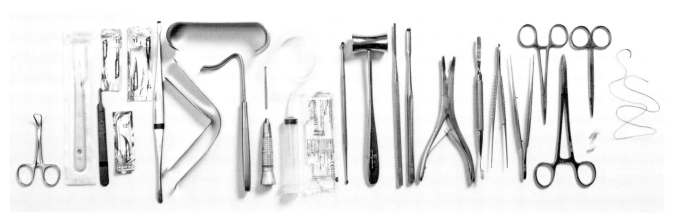

FIGURE 10.4
A selection of surgical instruments and items.

Tooth Impaction

Impaction is usually due to obstruction of the tooth's path of eruption by soft tissue, bone or adjacent teeth. The teeth most commonly impacted are third molars ('wisdom' teeth), followed by canines, second premolars and mandibular second molars. Impacted teeth may **erupt ectopically** and can cause considerable difficulties for the patient.

MANAGEMENT OF IMPACTION

The various approaches to the management of impactions are:

- Leaving them alone (observing them)
- Exposing them surgically to allow eruption (see below)
- Exposing them surgically and using orthodontics to help eruption into the correct position (see below)
- Extracting them.

A common procedure involves exposure of canines and second premolars whose eruption has been impeded. Upper canines are commonly impacted either labially or palatally, and second premolars in a palatal or lingual position. Exposure is usually undertaken in combination with orthodontic management, which ensures that there is adequate space for movement of the impacted tooth. Sometimes the tooth may require traction to help it erupt. Figure 10.5 shows the instruments required for bonding a gold

> **Term to Learn**
> **Ectopic eruption:** when a tooth erupts at an angle or in a location away from its normal position in the dental arch, that is it is displaced or incorrectly positioned. There are several causes for ectopic eruption, of which the most common are lack of available space and trauma.

249

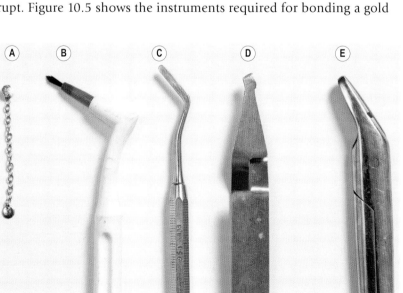

FIGURE 10.5
Instruments and gold chain required for uncovering an impacted canine and bonding the gold chain to it. (A) The gold chain; (B) brush for applying the acid for acid etching (see Chapter 11); (C) flat plastic; (D) bracket holder; (E) angled forceps.

chain to the exposed tooth. The chain is then attached to an orthodontic appliance (see Chapter 11) or an implant and gentle traction applied to pull the tooth into its correct location.

COMPLICATIONS OF IMPACTION

- Infection (pericoronitis)
- Caries of, or displacement of, adjacent teeth
- Dentigerous cysts (rarely).

Removal of impacted teeth may also cause significant morbidity, particularly:

- Temporary:
  - Pain and swelling
  - Haemorrhage or bruising
  - Trismus
  - Infection.
- Longer-lasting damage to the:
  - Nerves (usually the inferior alveolar and lingual)
  - The crown or roots of adjacent teeth
  - The periodontium of adjacent teeth
  - The maxillary antrum (**oro-antral fistula**).
- Displacement of roots, or sometimes the tooth, into adjacent soft tissue spaces, i.e. the floor of mouth, infratemporal fossa, or antrum.

Term to Learn
Oro-antral fistula:
when the oral cavity communicates with the maxillary sinus through an opening in the roof of the mouth.

IMPACTED BUT ASYMPTOMATIC WISDOM TEETH

In the past, unerupted third molars were routinely extracted even if they did not cause the patient any symptoms. However, nowadays, this is not done as research has found no evidence to support this practice (Box 10.3). NICE guidelines help the clinician decide on the fate of wisdom teeth. Many unerupted third molars remain asymptomatic for years, or for ever.

BOX 10.3 NICE GUIDELINES ON REMOVAL OF UNERUPTED THIRD MOLARS

- The routine practice of prophylactic removal of pathology-free impacted third molars should be discontinued in the NHS. The standard routine programme of dental care by dental practitioners and/or paraprofessional staff need be no different, in general, for pathology-free impacted third molars (those requiring no additional investigations or procedures).
- Surgical removal of impacted third molars should be limited to patients with evidence of pathology. Such pathology includes unrestorable caries, non-treatable pulpal and/or periapical pathology, cellulitis, abscess and osteomyelitis, internal/external resorption of the tooth or adjacent teeth, fracture of tooth, disease of the follicle including cyst/tumour, tooth/teeth impeding surgery or reconstructive jaw surgery, and when a tooth is involved in or within the field of tumour resection.
- Specific attention is drawn to plaque formation and pericoronitis. Plaque formation is a risk factor but is not in itself an indication for surgery. The degree to which the severity or recurrence rate of pericoronitis should influence the decision for surgical removal of a third molar remains unclear. The evidence suggests that a first episode of pericoronitis, unless particularly severe, should not be considered an indication for surgery. Second or subsequent episodes should be considered the appropriate indication for surgery.

ODONTOGENIC INFECTIONS

Odontogenic infections are infections that arise from teeth, particularly non-vital teeth. They also include pericoronitis (Chapter 5) and post-surgical infections. They are:

- Commonly polymicrobial (caused by a mixture of oral bacteria including both bacteria that grow without oxygen (anaerobes) and those that need oxygen (aerobes)
- Usually minor, and localised to the alveolus or sulcus, and resolve promptly with appropriate management – mainly this is drainage
- Sometimes severe and life-threatening, particularly if they are necrotising or if they spread. **Fascial space** infections endanger the airway and may spread to the chest. Infections may also spread via blood by entering into the blood vessels.

Term to Learn
Fascial space: the actual or potential spaces between the different layers of tissues in a particular body region, through which infection can spread rapidly.

Management

- Establish and maintain drainage of pus; this may be achieved via an incision, root canal treatment or tooth extraction.
- Remove the cause – often an unsavable tooth.
- Give supportive treatment as required, which often includes pain-killers (analgesics) such as paracetamol (acetaminophen) to lower any fever, and sometimes antibiotics, hydration and nutrition.
- Patients with *severe infections*, who have swelling, difficulty opening the mouth (trismus) and a fever (pyrexia) in excess of 39 °C may develop significant airway blockage which is potentially lethal; they thus require urgent specialist care.

ODONTOGENIC CYSTS

As defined in Chapter 5, a cyst is an abnormal sac-like structure that is usually filled with fluid. Odontogenic cysts are those that occur in the jaws. They are of several types:

- *Periapical cysts* – these arise in relation to non-vital (carious or traumatised) teeth; these are the most common type of odontogenic cyst.
- *Residual cysts* – these arise when periapical cysts are incompletely removed.
- *Dentigerous cysts* – these are the next most common type of odontogenic cyst and arise around some unerupted teeth.
- *Keratocysts* (keratocystic odontogenic tumours): these are less common but have a tendency to recur.

251

Management

- Enucleation – this involves scooping out the cyst (complete with its lining); it is done for most periapical, residual and dentigerous cysts.
- Keratocysts require more thorough removal. If they are large and perforating bone, or have recurred many times, they should be removed and the patient followed up long term.

PREPARATION BEFORE SURGERY
Scrubbing and Gowning

- Lather hands and forearms with soap or a special solution.
- Scrub with a brush for one minute, especially the nails and hands. Vigorous scrubbing is debated as bacteria may be brought out of skin pores and increase rather than reduce skin bacterial counts.
- Lather and rinse hands and forearms vigorously for a further five minutes – turn taps on with elbows.

- Rinse off soap, holding your hands at a higher level than the elbows.
- Dry with a sterile towel. It is important to prevent the towel touching unsterile skin at the elbow and then wiping the opposite hand with it.
- The sterile gown is unfolded and the arms pushed into the armholes; then the arms are held up. A nurse should then pull down the shoulders and body of the gown and tie it behind. It is inadvisable to pull the sleeves up yourself because of the risk of inadvertently touching the mask or collar.
- Gloves are donned (know your glove size), care being taken not to touch the outside with the skin of the opposite hand.
- Thereafter, observe a 'no touch' technique, keeping your hands near your abdomen or chest while waiting or moving around in theatre.

IDENTIFY AND LEARN

Donning gloves is probably the most important stage. Ask a senior colleague or a theatre nurse to show it you on your first day in theatre if you do not feel perfectly comfortable with your technique.

HOW LONG TO SCRUB AND WITH WHAT?

How long?

Surgical personnel have traditionally been required to scrub their hands for 10 minutes pre-operatively. However, studies have found that scrubbing for five minutes reduces bacterial counts as effectively. It may also help prevent skin damage associated with such lengthy handwashing.

With what?

Surgical handwashing protocols also used to require surgical staff to scrub hands with a brush, which can also damage skin and result in increased shedding of bacteria from the hands.

Some studies have indicated that scrubbing with a disposable sponge or combination sponge-brush is as effective. Other studies have indicated that neither a brush or sponge is necessary to reduce bacterial counts on the hands of surgical staff to acceptable levels.

A two-stage surgical scrub using an antiseptic detergent, followed by application of an alcohol-containing preparation has been demonstrated to be effective.

Handwashes

Immediate and persistent antimicrobial activity is the most important in determining the efficacy of a handwashing product. Agents used for surgical hand scrubs should:

- Substantially reduce micro-organisms on intact skin
- Contain a non-irritating antimicrobial preparation
- Have broad-spectrum activity
- Be fast and long acting.

Formulations with 60–95% alcohol alone or 50–95% when combined with limited amounts of a quaternary ammonium compound, or chlorhexidine gluconate, more effectively lower bacterial counts on the skin immediately after scrubbing than other agents. The next most active agents, in order of decreasing activity, are: chlorhexidine gluconate, iodophors, triclosan and plain soap.

See Subchapter 1.2 for a detailed discussion of handwashing.

Assisting

- Avoid damaging the patient, the surgeon or assistants, or yourself.
- Many surgical instruments, for example artery forceps and some suture holders, have a ratchet device to keep them closed. If you will be assisting, you will need to learn to be adept at opening and closing these with either hand.
- Scissors can be most accurately controlled if the thumb and ring finger are placed in the rings and the tip of the index finger is placed along the shaft.
- Ligatures or sutures should be cut with the ends of the blades: scissors seldom need to be opened more than 1 cm at the tip and the blades should be held at right angles to the skin.

> **KEY POINT** Take care! Scissors inexpertly wielded can be a danger both to the patient and the surgeon.

DAY CARE (DAY-STAY) SURGERY
Preparations
ADVANCE ARRANGEMENTS

- Booking a patient for day-care surgery depends on local protocols that have been set by the hospital administration, responsible consultant, secretary and senior departmental nurse.
- The patient is booked on the appropriate operating list, and a letter of information is sent to the patient confirming details of the agreed plan.
- Patients should be clearly instructed about:
  - The time they should arrive
  - What they should bring
  - What to do about medication they take.

Certain investigations (e.g. radiographs, blood tests, etc.) may be indicated, depending on the actual operation that will be done and the general health of the patient (see Subchapter 17.1 and below).

A pre-admission appointment in the week prior to the operation is a good opportunity for the clinicians to complete the medical history, obtain informed consent, finalise investigations, and give advance instructions and advice.

ADVANCE INSTRUCTIONS

Essential advice to patients having out-patient GA or conscious sedation (CS) should be in the form of verbal and written instructions (Box 10.4).

253

BOX 10.4 PATIENT INFORMATION ABOUT DAY-CARE SURGERY UNDER CONSCIOUS SEDATION OR GENERAL ANAESTHESIA

Some drugs that you will be given before and during the operation may affect you for the rest of the day and possibly longer. Therefore:
- You must NOT eat or drink anything for six hours before the operation.
- You must bring a responsible adult escort, who should accompany you home and stay with you until the next morning.
- You must NOT, for the 24 hours after the procedure:
  - Drink alcohol or take recreational drugs
  - Ride a bicycle or motor cycle, or drive any vehicle
  - Operate machinery
  - Go to work
  - Do housework or cooking
  - Undertake any responsible business matters
  - Sign important documents.

Procedures

ROUTINE CHECKS BEFORE THE PROCEDURE

As a dental nurse, you must make the following checks:

- Patient's full name, date of birth, address and hospital number
- Nature, side and site of operation
- That any teeth marked for extraction agree with those entered in the:
  - Consent form
  - Patient's notes
  - Referring practitioner's notes
- Medical history, particularly of cardio-respiratory disease or bleeding tendency. Any relevant medical history must be drawn to the anaesthetist's attention
- Availability of suitable social support on discharge
- Consent has been obtained in writing from the patient or, in a person under 16 years of age (18 years in Australia), from a parent or guardian, and that the patient adequately understands the nature of the operation and sequelae. Ensure that the consent form has been signed by the patient or guardian and relevant clinician (member of staff)
- Necessary investigations are available. If permanent teeth are to be removed, check that radiographs showing complete roots are available
- Patient has had nothing by mouth for at least the previous six hours
- Patient has emptied their bladder
- Patient has removed any contact lenses
- Patient's dentures or other removable appliances are removed and bridges, crowns and loose teeth have been noted by the anaesthetist
- Necessary pre-medication and, where indicated, regular medication (e.g. the contraceptive pill, anticonvulsants) have been given
- Equipment and suction apparatus are working satisfactorily, correct drugs are available and drug expiry date has not passed
- Emergency kit is available and drug expiry date has not passed
- A responsible assistant is present
- Patient will be escorted by a responsible adult
- Patient has been warned not to drive, operate machinery, drink alcohol or make important decisions for 24 hours after an operation.

THE PROCEDURE

Theatre procedures during day-stay surgery do not differ from those relevant to in-patients (discussed below). The only difference is that the operation should be completed by early afternoon. Only then will the patient realistically be discharged safely on the same day. The procedures involved in intravenous sedation are discussed in Chapter 12.

AFTER THE OPERATION

- Complete the case notes and daybook immediately (must be dated and signed by the responsible member of clinical staff).
- Check patient, particularly for complete consciousness and clear airway (and speak to accompanying responsible adult) before discharge.
- Check the patient understands the post-operative instructions.
- Check the patient knows where and how to obtain advice in the event of emergency/complication.
- Give an advice sheet to complement the one given before the operation. This should once again outline the main instructions regarding drug effects, and possible adverse effects and complications.

254

- Consider whether analgesics and/or antibiotics need to be prescribed.
- Return any dentures, etc. to the patient.

IN-PATIENT CARE
Indications for Routine Admission for In-Patient Care
MAJOR OPERATIONS

- Cancer surgery
- Craniofacial, orthognathic or cleft surgery
- Surgery involving vascular lesions
- Some surgery related to:
  ○ Fractures
  ○ Orthodontics
  ○ **Pre-prosthetics**
  ○ Implants
  ○ Multiple or complicated extractions.

Patients with serious systemic disease are admitted to hospital when their condition may influence the following:

- Anaesthesia (e.g. cardio-respiratory disease, sickle cell anaemia, drug abuse)
- Disease control (e.g. unstable diabetes or epilepsy)
- Surgery (e.g. bleeding disorders)
- Dental treatment indirectly
- Immunity (e.g. HIV/AIDS, immunosuppressive therapy)
- Behaviour (e.g. some mental health disorders, some drug abusers).

OTHER REASONS

- Complicated investigations required
- Social reasons, e.g. some patients:
  ○ Living alone, or with irresponsible carers, or far from medical care
  ○ Having difficulty eating
  ○ Subject to abuse.

Exceptions to admission for routine in-patient care include patients with a communicable infection, or a recent history of contact with one, who should only be admitted if there is a good indication. In such cases, the occupational health department should be contacted for advice.

CHECKS AT A ROUTINE HOSPITAL ADMISSION

Patients are best admitted on the day of operation unless there are special pre-operative preparations or treatment needed. Patients should be admitted early enough for the consultant to see them on the ward round before operation.

As a dental nurse, you need to remember that:
- No admission is 'routine' to the patient or their partner or family.
- Patients need reassurance and, if they are admitted the night before the operation, may well benefit from being given a sedative. Reassure them (and partner or family) about the various pre-operative and post-operative procedures, particularly if the patient is to recover with bruising and swelling, in a strange ward (e.g. intensive care), or if **nasogastric tubes**, intravenous infusions, **catheters**, etc. will be used.
- Check the patient has given informed consent to the operation.
- Check that any necessary investigations have been performed, and the results are available.
- Check that the necessary dental items are in theatre for the operation.
- Check the patient has appropriate social support for discharge.

Term to Learn
Pre-prosthetics: in some patients who require dentures, the edentulous arch presents problems that would make wearing a denture difficult. Pre-prosthetics refers to surgical procedures that are carried out to improve the state of the arch so that fitting a denture becomes possible.

255

Terms to Learn
Nasogastric (NG) tube: a tube that is passed through the nose and goes into the stomach; it is used for feeding.
Catheter: a thin, flexible plastic tube that is inserted into a blood vessel or a body cavity or duct to allow, for example, administration of some drugs or fluids (normal saline or blood).

Working with Patients, Partners and Relatives

PATIENTS' REACTIONS TO HOSPITALISATION AND ILLNESS

Any operation is a worrying, stressful and usually new prospect to most patients. They feel vulnerable and at a disadvantage. At the very least, their routine has been upset; they have left the security and privacy of their own homes and comfort of partners or relatives for an alien world, which they may often regard with fear. Many people who have been waiting to come in to hospital know that, in the next few days, they have before them discomfort and perhaps danger.

The most normal and self-sufficient individual would find all this daunting: the vulnerable, the older patient, and the very young may become overwhelmed and distressed. Patients of different cultural and ethnic backgrounds vary in their emotional response to separation from their family, and to illness, pain, operation or hospitalisation. For the patient it may well be one of the most important and stressful experiences of their life.

KEY POINT Patients may well remember for a long time everything you say or do at this stage, including your body language.

Try to be understanding and show empathy to the patient and family in every way. Even if you have no further role to play in the patient's management, being the first person they deal with, you will probably have the greatest effect on whether this experience is going to be a pleasant or haunting one for them.

Be patient, gentle, calm and confident, and try not to hurt or upset the patient in any way. The idea that the patients are happier if they do not know what is planned for them is misfounded. Patients are entitled to be told what is going to happen to them, and in a language they can understand. Give the patient and family as much information as they want, within your scope of knowledge, and reassure them that you will try to find out what you do not know.

The difficulty about talking to patients is how to explain things without frightening or confusing them. However, it is probably better to risk this than to have an apprehensive patient complaining about apparent secrecy.

KEY POINT Remember that most patients are not interested in technical details: all they want is a simple, honest explanation, and reassurance.

PATIENTS' RELATIVES AND PARTNERS

Relatives and partners are usually interested and concerned, although occasionally intrusive or abusive. Allow the patient time with their friends and relatives – this is usually important in helping them to cope.

PASSING ON INFORMATION ABOUT PATIENTS

Always remember the question of confidentiality (see Chapter 3) but, with this in mind, the date and time of the operation and discharge may well be needed by caring relatives or partners.

Nursing staff usually handle phone calls from relatives and partners in the first instance. Be careful and tactful in what you say and never give personal or medical details by phone or email, or on an answerphone.

Clerking in the Patient

Patients must be clerked on the day of admission. Unclerked patients should not be on the ward for more than a very short time (an hour or so, at the most).

Admitting a Patient

URGENT ADMISSIONS

Ensure everyone is informed about the admission. The responsible specialist, or their deputy, must always be informed if a patient is admitted under their care. The appropriate arrangements for a bed must be made, usually via the surgical bleep-holder (a senior hospital nurse), and the relevant ward sister must be told.

NON-URGENT (ROUTINE) ADMISSIONS

Ensure everyone is informed about the admission. It is courtesy to communicate with all the healthcare professionals involved in the care of the patient, unless you are certain they are well aware of the situation.

Investigations

- All patients admitted for a procedure under GA should have the following checked:
  - ○ Temperature
  - ○ Pulse
  - ○ Blood pressure
  - ○ Respiratory rate
  - ○ Urine.
- Most patients will also require a full blood picture (FBP) and test for haemoglobin level (Hb) to exclude anaemia.
- Patients of over 50 years of age and any patient with a history of heart disease should have an electrocardiogram (**ECG**) taken to exclude coronary artery disease.
- Patients with a possible high alcohol intake should have a chest X-ray (often called CXR) to exclude tuberculosis and liver function tests (often called LFTs) to exclude liver cirrhosis.
- Patients from some ethnic groups may need special investigations (e.g. SickleDex, for sickle cell anaemia in some black patients; see Subchapter 17.1).
- Investigations relevant to the procedure may also be indicated.

> **Term to Learn**
> **ECG:** a test that records the electrical activity of the heart, the rate and regularity of the heart beat, through electrodes attached to the skin. The result of the test is printed out in the form of a continuous line of waves on a graph. The shapes of the waves are interpreted by the doctor and indicate if there are any problems.

257

FIND OUT MORE

Why do people with a high alcohol intake require LFTs in particular before surgery?

Checks before In-Patient Dental Treatment Under GA

As a dental nurse, you must make the following checks:

- Patient's full name, date of birth and hospital or case number
- Nature, side, and site of operation
- Medical problems, particularly any cardiac or respiratory disease or bleeding tendency, should be highlighted and everyone involved should be aware of these
- Consent has been obtained in writing from the patient or, in a person under 16 years of age (18 years in Australia), from a parent/guardian, and that the patient adequately understands the nature of the operation and its sequelae
- The theatre is booked, and any special equipment needed has been prepared
- Necessary dental items such as splints, X-rays and models are available in the correct theatre
- The patient has had nothing by mouth for at least the previous six hours
- The patient has an empty bladder
- The patient has removed any contact lenses
- Dentures and other removable appliances have been removed, and bridges, crowns and any loose teeth have been noted by the anaesthetist

- Necessary pre-medication (see following section) and, where indicated, regular medication (such as the contraceptive pill, anti-convulsants or anti-depressants) has been given
- Any particular arrangements for patients with special requirements have been made
- Necessary investigations (blood tests etc.), if needed, have been completed.

Checks before Maxillofacial Surgery

In addition to the checks needed before in-patient dental treatment under GA, the following are required pre-operatively. Ensure that:

- The patient, partner and relatives are made aware that the patient may wake up in the intensive care unit after the operation, and in addition that they may have:
  - Swelling and possible bruising
  - A nasal tube fitted
  - Intravenous cannulae inserted
  - Facial sutures
  - A tracheostomy
  - **Intermaxillary fixation**
  - Hair shaved.
- A bed is booked in intensive care (if indicated)
- Blood is available (if indicated)
- A CXR is available. If the GA is likely to be prolonged, this is useful as a baseline in the event of post-operative complications
- An ECG (if indicated) is available
- The Hb level is known
- Urea and electrolytes (U&Es), and urinalysis have been done
- Investigations relevant to the surgical procedure are available:
  - Radiographs (and tracings)
  - Photographs
  - Models and templates
- You are conversant with the post-operative management
- The ward, consultant, theatre, anaesthetist, partner and relatives are informed if the patient is returning to a different ward (also inform the new ward of the patient's details and management).

Term to Learn
Intermaxillary fixation: The process of stabilising the mandible against the maxilla by running stainless steel wires or elastic bands between the two jaws, for example when the mandible has been fractured following trauma. The jaws are temporarily fixed together, which obviously makes eating and speaking a challenge.

258

IDENTIFY AND LEARN

Try to identify a template used for maxillofacial surgery in your workplace. If this is not available, try to find out why it is necessary for the surgery.

Pre-Medication

The aims of giving pre-medication are to:

- Allay anxiety
- Reduce cardiac excitability and the possibility of arrhythmias
- Reduce bronchial secretions
- Reduce gastro-intestinal complications
- Provide some analgesia (pain relief)
- Aid the induction of GA
- Provide some amnesia.

The responsibility for pre-medication usually rests with the anaesthetist. They will often have their own regimen.

Pre-medication (pre-med) details should be arranged with the anaesthetist and ward sister. Problems of heart rhythm irregularities are most common in infants and young children, and thus most children younger than 12 years require pre-medication before in-patient GA.

> **KEY POINT** Remember that not every patient needs pre-medication; every drug has potential problems including adverse effects, hypersensitivity, prolonged sedation, drug interactions, etc.

TIMING OF PRE-MEDICATION

- Pre-medication is effective for about four hours; therefore, do not give it too early.
- Do not give pre-medication too late; if only 30–60 minutes are available before the operation, the anaesthetist will instead give suitable drugs intravenously before induction. Atropine given intramuscularly takes effect within 30 minutes; morphine takes about one hour.
- If the operation is delayed for more than three hours, the doctor will usually request a repeat prescription of atropine.

CONTRAINDICATIONS AND ADVERSE REACTIONS TO PRE-MEDICATION

- Atropine is contraindicated in glaucoma (increased pressure in the eyes).
- Hyoscine may cause confusion and should be avoided in older people.
- Atropine and hyoscine may cause drowsiness, blurred vision, urine retention and dry mouth.
- Morphine is contraindicated in patients who have a head injury or respiratory disorders.
- Benzodiazepines are contraindicated in glaucoma and respiratory disorders.

259

POINTS TO REMEMBER ABOUT THE REGULAR THEATRE OPERATING LIST

- The operating list should not be made too long.
- For each operation, time must be allowed for induction of anaesthesia (usually about 15 minutes per patient), any over-running and breaks.
- Arranging the patient sequence for operation is decided as follows:
  - 'Big' cases done first
  - Diabetic, highly anxious patients, or those unable to cooperate are put early in the list
  - 'Day' cases should be completed before 15.00 hours
  - 'Dirty' cases (e.g. draining an abscess) should be done at the end
  - Patients with blood-borne infections (e.g. hepatitis or HIV/AIDS) should be done last of all
  - The surgeon's preference.
- The list should note the:
  - Patient's full name, hospital number, ward, operation, side/site of operation (in block capitals) and type of anaesthetic to be given
  - Name of the operator, responsible consultant surgeon and anaesthetist
  - Start time
  - Theatre number or name.
- The list should be sent to the theatre, ward, anaesthetist, surgeon and house officer on duty.
- If the order of the list changes, all must be informed – including the patient, partner and relatives.

In Theatre

Ensure that last minute jobs have been done, such as checking that everything for theatre is ready, and that all necessary phone calls are made. Ensure someone can answer necessary calls on your page/bleep, or mobile telephone. Then scrub and gown.

PREPARING THE PATIENT
Painting

- The eyelids should be carefully closed by the anaesthetist and covered with gauze pads, smeared with a little Vaseline, and secured with micropore or strapping prior to antiseptic preparation of the face. Many centres also use plastic or other eye guards.
- The operation site and several centimetres around in all directions should be painted with an antiseptic, dried with a sterile swab and then painted with a bactericidal agent.
- Cetrimide solution or povidone iodine solution (provided there is no iodine sensitivity) are most suitable for preparing the face. It is not essential to paint inside the lips and mouth prior to oral or maxillofacial surgery, although some do.
- Spirit solutions must *not* be used to prepare the skin around the eyes.

Draping

- The anaesthetist will disconnect the air-line and lift up the head.
- Two towels are passed under the head and pulled down behind the neck.
- The top towel is folded over the patient's forehead or face if only the neck needs to be exposed, and secured with a towel clip. It is important to cover all areas that do not need to be exposed during the operation, as this seals off potential sources of micro-organisms.
- The lower towel is then drawn down over the shoulder on both sides, and the chest covered by another towel.
- Keep the towel edge, which will be next to the exposed skin, in view at all times by holding it between the two hands, allowing the rest of the towel to trail.

DIATHERMY

Monopolar diathermy is frequently used for cutting through muscles and coagulating blood vessels. The diathermy point carries a positive electric charge, which runs to earth through the patient. Unless the patient is earthed by means of a large electrode bandaged to the thigh the tissue may become overheated by the electric current passing through it, leading to a severe burn. *It is essential that no other part of the patient is in contact with a conductor,* since the current will often flow through and burn the skin at this point.

Before draping, therefore, all theatre staff must ensure that no part of the patient is touching metal fittings or the metal tabletop.

Bipolar diathermy does not need earthing, and may also be used for coagulation of small blood vessels. Although less effective, it is less destructive and is preferred in operations of the face.

Diathermy is absolutely contraindicated if any explosive anaesthetic agents are used, or if the patient has a cardiac pacemaker.

Assisting at Operations
GENERAL POINTS

- To assist well requires an informed knowledge of the steps in the operation, concentration, stamina and tact.
- Try not to talk unless so encouraged.
- The operating theatre is a serious place and joking is inappropriate, as are comments about the patient. Surgeons have been brought before the General Medical Council by patients who could hear what was being said during their operation, despite appearing to be unconscious!
- If you are swabbing, take care that you do not re-introduce into the mouth (and hence the larynx) any swab on which extracted roots, teeth, etc. may have been placed for disposal.

OPERATION RECORDS

- Operation records are made in ink (red ink has traditionally been favoured for this purpose, but it copies poorly, so check local preference).
- The following are recorded in the case notes:
  ○ Names of the operator and assistant
  ○ Name of the anaesthetist
  ○ Name of the nurse
  ○ Date, time and place of operation
  ○ Overall description of the operation and, especially, any deviations from routine or any complications
  ○ Any blood loss
  ○ Post-operative instructions given.

Post-Operative Care

- The *early post-operative period* is one of the most dangerous times for the patient who is recovering from GA or CS. This is because the patient's reflexes are impaired at this time.
- It is imperative to ensure that the patient's airway is protected until the patient fully recovers their reflexes. The patient must be kept in the tonsillar or head injury position with an airway in place and constantly attended by a trained person, until the cough reflex has fully recovered.

FIND OUT MORE

Ask any senior colleague in your workplace to demonstrate the tonsillar or head injury position to you.

261

If the patient is slow to regain consciousness the anaesthetist should be, and remain, present. The following checks must be carried out:

- Airway and respiration
- Pulse and blood pressure
- Pupil diameter and reactivity.

Consider whether there has been a myocardial infarction or other medical complication.

When the patient's reflexes have returned:

- Remember to return any medication the patient should usually receive daily (e.g. anti-convulsants).
- Monitor the temperature, pulse, respiration and blood pressure.

About 50% of patients have transient and self-resolving drowsiness, hangover, nausea, sore throat (after intubation and/or packing), aches and pains (from **suxamethonium**).

Term to Learn
Suxamethonium (Scoline): a drug used to paralyse muscles temporarily in order to help induce GA.

LEAVING THEATRE

Even after the reflexes have recovered, a post-operative patient usually needs to spend some time (usually at least an hour) in the recovery area to ensure that the anaesthetist and surgeon have quick access to them, if need be. Airway compromise (e.g. airway collapse due to aspiration of large blood clots), or rapidly progressing swellings (e.g. haematoma due to arterial bleed under a surgical flap) need urgent attention by the anaesthetist and the surgeon.

POST-OPERATIVE COMPLICATIONS

See also Chapter 16.

Systemic Post-Operative Complications

The most important systemic post-operative complications are *deep vein thrombosis* (DVT), and *pulmonary embolism*.

DVT

DVT refers to the formation of blood clots in the veins that lie deep within tissues, most commonly in deep veins of the legs. The clots can break off and travel in the blood to reach the lungs (pulmonary embolism) or brain where they can block the flow in smaller blood vessels, which can lead to paralysis of a part of the body or even death.

Predisposing Factors

- Major operation with immobility of legs.
- Older age.
- Obesity.
- Pregnancy or patient taking the contraceptive pill.
- Inherited tendency to thrombosis.

Prophylaxis

Prophylactic treatment may be indicated in:

- Long major operations
- Patients likely to be immobilised after operation
- Older patients
- Obese patients
- Pregnant patients
- Patients with a history of DVT
- Patients with an inherited tendency to thrombosis.

Prophylactic treatment for DVT consists of:

- Avoiding **oestrogen**-based drugs (e.g. contraceptive pill)
- Using leggings for intermittent pressure
- Giving anticoagulation medication: low-dose subcutaneous heparin or low-molecular-weight heparin.

Diagnosis

A tender, warm and oedematous leg is indicative of DVT.

Investigations

- Venography.
- Doppler ultrasound.
- Radio-iodine fibrinogen uptake.

FIND OUT MORE

Look up the terms venography, Doppler ultrasound and radio-iodine fibrinogen uptake on the internet.

Possible Consequences

- Local pain and swelling (of the calf usually)
- Pulmonary embolism (which may be lethal)
- Late development of **varicose veins**.

Management

- Anti-coagulation medication (see Prophylaxis above)
- Bed rest until pain and oedema resolve
- Leg exercises
- Leg bandaging.

If pulmonary embolism is suspected, that is, the patient has breathing difficulty or chest pain:

- Give 100% oxygen
- Consult the surgeon.

POST-OPERATIVE JAUNDICE

This may be due to:

- Liver disease:
  - Halothane hepatitis – this may occur if there are repeated administrations of halothane
  - Gilbert syndrome – an inherited enzyme defect in which jaundice may follow use of GA, ingestion of alcohol or starvation
  - Viral hepatitis (uncommon) – may follow blood transfusion.
- Other reasons:
  - Sepsis
  - Hepatotoxic drugs
  - Haemolysis (haemolytic anaemias or incompatible transfusion)
  - Incidental hepato-biliary disease (e.g. gallstone disease).

263

PROBLEMS WITH EATING

Apart from nausea and dysphagia and possibly transient anorexia, some patients, especially those with intermaxillary fixation, may need a special soft or liquidised diet. Consult the dietician.

Special diets may also be required for other reasons including:

- Religious or cultural grounds
- Ethical grounds (vegetarians and vegans)
- Diabetes mellitus
- Medication: monoamine oxidase inhibitors (used for certain mental health disorders)
- Severe kidney disease
- Severe liver disease
- Food fads.

Patients with difficulty eating should be weighed daily; they need to be fed:

- Through a nasogastric (NG) or orogastric tube, or through a special method called percutaneous endoscopic gastrostomy (PEG). Continuous infusion of a liquid feed is preferred, since intermittent feeding can cause diarrhoea.
- Parenterally, i.e. via an intravenous catheter in the veins called the subclavian and jugular veins. This is called total parenteral nutrition or TPN. TPN is best avoided but, if it is necessary, the fluid balance, blood glucose, urea and electrolytes, and liver function need regular monitoring.

SHOCK

Shock (see also Chapter 2) is defined as the condition in which there is:

- Low blood pressure
- **Acidosis**
- **Oliguria.**

Shock may follow a major operation, because of severe haemorrhage, infection, allergy, etc.

If untreated, shock may lead to cerebral (brain) hypoxia, acute kidney failure and death.

Management

- Lay the patient flat with legs raised
- Maintain airway; give oxygen (10–15 L/min)
- Monitor the pulse and blood pressure
- Consult a doctor.

Local Oral and Dental Complications

These are covered in Chapter 16.

DISCHARGE OF HOSPITAL PATIENTS

Routine Discharge

- The patient, partner and relatives should be forewarned as accurately as possible of the date and time of intended discharge.
- Inform the Admissions Officer and, if transport is needed, also the Ambulance Officer, well in advance of the planned discharge (one to two days at least, where possible). The ward sister may do this for you.
- On, or before, the day of discharge, ensure that the discharge letter has been prepared and given to the patient for delivery to their general practitioner (GP).
- Arrange for community care, where necessary, with the district nurse.
- Arrange an out-patient follow-up appointment.
- Arrange for the patient to take or collect from their dentist or GP any necessary long-term medication.
- Give a sick note if required.
- Tell the patient what they should expect; for example, how long any pain or swelling is likely to persist, and what they should do if there are complications or uncertainty.

PURPOSE OF THE DISCHARGE LETTER

The discharge letter briefs the GP on the patient's condition and treatment given. It includes the following information:

- Date of admission
- Diagnosis on admission
- Operation carried out (and date)
- Subsequent progress
- Date of discharge
- Condition on discharge/medications
- Follow-up treatment required (e.g. suture removal)
- Any special points of note (e.g. complications)
- Date of follow-up appointment at out-patients.

Convalescence

Recommendation for convalescence is the responsibility of the consultant in charge of the patient and should be made as early as possible. Referrals are usually made in consultation between the ward sister and the convalescence secretary or medical social worker.

The medical information given to the convalescence secretary must be up to date with details of all treatment, and must include particulars of any **co-existing disease**. All drugs needed must be listed and sent with the patient to the convalescent home.

Irregular Discharge

- It is not part of a dental nurse's duty to detain patients who are mentally well against their will. However, if a patient wishes to take his or her own discharge against medical advice, you should explain the consequences politely to them, in the presence of a witness. This should then be duly recorded in the case notes.
- If the patient insists on leaving, try to contact your immediate senior to see if they can be more persuasive. If you are concerned because, for example, the patient has had an operation and is not in a fit state to discharge themselves, speak immediately to the responsible specialist.
- If the patient still insists on leaving, ask them to sign a statement accepting responsibility for their own discharge, in the presence of a witness. Record the event in the case notes.
- Occasionally the patient may take their own discharge but refuse to sign such a declaimer. Again record the events in the case record, and also ask the witness to sign the case notes, stating that the patient is 'leaving against medical advice'.

URGENT HOSPITAL ADMISSION OF THE DENTAL PATIENT

Urgent hospital admission of the dental patient may be required for a number of reasons.

Trauma

An injured patient may have:

- Loss of consciousness
- Shock
- Head injury
- Cervical spine injury
- Other serious injuries
- Laryngeal trauma
- Fractured jaws:
  - Middle facial third fractures
  - Mandibular fracture (simple or **undisplaced** may not require urgent admission)
  - **Zygomatic** fractures with danger of eye damage.

Inflammatory Lesions and Infections

- Cervical/facial fascial space infections.
- Oral infections if patient is 'toxic' or severely immunocompromised.
- **Necrotising fasciitis.**
- Tuberculosis (some patients).
- Some deep fungal infections (mycoses).
- Severe viral infections, especially in the severely immunocompromised.
- Severe **vesiculo-bullous disorders** (pemphigus and Stevens–Johnson syndrome).

KEY POINT Discharge patients only with the express consent of the specialist responsible.

Term to Learn
Co-existing disease: diseases that occur together. Many people have more than one condition at a time. The term co-morbidity is also used.

Terms to Learn
Undisplaced fracture: Where the two segments of a fractured bone are still in their normal positions.
Zygomatic: Refers to the cheek bone called the zygoma, which makes up the sides of the face (see Subchapter 4.2).

265

Terms to Learn
Necrotising fasciitis: infection of the deeper layers of the skin and tissues that lie under the skin (subcutaneous tissues) that results in necrosis and can spread through the fascial planes; also called flesh-eating disease.
Vesiculo-bullous disorder: a disease that is characterised by the presence of blisters on the skin and sometimes the mouth.

Blood Loss

- Severe or persistent haemorrhage (particularly if bleeding tendency).
- Less severe bleeding but in a highly anxious patient.

Other Reasons

- Collapse of uncertain cause.
- Airway obstruction.
- Vulnerable patients who have no social care or support.
- Disturbed, severely depressed or some other psychiatric patients.
- Children or others who are, or might be, being abused.
- Diabetics out of control because of oral pain or infection.

Emergency Theatre List

Emergency lists usually run 24 hours a day but, at night, surgeons usually operate only for *real* emergencies. It is the duty of the foundation officer to book an emergency case in theatre as soon as:

- They know what the planned management is
- After the senior surgeon in charge and the anaesthetist have been consulted
- A ward bed has been arranged.

It is rare for maxillo-facial operations to be done early for life-saving reasons.

REFERRAL

Referral of patients with surgical problems to either a specialist practitioner or a hospital consultant depends on several factors:

- The dentist's knowledge and ability to treat patients, which varies considerably
- The patient's desire to see a specialist or undergo specialist treatment
- The age and general health status of the patient
- The complexity of treatment required.

FIND OUT MORE

For more information on care of the patient before, during and after surgery, visit the emedicine 'Perioperative Care Articles' webpage (http://www.emedicine.com/med/PERIOPERATIVE_CARE.htm).

CHAPTER 11

Correction of Malocclusion: Orthodontics

CHAPTER POINTS

- This chapter covers the requirements of the NEBDN syllabus Section 11: Orthodontic procedures. For the examination, you need to gain knowledge of removable, fixed and functional orthodontic appliances.

- In addition this chapter briefly covers orthognathic surgery and cleft lip and palate. This is because patients may have had or heard about or require treatment in these areas. Therefore you need to be aware about them.

INTRODUCTION

Orthodontics (from the Greek *ortho* = straight; and *odons* = tooth) is the specialist branch of dentistry that aims to produce: (i) ideal tooth positioning in relation to the lips, teeth and jaws within the face and (ii) improved **occlusion**. All these ultimately aim to achieve improved facial aesthetics (appearance) and function.

REASONS FOR DOING ORTHODONTIC TREATMENT

Orthodontic treatment is carried out largely for aesthetic reasons, and it can have significant psychological benefits. It is also required for:

- Reduction of the risk of traumatic injuries to prominent incisors (by reducing their prominence)
- Alignment of teeth
- Correction of **crossbites**
- Correction of deep traumatic **overbites**
- Correction of anterior **openbite** or Class III incisor relationship (see below) to improve incising function
- To enhance the results of restorative treatment by ensuring that the teeth are positioned correctly before they undergo restorative treatment (multidisciplinary care).

Most orthodontic patients are children or teenagers, but adults are increasingly seeking orthodontic treatment and even older individuals may seek it. Teenagers and adults are also often more interested in cosmetic alternatives such as lingual orthodontics or aesthetic brackets, to traditional orthodontic appliances.

There is often a conflict between the real need for, and a person's wish to have, orthodontic treatment. To put things in perspective the Index of Orthodontic Treatment Need (IOTN) was developed.

Term to Learn
Occlusion: this is the dental term for 'bite', that is, the way the upper and lower teeth bite together on closing the mouth.

267

Terms to Learn
Crossbite: the condition in which teeth bite the wrong way round, for example the upper incisors *behind* the lower incisors when the person bites.
Overbite: the amount of overlap of the lower anterior teeth by the upper anterior teeth when a person bites. It is normally 1–2 mm.
Overjet: the amount the upper teeth project beyond the lower.
Openbite: the condition in which there is no overlap or even a space between some of the upper and lower teeth when the person bites.

INDEX OF ORTHODONTIC TREATMENT NEED

The IOTN is a tool used by the clinician to help decide which patients really need orthodontic treatment, that is whether there will be a benefit to dental health by having treatment. The index is designed so that a malocclusion may be quickly assessed clinically or from dental models (see Figure 9.2). Because treatment needs to be justified on either dental health or aesthetic needs, there are two components to the IOTN:

- Dental Health Component (DHC)
- Aesthetic Component (AC).

The DHC

The DHC has five categories ranging from 1 (no treatment need) to 5 (great need). Examples of patients in grade 1 are those with minor tooth displacements. In contrast grade 5 patients are, for example, those with cleft lip and palate or multiple missing teeth.

To measure the DHC of a patient, the clinician uses a simple ruler and notes the single worst feature of the malocclusion. The features are looked for in the following order:

1. Missing teeth
2. **Overjet**
3 Crossbites
4. Displacement of contact points
5. Overbite

The acronym MOCDO can be used to remember the hierarchical scale.

The AC

The aesthetic component of the IOTN consists of a 10-point scale. The 10 points are represented by photographs of teeth in worsening alignment from 1 to 10. The patient's teeth are compared with the photographs to see which one they match with to get a score. (The photographs were rated for attractiveness by a panel of **lay people** during the development of the index. The degree of worsening of the attractiveness is the same between each set of photographs, that is, between 1 and 2 and 2 and 3, and so on.)

Term to Learn
Lay people: those who are not trained in the condition that is being looked at.

268

FIND OUT MORE

Look at a hard copy of the Aesthetic Component of the IOTN kept in your workplace.

MALOCCLUSIONS

Malocclusion is the term used for the misalignment of teeth and/or incorrect relationship between the maxillary and mandibular teeth. The most common malocclusions requiring orthodontic treatment are:

- *Anteroposterior discrepancies* – these are deviations between the maxillary and mandibular teeth in the front to back direction. For example, the maxillary teeth can be too far forward relative to the mandibular teeth ('increased overjet'). Depending on the severity of the problem, this can be treated using: removable functional appliances, headgear, fixed appliances or orthognathic surgery to reposition the jaw bones (in the most severe cases). All these terms are explained later in the chapter.
- *Crowding* – this usually occurs due to insufficient room in the jaw for the normal complement of adult teeth. A few teeth (usually premolars) may need to be extracted to make room for the remaining teeth.
- *Asymmetry* – this is when the centre lines of the upper and lower anterior (front) teeth do not match.

- *Deep bite* – this is when the maxillary teeth cover the mandibular teeth too much when the patient bites on their posterior (back) teeth.
- *Reverse bite* – this is when the maxillary incisor teeth bite (occlude) inside the mandibular incisor teeth.
- *Anterior openbite* – this is when there is a gap between the anterior upper and lower teeth when the patient bites on their posterior teeth.
- *Impacted teeth* – this is when teeth fail to erupt due to a mechanical obstruction or simply a failure in the mechanism that is responsible for tooth eruption. An example of obstruction is that the root of another tooth may be too close and the impacted tooth may get stuck against it.

Malocclusion can be accompanied by disharmony between the jaw bones themselves, that is, where the relationship between the upper and lower jaw is not appropriate. In these patients, the dental problem of malocclusion is usually due to the skeletal disharmony.

IDENTIFY AND LEARN
Take a set of adult upper and lower models and identify the anterior buccal cusp of the first permanent molar and anterior buccal groove of the lower first permanent molar.

CLASSIFICATION OF MALOCCLUSION
The Angle classification is the most common classification of malocclusion. It is based on the relative position of the maxillary first molar to the mandibular first molar as measured from front to back (the sagittal plane).

There are three categories in this classification. The Class II malocclusion has two subdivisions.

Angle Class I Molar Relationship
This is the 'ideal relationship' in which the anterior buccal cusp of the upper first permanent molar should occlude with the anterior buccal groove of the lower first permanent molar.

Angle Class II Division 1 Molar Relationship
- The anterior buccal cusp of the upper first permanent molar occludes anterior to the buccal groove of the lower first permanent molar.
- The lower incisor edges lie posterior to the **cingulum** of the upper incisors, but the upper incisors are normally inclined or they are **proclined**.
- There is an increased overjet.
- The overbite is also frequently increased.

Angle Class II Division 2 Molar Relationship
- The molar relationship is the same as in Class II division 1.
- The lower incisor edges lie posterior to the cingulum of the upper incisors.
- The upper central incisors are retroclined but the upper lateral incisors may be proclined.
- The lower anterior teeth are frequently **retroclined**.
- There is an increased overbite. In severe cases the lower incisors may occlude with and damage the palatal mucosa (traumatic overbite).

Angle Class III Molar Relationship
- The anterior buccal cusp of the upper first permanent molar occludes posterior to the buccal groove of the lower first permanent molar.
- The lower incisor edges lie anterior to the cingulum of the upper incisors.
- Frequently there is a 'reversed overjet'. This means the lower anterior teeth lie in front of the upper anterior teeth.
- The upper incisors are often crowded and usually proclined.
- The lower incisors are retroclined.

269

Terms to Learn
Cingulum: the bulging out portion of the lingual/palatal surfaces of the crown of anterior teeth, closest to the root.
Proclined/retroclined: protruding excessively/ excessive lingual or palatal tilting.

KEY POINT When referring to the Angle classification, the class is always given in Roman numbers. The subdivisions of Class II are always written as Arabic numbers.

ORTHODONTIC ASSESSMENT

Apart from a full clinical assessment as usual, the following are taken:

- Photographs
- Impressions for study models
- Radiographs.

Study models (also called casts) of the upper and lower teeth are used to analyse the tooth and jaw relationships in detail. Thus they must be of good (diagnostic) quality. For this reason:

- The liquid plaster of Paris is carefully poured into the impression (mould) so that no large voids or bubbles are present.
- The models are adequately trimmed (without extra bits of plaster jutting out from the sides). A way to check this is that when the models are put together and placed on their heels, the upper and lower teeth should remain in touch at the maximum possible points (in the mouth this is called centric occlusion).
- They are labelled and kept in protective model boxes to ensure they do not break.
- The models and boxes are labelled with the patient's name and model box number and stored in a safe place.

Study models are part of the patient record and thus must be kept until:

- The patient's 25th birthday
- If the patient was 17 or over at conclusion of treatment, until their 26th birthday
- Until eight years after the patient's death if sooner.

270

Radiology

Term to Learn
Serial films: films of the same person taken in the same position over intervals of months or years.

The British Orthodontic Society (BOS) has issued guidelines on the legal background of orthodontics, applications of different radiological techniques and selection criteria for the techniques. These are described in Chapter 14. Here we limit the discussion to radiographs specifically taken for orthodontic purposes.

Cephalometrics is the study of lateral skull radiographs taken under standardised conditions. The patient is placed carefully in a machine called a cephalostat, which positions the head in a standardised, reproducible manner. The film is placed 381 mm (15 inches) from the head, a standard distance for all cephalometric radiographs taken worldwide. Features seen on the X-ray film are then traced, and various standard landmarks, lines and angles are measured and recorded (e.g. Eastman Analysis). Comparisons are made with normal values to give the diagnosis, and an assessment of growth and/or effects of treatment can be done by comparing **serial films**. Figure 11.1 shows a cephalogram and its tracing.

KEY POINT Normal values in cephalometrics can vary slightly from population to population and between ethnic groups.

THE TIMING OF ORTHODONTIC TREATMENT

Malocclusion often becomes noticeable as a child's permanent teeth erupt, between the ages of 6 and 12 years. Treatment that begins while a child is still growing helps produce most favourable results. Thus most children should have:

- Orthodontic evaluation no later than age 7 years, by when they have a mix of primary teeth and permanent teeth
- Orthodontic treatment if required, beginning between ages 8 and 14 years.

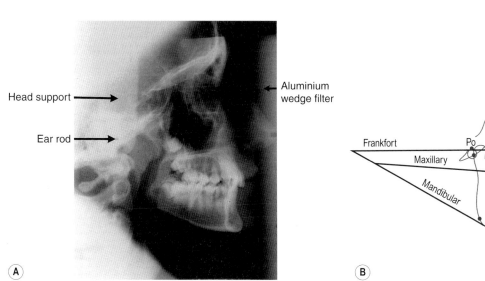

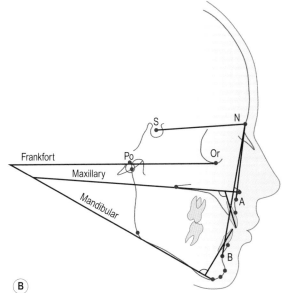

Head support

Ear rod

Aluminium
wedge filter

FIGURE 11.1
(A) A lateral cephalogram; (B) cephalometric tracing made from the cephalogram.

Although the treatment plan is customised for each patient, most will need braces for one to three years, depending on what needs correcting. Treatment is followed by a period of wearing a retainer.

271

> **IS ORTHODONTIC TREATMENT PAINFUL?**
>
> A little discomfort may be expected during normal orthodontic treatment. Overly rapid tooth movement may cause pain and may even cause root resorption or death of a tooth. Newer materials can apply a more constant, gentle force to move teeth and usually require fewer regular adjustments.

ORTHODONTIC TREATMENT

The main goals of orthodontic treatment were described on p. 267. This can involve the use of:

- Fixed appliances – sometimes called 'braces' or 'train tracks' (Figure 11.2).
- Removable appliances (ROAs) – these are used for correcting simple problems, such as moving a single tooth or expanding the dental arch. They have an acrylic baseplate with wires and springs attached (see the ROA in Figure 11.6 below).
- Functional appliances – these are usually removable appliances that are sometimes used to influence jaw growth and improve the way the maxillary and mandibular teeth meet.
- Retainers – these are used *after* treatment, to keep the teeth in their new positions.

FIGURE 11.2
A fixed orthodontic appliance. Note the brackets on the anterior teeth and the bands with welded attachments on the molars, the archwire running through the bracket and the elastics.

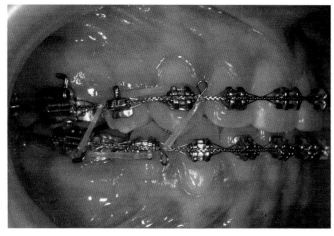

Fixed Appliances

KEY FEATURES

- Fixed appliances consist of brackets and archwires (Figure 11.2), which are tied into the bracket slots using elastic rings (often coloured) or metal ligatures (Figure 11.3).
- The brackets are made from metal, plastic or ceramic materials. The ceramic brackets are clear or tooth coloured so are less visible and usually used in adults. Usually brackets are placed on the labial and buccal surfaces of teeth. However, they can also be bonded to the lingual/palatal surfaces of the teeth (this is called 'lingual orthodontics').
- The brackets are most commonly attached to the teeth by bonding with resins. This requires acid etching of teeth.
- Composite resin is applied to the bracket base and works as the adhesive that bonds onto the acid-etched tooth (see Chapter 12). The teeth must be kept dry during placement of the brackets to ensure successful bonding.

IDENTIFY AND LEARN

If your workplace provides orthodontic treatment, look at some brackets. Otherwise find a dental catalogue, and check out the aesthetic difference between metal and ceramic brackets and note the slot in which the wire is placed. Also note the 'wings' that hold the elastic ring or ligatures in place.

FIND OUT MORE

What kind of brackets are usually used on the last tooth in the arch – usually the first or second molar? What are they called?

272

- Brackets can also be welded onto steel bands (Figures 11.2 and 11.4) that are then fixed onto the teeth using glass ionomer cement.
- Bands are commonly placed on posterior teeth, where the forces (e.g. during chewing) can be high. They are also sometimes used for restored teeth (when the acid-etch technique may be less successful).

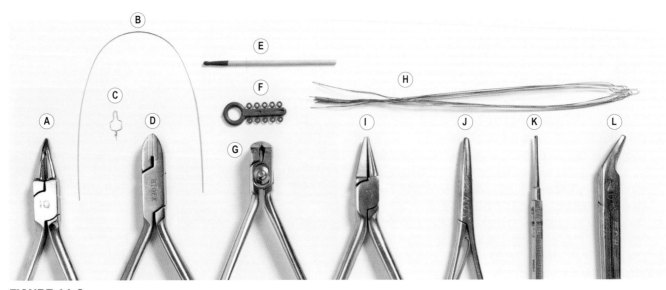

FIGURE 11.3
Selection of orthodontic instruments: (A) Weingart pliers; (B): archwire; (C) a 'quick' ligature (quick-lig); (D) ligature cutter; (E) disposable archwire marking pencil; (F) elastic modules; (G) distal-end cutter; (H) long ligature (long-lig); (I) light wire pliers; (J) Mathieu needle holder; (K) end tucker; (L) band (tape cutter).

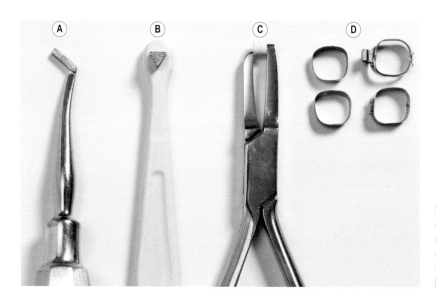

FIGURE 11.4
(A) Anterior band pusher;
(B) posterior band pusher;
(C) posterior band remover;
(D) selection of orthodontic bands.

- Use of bands may require placement of *separators* (Figure 11.5) between the posterior teeth one week before band placement in order to lessen the tight tooth contact between them and allow the band to be passed easily between them.

STEPS IN TREATMENT

- Orthodontic archwires once tied into the brackets generate forces necessary to move teeth gently into their desired position. They are made from several different materials (e.g. nickel-titanium, stainless steel) and are supplied in different cross-sectional shapes (round or rectangular) and dimensions.
- The first wire to be used is usually a very thin round nickel-titanium archwire (0.014 inch diameter). This wire creates light forces and is very springy. So it is ideal for tying into brackets on crowded and rotated teeth.
- Once the first wires have worked, that is, produced reasonable alignment of the teeth in the arch, the archwires are progressively changed. This is done until it is possible to place a stiff stainless steel archwire that allows teeth to be moved without excessive tipping. This is called bodily tooth movement.
- Typically, archwire changes or other adjustments are undertaken every five to six weeks. This usually involves placing slightly stiffer wires, which gives the patient the feeling 'that the brace has been tightened', and can result in some discomfort for three to four days following adjustments.

273

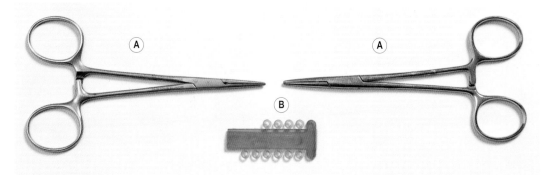

FIGURE 11.5
(A) Mosquito artery forceps;
(B) orthodontic separators.

- In the final stages of treatment, patients may also be asked to wear elastics (see Figure 11.2). These deliver additional forces to move the teeth further into the desired positions. Elastics of different diameters and strengths are available to help:
  - ◦ Close spaces between teeth
  - ◦ Close openbites
  - ◦ Shift the dental midline.
- The average duration of orthodontic treatment is about 18 months.

Removable Appliances

KEY FEATURES

- Removable orthodontic appliances (ROAs) are also called plates. They can be of various types and an example is shown in Figure 11.6.
- The advantages of ROAs are:
  - ◦ They are cheaper than fixed appliances
  - ◦ They can be removed for cleaning the teeth.
- The main disadvantages are:
  - ◦ The patient must remember to wear them
  - ◦ They can only apply a tipping force – meaning they are most suitable for treatment of some simple Class I and mild Class II and III malocclusions – and mostly in the upper arch.
- Nevertheless, ROAs can be helpful in addressing many patients' needs and, in some cases, have advantages over fixed appliances.
- Certain removable appliances (e.g. Invisalign) are also used in mild cases as an aesthetic alternative to fixed appliances in patients who feel conscious about wearing braces.
- The most familiar ROA is the retainer, the Hawley or Essix device.
- Like fixed appliances, ROAs require adjustment and monitoring every five to six weeks. This may involve adjusting the wires or cutting away of the acrylic plate. Figure 11.6 shows the instruments required for adjusting ROAs – both when used as a retainer or for moving the teeth.

274

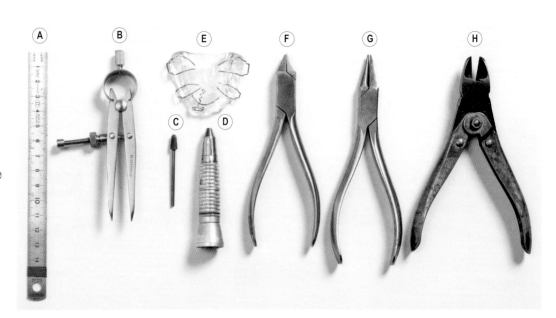

FIGURE 11.6
Tray set up for a removable orthodontic appliance patient: (A) metal ruler; (B) dividers; (C) acrylic trimmer; (D) straight handpiece; (E) removable appliance; (F) Adams' universal pliers; (G) spring forming pliers; (H) Mauns' wire cutters.

Headgear

Sometimes the clinician wants to use the head as an 'anchor' against which to move the teeth. This requires the use of a device called the headgear (Figure 11.7). The headgear has two components: (i) the 'facebow' which is the part that attaches the fixed or removable appliance to (ii) the strap that goes round the head. Headgear is usually only worn at home and at night while sleeping.

A headgear can also be used as a dental orthopaedic appliance.

Orthodontic Tooth Movement

Tooth movement happens due to the **remodelling** of the alveolar bone and alterations in the blood supply to the periodontal ligament. These are triggered by the forces that are applied to the teeth by the orthodontic appliances. The amount of bone remodelling depends on the magnitude, direction and duration of the applied force. Eventually, the supporting bone architecture is re-established and the teeth settle down in their new positions.

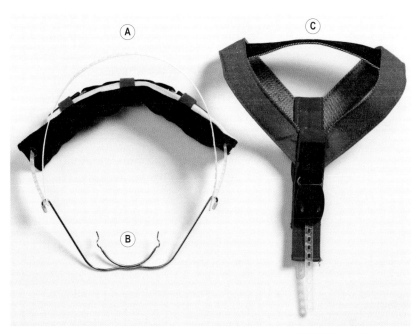

FIGURE 11.7
Headgear: (A) safety strap; (B) facebow; (C) headgear strap.

Retention

- Teeth that have been moved orthodontically have a natural tendency to move back to their original positions. In addition, teeth continue to move throughout life as a response to normal facial growth and changes in the soft tissues that cover the face. Therefore, after orthodontic treatment, patients have to wear retainers to maintain the corrected tooth positions.
- Retainers may be removable or fixed.
- They are typically worn daily for one year following fixed appliance treatment and then ideally for a few nights per week indefinitely if the teeth are to be maintained in their corrected positions.
- There are several designs of removable retainer (e.g. Hawley, Begg and Essix retainers); each has advantages and disadvantages in terms of durability and aesthetic appearance.
- An advantage of a fixed retainer, a wire bonded permanently to the lingual tooth surfaces, is that the patient does not have to remember to wear the appliance; but a disadvantage is that it can be difficult to clean around the wire.

> **Term to Learn**
> **Remodelling:** the process by which bone is constantly being removed and deposited to maintain its form. For example, during growth or when the teeth are moved.

275

IDENTIFY AND LEARN

Identify a Hawley and Essix retainer in your workplace. If not available, search for images on the internet.

Complications of Orthodontic Treatment

- Patients wearing braces should not use chewing gum or eat sticky or hard foods, such as toffee and nuts because they can damage the braces.
- Braces can also be damaged when playing sports – so it is important for patients to wear a *mouthguard* when playing sports.
- Braces and ROAs can cause ulcers in the mouth. This happens because of, for example, rubbing of a wire or bracket against the cheeks and lips. However, these heal in a few days. In the meantime the patient can use orthodontic wax or dental silicone to cover the offending part of the brace until the ulcer heals.

- A wire end at the back of the mouth can also stick out and rub against the mucosa. This can cause mild to severe ulcers and pain. Patients with such problems should again use the wax or contact the dental surgery as it may be necessary for the clinician to carefully bend the edge of the wire or clip it.

IDENTIFY AND LEARN
Find some orthodontic wax and dental silicone and ask your supervisor to show you how a patient should use this.

- Some people believe that orthodontic treatment may be followed by dysfunction of the temporomandibular joints (TMJs; see Subchapter 4.2) but there is no scientific evidence to prove this.

Other potential complications of orthodontic treatment apart from mild discomfort are:

- Decalcification – when the mineral in the tooth surface under the brackets or bands gets dissolved due to poor oral hygiene and accumulation of food and plaque. It appears as whitish areas when the brackets are removed.
- Caries – if the decalcification is allowed to continue, it can eventually lead to caries (see Chapter 5).
- Gingivitis – poor oral hygiene means the plaque can irritate the gingiva as well.
- Root resorption – shortening of the length of the root as the tooth moves.

Although these complications are rarely serious, dental plaque easily accumulates on and around appliances. So it is crucial to give dietary and other advice to the patients to maintain their oral hygiene by brushing and flossing thoroughly (Box 11.1 and Chapter 7).

DENTAL ORTHOPAEDICS
The term *dental orthopaedics* is sometimes used for treatment involving the use of 'orthopaedic appliances' for growth modification. Such appliances include functional appliances, headgear and facemasks. They are used in some growing patients (age 5 to 13 years) with the hope of modifying jaw growth to correct the occlusion. This treatment may help improve aesthetics and function, but following such treatment, fixed appliances are often needed to align the teeth and perfect the occlusion.

IDENTIFY AND LEARN
Identify a functional appliance and orthodontic face mask either in your workplace or in a dental catalogue.

FIND OUT MORE
Which are the two most commonly used functional appliances in the UK?

BOX 11.1 CARE OF MOUTH WHEN USING ORTHODONTIC APPLIANCES
- Maintain good oral hygiene.
- Avoid sugary foods, sweets, fizzy drinks and chewing gum.
- Use a fluoride mouthwash (daily or weekly preparations are available).
- Brush teeth after every meal, using a fluoride toothpaste.
- Clean appliance and/or teeth at night, around brackets and beneath archwires, using inter-dental brushes (see Figure 8.1).
- Attend all dental appointments.

ORTHOGNATHIC SURGERY

Patients who have a severe mismatch (discrepancy) of the relationship of the maxillary teeth and jaw with the mandibular teeth and jaw may require oral and maxillofacial surgery of the jaws (orthognathic surgery). This is because fixed appliance treatment alone cannot correct some kinds of severe discrepancies. Orthognathic surgery has similar aims to orthodontics: to provide an ideal occlusion within a pleasing facial form, that is improving both aesthetics and masticatory function.

Orthognathic surgery can also be used in patients with:

- Breathing problems that disrupt their sleep because transient airway blockage impedes breathing (sleep apnoea)
- Congenital conditions such as cleft lip and palate (see p. 278).

Planning for Orthognathic Surgery

Planning for orthognathic surgery usually involves many specialists who together form the *multidisciplinary* team (MDT). An MDT typically includes an oral and maxillo-facial surgeon, an orthodontist, a dental hygienist, the patient's general dentist, dental nurses and often a liaison **psychiatrist**. A psychiatrist is a useful member of the team as a psychological assessment is often needed to assess the patient's need for and potential reaction to surgery and its consequences. Cephalograms, dental radiographs, study models, photographs and computer modelling are all used to predict the patient's facial appearance after the operation. Owing to the significant changes that can occur in the appearance of the patient after the operation, it is crucial to obtain informed consent (see Chapter 3).

> **Term to Learn**
> **Psychiatrist:** a specialist medical practitioner who deals with mental health issues and problems.

Pre-Surgical Orthodontics

Pre-surgical orthodontics is the term used for the orthodontic treatment that is carried out in the 12–18 months prior to orthognathic surgery. The aim is to ensure:

- The teeth are correctly positioned within each jaw so that after the surgery the occlusion is improved
- Correct alignment of the dental arches
- There is root divergence adjacent to surgical sites, that is, there are no tooth roots in the line of the planned area of surgery.

> **Term to Learn**
> **Mini-plate:** small, flat pieces of metal with screw holes. The plate is placed over the ends of the two parts of a cut or fractured bone and screwed into the bony pieces. This holds the bony segments together to allow healing and joining together.

Orthognathic Procedures

Either one or both the jaws may be treated during the same surgical procedure. Incisions are made usually within the mouth to gain access to the jaw(s). The bones can be cut (osteotomy) and re-aligned and then held in place with surgical **mini-plates** and screws. The bone cutting is usually done using special electrical saws, burs and chisels.

IDENTIFY AND LEARN

Identify three instruments or materials used in orthognathic surgery either in your workplace or in a dental catalogue.

A wide range of orthognathic procedures are possible:

- Le Fort I osteotomy – to re-align the maxillary bone.
- Sagittal split osteotomy – the commonest procedure used in the mandible.
- Sliding genioplasty – an additional procedure to correct chin deformity.

> **KEY POINT** Any surgery can be followed by complications such as bleeding, swelling, and infection. There also could be some numbness in the face due to unavoidable nerve damage.

If the surgery is done on both jaws at the same time it is called a *bi-maxillary osteotomy* or *maxillomandibular surgery*.

277

Post-Surgery Procedures

After surgery, orthodontic treatment may be required again for six to 12 months to finalise occlusal adjustments.

Distraction Osteogenesis

Distraction osteogenesis is a type of orthognathic surgery. Its aim is to expand or elongate the jaw bone, most commonly for the correction of severe jaw deformities. This treatment induces new bone to form by applying controlled traction (pulling pressure) to the bone via a special mechanical device called a *distraction device*. The device is surgically inserted into the jaw. Most devices have a small screw, which is turned daily to apply distraction.

- Upper jaw distraction uses a rigid external halo frame that produces minimal scarring, which is hidden in the hairline.
- Lower jaw distraction can be done using either an intra-oral or an extra-oral approach.

After osteotomy, the patient is shown how to use the device and advised on how much distraction to apply every day. After the bone has been expanded as required, the distraction device is left in situ for about 60–90 days, to fix the position of the newly formed bone, before it is removed.

CLEFT LIP AND PALATE

Cleft lip and cleft palate, which can occur separately (Figure 11.8) or together are variations of a type of congenital deformity that occurs while the various facial structures are developing inside the fetus.

- A cleft lip occurs when the parts of the soft tissue that form the upper lip do not fuse (join) together as they should. The term *hare lip* is sometimes used to describe cleft lip because of the resemblance to a hare's lip.
- A cleft palate occurs when the two bony plates of the fetal skull that form the hard palate (roof of the mouth) are not completely joined. When cleft palate occurs, the soft palate (uvula) is also usually split. Cleft palate can be complete (soft and hard palate; Figure 11.8) or incomplete (there is a 'hole' in the roof of the mouth, usually as a cleft soft palate). A submucous cleft has no hole in the soft tissues but the uvula may be split into two (bifid uvula).

FIGURE 11.8
A cleft palate.

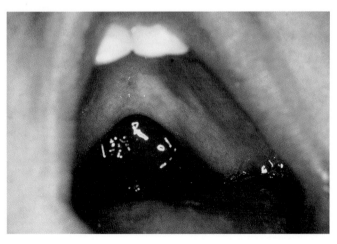

Cleft lip/palate occurs in about 1 in 800 live births worldwide. There are many causes for the disturbance in facial development and they can be broadly categorised into genetic and environmental. A maternal diet low in folic acid and vitamins, and exposure of the pregnant mother to toxins (pesticides, retinoids, anticonvulsants, alcohol, cigarettes, nitrates, organic solvents, lead, and illegal drugs e.g. cocaine, crack cocaine, heroin) may be responsible.

The abnormal connection between the mouth and nasal cavity causes air to leak into the nose (called velopharyngeal insufficiency), resulting in a hyper-nasal voice and impaired speech.

278

TABLE 11.1 Schedule for Management of Patients with Cleft Lip and Palate

Approximate Age	Schedule*
Birth	Assessment
	Discuss with team and parents
	Feeding advice
	Possible pre-surgical orthodontics
3 months	Repair cleft lip
9–18 months	Repair cleft palate
	Oral hygiene instructions given to parents
30 months	Assess speech
4 years +	Consider surgery to correct the lip and/or palate
5 years +	Consider surgery for correction of speech defects
	Speech therapy
	Preventive dentistry
8 years +	Simple orthodontics
10 years +	Alveolar bone graft to fill the bony gap in the palate
12 years +	Definitive orthodontics
16 years +	Maxillofacial surgery if needed for correcting maxillary hypoplasia or nasal deformity
	Restorative dentistry

Preventive dental care is required throughout.

The aim of treatment is to improve the aesthetics and function, particularly speech. An MDT is required with oral and maxillo-facial, ENT and plastic surgeons, orthodontist, restorative dentist, hygienist and speech therapist. One example of a schedule that is followed for treating a patient with a cleft of the lip or palate is shown in Table 11.1.

MALOCCLUSION AND REFERRAL

Referral of patients with orthodontic problems, to either specialist practitioners or hospital consultants, depends on several factors:

- The general dental practitioner's knowledge and ability to treat malocclusion
- The patient's desire to see a specialist or undergo specialist treatment
- The age and general health status of the patient.

FIND OUT MORE

To find out more about orthodontic treatment, see *Orthodontics at a Glance* (D Gill, published by Wiley Blackwell, 2008).

To find out more about taking radiographs for orthodontic treatment, see *Orthodontic Radiographs – Guidelines*, 3rd edition (KG Isaacson, AR Thom, K Horner & E Whaites, published by the British Orthodontic Society, 2008).

CHAPTER 12

Dental Drugs, Materials, Instruments and Equipment

> **CHAPTER POINTS**
> * This chapter covers the requirements of the NEBDN syllabus Section 12: Dental drugs, materials, instruments and equipment.

INTRODUCTION

The hazards associated with materials commonly used in dentistry are also discussed in Subchapter 1.1. Oral health products are discussed in Chapter 8.

The many different drugs and materials used in dentistry greatly benefit the patient. Some, however, can occasionally harm the patient, dental staff or the environment.

With all drugs and materials, ensure that the expiry date has not passed.

DENTAL DRUGS AND PRODUCTS

Toothpastes, fluorides, anti-plaque and other mouthwashes, etc. are discussed in Chapter 8. Whitening agents, antiseptics and disinfectants (decontaminating agents), the other products used in oral healthcare, are discussed here. The most common drugs used in dentistry are anaesthetics, sedatives, analgesics and anti-microbial drugs.

Whitening Agents

Tooth-whitening products include strips, gels and varnishes containing hydrogen peroxide (H_2O_2) and are used for bleaching. H_2O_2 has been used for more than 70 years for oxygenating mouthwashes and to bleach teeth. The most common source of H_2O_2 used for whitening is carbamide peroxide which typically contains between 10% and 30% peroxide (15% is recommended), roughly equivalent to 3–10% hydrogen peroxide.

There are two methods of bleaching or whitening teeth:

* External
* Internal.

EXTERNAL BLEACHING

External bleaching can be done in two ways:

* *Laser bleaching* uses laser light energy to accelerate the bleaching using high-concentration agents (30% peroxide) in gels in the dental office.
* *At-home whitening* is usually done with low-concentration oxidising agents in a whitening strip or a thin mouthguard. These hold a relatively low concentration of the

281

Terms to Learn
Enamel porosities:
gaps in the mineral structure (hydroxyapatite) of enamel.
Inter-prismatic:
The mineral deposits in enamel are laid out in bundles called enamel prisms. The spaces between these prisms are called inter-prismatic spaces.

bleaching agent next to the teeth for long periods of several hours a day and they are usually used for from five to 14 days. During this period, the oxidising agent penetrates **enamel porosities** and oxidises **inter-prismatic** enamel stain deposits (dentine is also bleached).

Bleaching is not recommended in:

- Children under the age of 16
- Pregnant or lactating women.

Problems with External Bleaching

- Temporary soft tissue irritation and increased tooth sensitivity, which disappear within one to three days of stopping or completing the whitening.
- Over-bleaching ('over-white teeth' or 'hyperodonto-oxidation').
- Chemical burns – this is a more serious problem and occurs if a high-concentration oxidising agent contacts unprotected tissues.
- Direct exposure of skin or eyes to hydrogen peroxide may cause irritation or burns, while ingestion may be irritating to the oesophagus and stomach.

KEY POINTS The effects of bleaching can last for several months, but may vary depending on the patient's lifestyle.

Some teeth may lose the bleached effect with time (rebound effect).

INTERNAL BLEACHING

Internal bleaching is performed on teeth that are discoloured due to *internal staining*. This usually happens in teeth that have become non-vital from trauma or caries (see Chapter 5). Internal bleaching involves drilling a hole to the pulp chamber, cleaning and filling the root canal, and sealing a hydrogen peroxide gel into the pulp chamber for some days, and replacing this as needed (so called 'walking-bleach' technique).

Antiseptics and Decontaminating Agents

Antiseptics and decontaminating agents should be used carefully as they can produce adverse reactions.

ADVERSE EFFECTS

Term to Learn
Dermatitis:
inflammation of the tissues of the skin.

Decontaminating agents such as hypochlorite, glutaraldehyde, hexachlorophene, benzalkonium chloride, formaldehyde, chlorhexidine, and alcohols can cause **dermatitis**. Furthermore:

- Hand-cleansing now usually involves the use of alcohol gels (see Chapter 1)
- Commercial alcohol-based agents, however, bind blood and protein to stainless steel and thus should not be used on surgical instruments
- Alcohols such as ethanol or isopropanol damage gloves so therefore, alcohol rubs/gels should not be used to decontaminate gloves
- Alcohol-impregnated wipes can be used for cleaning surfaces
- Alcohol-impregnated wipes are not effective in hand decontamination.

KEY POINTS Hypochlorite may corrode metal.

Mouthwashes containing chlorhexidine occasionally cause stomatitis (sore mouth) or even rarely, severe allergies.

Metal instruments can be decontaminated using aldehydes, chlorhexidine or hypochlorite.

Local Anaesthetics

Local anaesthetics (LAs) most commonly used for dental procedures belong to a group of drugs called amides (for example lidocaine, prilocaine, articaine and mepivacaine). Most LA dental cartridges also contain a vasoconstrictor, either adrenaline or felypressin (see Chapter 13).

> **KEY POINT** Reactions to these LAs are *very* rare.

Oral Sedation Agents

For oral sedation, drugs called benzodiazepines (BZPs) are used. These include alprazolam, diazepam, oxazepam, temazepam and lorazepam. The most commonly used are diazepam and temazepam.

Most benzodiazepines take effect within one hour after they are taken. There is often little to choose between them in terms of **anxiolytic** effect and, in prolonged use, all (especially lorazepam) may produce dependence. All impair memory and judgement at least for a while. Alcohol and other drugs that depress central nervous system (CNS) function (e.g. antihistamines, anti-convulsants, tranquillizers) must be avoided as fatalities have occurred (Chapter 13).

Term to Learn
Anxiolytic: a substance that helps reduce anxiety.

Intravenous Conscious Sedation Agents

Again, benzodiazepines (especially midazolam) are the main agents used in conscious sedation. Midazolam is commonly used for intravenous sedation and occasionally for **intra-nasal** administration.

Adverse effects of benzodiazepines include confusion, slurred speech, lack of co-ordination, dizziness, headache, and nausea. In children, benzodiazepines can cause unusual behavioural reactions.

Flumazenil is a specific benzodiazepine **antagonist**, which allows rapid reversal of conscious sedation with benzodiazepines.

Term to Learn
Intra-nasal: through the nose.

Term to Learn
Antagonist: a drug that counteracts or reduces the effects of another drug.

283

Inhalational Sedation Agents

For inhalational sedation, sometimes termed relative analgesia or RA, two medical gases, nitrous oxide (N_2O) and oxygen, are used. These gases are stored in specifically coloured cylinders (Tables 12.1 and 12.2). At least 20% and more usually 30% oxygen is given.

Gases used in sedation/anaesthesia are usually supplied under high pressure either in cylinders or as a piped gas supply. The cylinders are made from molybdenum steel, in which gases and vapours are stored under pressure. The shape and colour of the plastic disc around

Term to Learn
ISO: stands for International Organization for Standardization, the body that is responsible for setting standards for a range of products worldwide.

TABLE 12.1 Medical Gases Used in the UK

Medical Gas	ISO Cylinder Colour	Pressure Stored at	Physical State in Cylinder
Oxygen	Black with a white collar	13 700 kPa	Gas
Nitrous oxide	Blue	4400 kPa	Liquid

TABLE 12.2 Gases Used in Anaesthesia/Sedation Machines

Size of Cylinder	Capacity (litres)	
	Oxygen	Nitrous Oxide
E	680	1800
J	6800	18000

the neck indicates when the cylinder was last examined. The most commonly used types/sizes are:

- H – these are free-standing and attached to the anaesthesia/sedation machine by a flexible hose. These are most economical, but reduce the mobility of the machine. Gas-specific connectors are used that make it impossible to attach the wrong regulator or fitting to the cylinder.
- E – these are attached directly to the machine via a yoke. A gas-specific pin-index system is provided on cylinders: pins on the yoke of the machine mate with holes drilled in specific positions on the valve of the cylinder. This provides a mechanical means of preventing incorrect connection.

FIND OUT MORE

What is molybdenum steel and why is it used for these gas cylinders?

Nitrous oxide (N_2O) is contraindicated for patients with:

- Bowel obstruction
- **Pneumothorax**
- Middle ear disease
- Sinus disease.

It is also contraindicated:

284

Terms to Learn
Pneumothorax:
abnormal collection of air in the space between the chest wall and the outer surface of the lung.
Intra-ocular pressure:
the pressure exerted by the fluids within the eye.

- Following eye operations (the use of nitrous oxide during general anaesthesia in gas-filled eyes may have serious side-effects because of gas expansion and increased **intra-ocular pressure**).
- In the first two trimesters of pregnancy (because of the effect of nitrous oxide on DNA production and the experimental and epidemiological evidence that nitrous oxide causes undesirable reproductive outcomes).
- In immunosuppressed patients or in patients requiring multiple general anaesthetic inductions, since nitrous oxide affects white blood cell production and function.

Analgesics (Pain Killers)

Pain is probably the most important symptom suggestive of disease. However, the absence of pain does not mean a patient may not have disease. Different people respond differently to pain. The threshold for tolerance is lowered by tiredness, psychological factors, etc.

WHY DOES PAIN OCCUR?

Pain occurs when there is tissue damage that leads to the release of chemicals such as prostaglandins. These chemicals are produced via an enzymatic pathway involving a chemical called cyclo-oxygenase (COX). Certain drugs such as non-steroidal anti-inflammatory drugs (NSAIDs, for example aspirin) block COX and thus prostaglandin synthesis.

NSAIDS

The NSAIDs:

- Produce a bleeding tendency
- Produce gastric irritation and sometimes ulceration
- Can cause deterioration of kidney function
- May worsen asthma and cause fluid retention as well as nausea, diarrhoea or **tinnitus** (buzzing in the ears)
- Interfere with the action of anti-hypertensive drugs and **diuretics**.

Aspirin, however, has long been in use, and its efficacy and adverse effects are well recognised. This is however, not so of the newer NSAIDs. Nevertheless, aspirin is contraindicated in:

- Children under the age of 12 years (because it possibly causes Reye syndrome – a serious liver disease)
- Mothers who are breastfeeding (again, because it possibly causes Reye syndrome)
- Patients with gastric disease
- Patients with bleeding tendency.

Paracetamol is preferred in these situations.

Terms to Learn
Tinnitus: the perception of a ringing-type sound in the ears when there is no sound.
Diuretic: a drug that increases urinary flow and so reduces the amount of fluids in the body when they are in excess.

FIND OUT MORE

Why is aspirin avoided in people with a bleeding tendency?

PARACETAMOL

- Paracetamol, also called acetaminophen, is the first choice analgesic for management of mild transient pain, especially in children and old people. It also reduces fever.
- It is not an NSAID but has similar analgesic properties to aspirin. However it is less irritant to the stomach than is aspirin.
- Paracetamol overdose – or repeated doses – lead to liver damage (hepatotoxicity). Paracetamol may be given in the short term to any patient with a healthy liver, but it should not be given to a heavy alcohol drinker or one who has stopped alcohol after chronic intake.
- Compound preparations (co-codamol) of paracetamol with codeine have no significant advantages; in fact codeine has no place in dental analgesia since it can be very constipating and may occasionally cause dependence.

PATIENT-CONTROLLED ANALGESIA (PCA)

- PCA means using a special machine that allows the person in pain to control the amount of drug they are using for relief of the pain. PCA is increasingly used when pain is severe, for example cancer pain. Much stronger analgesics, such as morphine, are used in PCA.

Anti-Microbials

Anti-microbials is a term that includes anti-bacterial (antibiotics), anti-fungal and anti-viral drugs. Indications for the use of antibiotics include:

- Odontogenic infections in ill, toxic or susceptible patients (e.g. immunocompromised patients)
- Acute ulcerative gingivitis

- Severe jaw or neck infections
- Some instances of:
  - Pericoronitis
  - Dental abscess
  - Dry socket.
- Prophylaxis in surgery:
  - In major procedures (e.g. osteotomies or tumour resection)
  - In immunocompromised or debilitated patients, or following intravenous **bisphosphonate** therapy, or after radiotherapy to the jaws.

> **KEY POINT** Anti-microbials will not remove pus. Drainage is therefore essential if there is pus.

ANTI-BACTERIAL DRUGS

- The bacteria causing most odontogenic infectious are *penicillin* sensitive.
- Pus (as much as possible) should be sent for **culture and sensitivities**, but anti-microbials should be started immediately if they are indicated.

- Anaerobic bacteria are implicated in many odontogenic infections: they often respond to penicillins or *metronidazole*.
- Very high blood levels of the drug can be achieved with oral *amoxicillin*; also patients usually comply well with this treatment (see below).
- Another anti-microbial should be used if the patient is allergic, or has had penicillin within the previous month (resistant bacteria).

ANTI-FUNGALS

Anti-fungals, for example miconazole, are used to treat oral or oropharyngeal fungal infections. However, before starting with anti-fungals the clinician will check why the patient is having the infection (see below). It is important to treat this underlying cause along with anti-fungal treatment.

ANTI-VIRALS

Most anti-virals, for example aciclovir, will be of maximum benefit if given early in the disease. They are indicated mainly for patients who have an immune defect.

ADVERSE EFFECTS OF ANTI-MICROBIALS

- Anti-bacterials predispose to candidosis (see Chapter 5).
- Tetracyclines are contraindicated in pregnancy and children younger than 7–8 years. This is because they can cause tooth discoloration (see Chapter 5).

ANTI-MICROBIALS AND FOODS

Erythromycin, penicillins (some), rifampicin and tetracyclines (except doxycycline) should be taken at least 30 minutes *before* food. This is because their absorption is otherwise delayed. Metronidazole may cause headaches if taken with alcohol.

ANTI-MICROBIAL AND DRUG INTERACTIONS

- Metronidazole, erythromycin, some anti-fungals such as miconazole, and occasionally amoxicillin, can enhance the action of warfarin, causing bleeding.

Haemostatic Agents

- Haemostatic agents act to stop bleeding. They act at differing sites in the complex pathways of blood coagulation and fibrinolysis.
- Most haemorrhage will cease with the use of topical haemostatic agents.

- Blood and blood products such as blood-clotting factors are required if there is serious bleeding. In the past, these were typically derived from human or animal material. This carried a potential risk of transmission of infections (e.g. HIV, hepatitis B virus infection, prion disease – see Chapter 5). Nowadays, drugs called recombinant factors are widely available, which avoid these risks and the religious objections to certain treatment (e.g. among Jehovah's Witnesses).
- Occasionally drugs such as desmopressin (which promotes release of some blood-clotting factors), tranexamic acid (anti-fibrinolytic agent), aprotinin (inhibitor of proteolytic enzymes plasmin and kallikrein) or etamsylate (corrects abnormal adhesion of platelets) are needed.

Topical Haemostatic Agents

- Haemostatic agents are often of animal source (Table 12.3) and, unless they are of synthetic origin, may thus be contraindicated in some patients on cultural/religious grounds.
- Floseal and fibrin sealants are the most effective.
- Gelfoam swells, so a lot of the effect is a mechanical effect.
- Surgicel has a relative anti-microbial effect compared with other haemostatic agents.
- Avitene has the worst foreign body reaction of all of these particular agents.

Floseal, Avitene and fibrin sealants are expensive. Gelfoam, Surgicel and collagen sponges are relatively inexpensive.

DRUG SAFETY
Adverse Drug Reactions

Almost any drug may produce unwanted or unexpected adverse reactions, some of which are life-threatening – such as anaphylaxis (Chapter 2). These reactions are often predictable. However, some are rarely predictable unless the person has previously reacted adversely.

Patients should be warned if serious adverse reactions are predictable and likely to occur (e.g. weight gain, hypertension and diabetes with systemic corticosteroids). They should also be provided with the appropriate warning card to carry.

The real number of adverse drug reactions that occur is not known, and many adverse reactions are probably not, at present, recognised as drug related.

Adverse drug reactions should be reported using the 'Yellow card' system.

TABLE 12.3 Some Topical Haemostatic Agents

Agent	Main Constituent	Origin
Avitene	Collagen	Bovine
Colla-Cote	Collagen	Bovine
Floseal	Thrombin	Bovine
Gelfoam	Gelatin	Bovine
Helistat	Collagen	Bovine
Instat	Collagen	Bovine
Thrombinar	Thrombin	Bovine
Thrombogen	Thrombin	Bovine
Thrombostat	Thrombin	Bovine
Beriplast	Fibrin	Various
Cyclokapron	Tranexamic acid	Synthetic
Surgicel	Cellulose	Synthetic

Term to Learn
Schedule: under the Controlled Substances Act (CSA), all controlled drugs are classified into five groups called schedules. Schedule I drugs are recreational drugs not meant for medical use (e.g. heroin); schedule II drugs also have a potential for misuse but are used as medicines also (e.g. cocaine and morphine); schedule III, IV and V are drugs with decreasing potential for misuse but which are useful medicines.

Using Controlled Drugs

- Some prescription medicines contain drugs that are controlled under the Misuse of Drugs legislation. These medicines are called controlled medicines or controlled drugs. A clinician can prescribe privately any **Schedule** II or III controlled drug on an FP10PCD form as long as the drug meets the dental needs of the patient. The forms are available from primary care trusts (PCTs).
- NHS and private controlled drug (Schedule II, III or IV) prescriptions are valid for 28 days. Invoices for controlled drugs must be kept for a minimum of two years. All Schedule II, III, and IV (part 1) controlled drugs must be denatured or rendered irretrievable before they are disposed.
- Patients, or their representatives collecting Schedule II and III controlled drugs must sign for them when collecting from the pharmacy.
- Midazolam and temazepam are UK Schedule III controlled drugs. Midazolam does not need to be kept in a controlled drug cabinet and records do not have to be kept in a controlled drug register.
- If temazepam (Schedule III) is held in a dental practice it must be stored in a controlled drug cabinet but no record in the controlled drug register is required.

FIND OUT MORE

Visit the website of the Medicines and Healthcare products Regulatory Agency (MHRA; http://www.mhra.gov.uk), the medicines safety watchdog, to read more about Yellow cards. The webpage 'Controlled drugs guidance for GP practices' (http://www.gp-training.net/protocol/therapeutics/cd.htm) gives useful information about what should be included in a controlled drugs register and how they should be stored.

Drugs, Products and Cultural Issues

Cultural issues may affect the use of and prescription of certain drugs and dental healthcare products. However, remember that some religions, though at first sight apparently objecting to some constituents of drugs, do not prohibit their use if the product is designed to enhance health. Alcohol and some animal products are the sources of most concern. Some cultures are characterised by the use of certain drugs, for example Rastafarians often use cannabis.

ESTABLISHING IF A DRUG IS OF ANIMAL ORIGIN OR CONTAINS ALCOHOL

- Check the drug label – 'porcine' may be written on it.
- Check the Summary of Product Characteristics.
- Check the patient information leaflet – but this does not always detail all the components.
- Contact the manufacturer and ask their medicines information department for specific details of the drug origin.

Terms to Learn
Active ingredient: the ingredients that are actually responsible for the effect produced by a substance.
Inactive ingredient: other ingredients in the substance that act as a vehicle for carrying the active ingredient or aid its absorption.

Oral Healthcare Products and Religious Issues

Most oral healthcare products are licensed only as 'cosmetics'. Cosmetic products are less rigorously tested than pharmacological products, although they must still be labelled with all **active and inactive ingredients**. Toothpastes fall into this category.

Some oral healthcare products are licensed as pharmacological products and must be labelled with all ingredients. For example, products such as alcohol-free chlorhexidine mouthwash, which are acceptable to all groups.

Product data sheets listing all ingredients should be available for all licensed products from the original manufacturer.

FIND OUT MORE

Where are the product data sheets kept in your workplace?

Oral healthcare products that may be of concern are:

- Mouthwashes – some contain colorants or excipients of animal derivation and many contain alcohol.
- Toothpastes – may contain 'glycerine', which further may be manufactured synthetically or derived from animal fat.
- Artificial salivas – some of these contain animal mucin (such as in Saliva Orthana). Products containing carboxy-methyl-cellulose (e.g. Glandosane or Luborant) may be preferred by some individuals.
- Other products of concern are:
  - Alginates
  - Analgesics
  - Anti-microbials
  - Bone morphogenic proteins
  - Bone fillers
  - Colorants
  - Drug capsules
  - Emulsifiers
  - Haemostatic materials
  - Periodontal membranes
  - Polishing (bristle) brushes
  - Prophylaxis pastes
  - Waxes.

> **KEY POINT** Always check the product data sheets. Bovine materials are also a concern because of prions (see Chapter 5), although there is no evidence of infection.

DENTAL MATERIALS

Dental Impression Materials

Dental impression materials are used to record the shape of teeth and alveolar ridges. There is a wide variety of impression materials available. Each has its own advantages and disadvantages. The ideal properties of an impression material are shown in Box 12.1.

Non-elastic impression materials such as zinc-oxide eugenol and impression compound ('compo') are occasionally used in edentulous patients. However, most commonly elastic impression materials are used. Common elastic dental impression materials are:

- Alginate-type hydrocolloids ('alginates'), and
- Synthetic rubber base impression materials ('rubber base' or 'elastomers').

BOX 12.1 IDEAL DENTAL IMPRESSION MATERIAL

An ideal dental impression material has the following characteristics:

- Non-toxic
- Non-irritant
- Acceptable taste
- Ease of mixing
- Good working time
- Good handling
- Good setting time
- Accurate
- Surface reproducibility
- Dimensional stability
- Compatibility with model materials
- Reasonable cost
- Reasonable shelf-life.

Advantages and disadvantages of the more common impression materials are summarised in Table 12.4.

ALGINATES

Alginate is an irreversible hydrocolloid. Alginates are used mainly for making impressions for:

- Removable complete and partial dentures
- Orthodontic appliances
- Making special impression trays for rubber base impressions for more precise procedures such as crowns and bridges.

TABLE 12.4 Advantages and Disadvantages of the Different Dental Impression Materials

Material	Advantages	Disadvantages
Alginate	Non-toxic Non-irritant Good surface detail Easy to mix and use Setting time can be controlled with water temperature Cheap Good shelf-life	Messy to work with Setting time dependent on operator handling Poor dimensional stability Incompatible with some dental stone plasters
Polysulphide	Extended working time High tear resistance Easily read margins Moderate cost	Extended working time Needs custom tray Stretches and distorts Hydrophobic Messy Unpleasant smell
Polyether	Fast setting Clean but has foul taste Least hydrophobic Good stability Easy to read margins Shelf-life at least two years	Sets too fast for multiple preparations Stiff Absorbs water Leaches components High cost Burning sensation in soft tissue
Condensation silicone	Clean and pleasant Adequate working time Easily read margins Low to moderate cost	Shrinkage Low tear strength Not dimensionally stable Hydrophobic (does not like water) Short shelf-life
Addition silicone (or vinyl polysiloxane)	Accurate Excellent surface detail Easy to use Fast setting Dimensionally stable Moderate tear strength No gas evolution Non-toxic and non-irritant Good shelf-life	Difficult to mix Sometimes difficult to remove impression from the mouth Too accurate in some circumstances Hydrophobic Tears easily Poor flow on soft tissue Putty wash separate Poor tray adhesive Difficult to pour models

Alginates are supplied in powder form to be mixed with water at room temperature. Alginate is a salt of alginic acid (from seaweed) (potassium alginate or sodium alginate) with a reactor (calcium sulphate). The reactor causes the alginate to change from a **sol form** when mixed with tap water to a gel form by an irreversible chemical reaction. Alginates also contain a retarder (sodium or potassium sulphate, oxalate, or carbonate) to give enough working time. Fillers increase the strength and stiffness of the gel. With time, the gel can lose water (syneresis; which results in shrinkage) or it can take up water (imbibition; which results in expansion) or other fluids. This affects the usability of alginates as the impression may change shape after setting.

See Chapter 9 for clinical aspects of alginates.

> **Term to Learn**
> **Sol form:** liquid form.

RUBBER BASE IMPRESSION MATERIALS (ELASTOMERS)

Elastomers are hydrophobic rubber-based materials. They are used where high accuracy is needed, such as in inlay, crown and bridge and implant work. Their advantages over alginates are that they have good tear resistance and dimensional stability. They are supplied ranging from low to high viscosity materials. 'Light-bodied materials' may be used in wash impressions and over the areas where high detail is required; they are used over a 'medium' or 'heavy'-bodied material. The materials can be used in two stages or in one stage.

There are three main types of rubber base impression materials – polysulphides, polyether and silicones – though only the last two are commonly used. See also Chapter 9.

Polysulphides

- Polysulphides were the first elastomeric dental materials.
- The two component parts are a base paste containing the polysulphide polymer and a filler of titanium dioxide and lithopone.
- In addition there is a plasticiser to give an acceptable viscosity, and a small amount of sulphur to enhance the reaction.
- The other paste, the reactor, contains lead dioxide, which takes part in the condensation polymerisation reaction.
- The bad handling properties, smell, taste and inability to provide adequate detail have seen the downfall of polysulphides.

Polyethers

- Polyether materials (e.g. Impregum) use a base paste which contains polyether and filler.
- The catalyst paste contains sulphonic acid ester (which enhances polymerisation and cross-linking) and inert oils.
- When mixed, the polymer and sulphonic acid ester react to form a stiff polyether rubber.
- Setting takes about five to six minutes.
- Heat and moisture speed this up.

Silicones

Condensation-cured silicones and addition-cured silicones (polyvinyl siloxane) are the two types of silicone impression materials. Addition-cured silicones have more advantages.

> **KEY POINTS**
> - An initiator in the earlier polyether impression materials could cause allergic reactions but the newer Impregum F has a reduced risk.
> - Polyethers are used in special or stock trays with an adhesive.
> - A one- or two-stage technique can be used.
> - Although dimensionally stable, the impression should be cast within 24 hours.

291

Condensation Silicones

- Condensation-cured silicones contain dimethyl siloxane, which undergoes a condensation polymerisation with the liberation of ethyl alcohol.
- The slow but steady evaporation of the alcohol is the cause of the shrinkage that can cause major problems.
- So these materials are not used in situations where high accuracy is required, for example an impression for a crown.

Addition Silicones (Polyvinyl Siloxanes)

- Addition-cured silicones (e.g. Xantropen, Extrude) are the most recently developed and most popular impression materials.
- They set by the *addition* of a base paste and filler, and by-products are not produced.
- This means they are highly accurate with little or no dimensional change on setting.
- They are supplied in two pastes, or in a gun and cartridge form, as light, medium, heavy and very heavy bodied types.
- One paste contains polydimethyl siloxane polymer.
- The other paste contains a pre-polymer plus a chloroplatinic acid catalyst.
- On mixing in equal proportions, cross-linking forms a silicone rubber.
- Setting takes about six to eight minutes.

Term to Learn
Flash point: the minimum temperature at which a material will blow up if it is exposed to a source of ignition.

292

FIND OUT MORE

Visit the freeware University of Birmingham website on Impressions for Prosthetic Dentistry for tips and useful information on impression materials (http://www.dentistry.bham.ac.uk/cal/impress/navmap.htm).

Acrylic Resin and Monomer

Acrylic resin is polymethyl methacrylate (PMM) acrylic monomer, the most common organic solution used in dentistry. It contains methyl methacrylate but often also other monomers, polymerisation inhibitors, plasticisers, ultraviolet light absorbers and activators.

KEY POINTS Many gloves are permeable to the monomer, and barrier creams may impede the setting of acrylic.

Overexposure to monomer can cause occupational asthma, chemical hepatitis and dermatitis in technicians. Monomer has a very low **flash point** (11 °C) and this has resulted in at least one dental technician dying in an explosion.

Methyl methacrylate monomer may cause transient nausea if inhaled in large quantities. Rarely it can cause dyspnoea and hypertension. It may also soften soft contact lenses. Handling of methyl methacrylate may occasionally cause transient finger and palmar paraesthesia ('pins and needles'), pain and whitening of the fingers in the cold and local neurotoxicity. Contact dermatitis is also a possibility, but is surprisingly rare.

KEY POINT Safe work practice means exposure to monomer should be kept to a minimum. Acrylic should be mixed under a glass screen with extraction, and skin contact avoided or minimised.

There is no evidence that methyl methacrylate is toxic to the fetus. Nor is it known to have any permanent toxic or carcinogenic effects under conditions of normal use.

IDENTIFY AND LEARN

Identify acrylic monomer and polymer in your workplace.

Dental Cements

Cements are used for lining cavities and cementing restorations. They include, from weakest to strongest (Table 12.5):

- Calcium hydroxide
- Zinc oxide eugenol (ZOE)
- Zinc phosphate

TABLE 12.5 An Overview of Dental Cements

Material	Properties	Main Uses	Mix
Calcium hydroxide	Not as strong as many cements Not irritant to pulp Setting accelerated by moisture	Lining for shallow cavities Sub-lining of deep cavities	Glass slab/paper pad (Figure 9.11) using a thymozine probe or Dycal applicator (Figure 12.2)
Composite	Strong and adheres to acid-etched tooth surface and cavities	Cement for ceramic restorations and orthodontic brackets	On paper pad with ceramic-tipped spatula. Depends on manufacturer
Glass ionomer	Strong and adheres chemically to tooth structure Best placed where there has not been excessive drying of the preparation Sensitive to moisture immediately following mixing and during setting	Cement, lining, non-load-bearing restorations Cement for composite restorations Releases fluoride Valuable in treatment of root caries	Glass slab or waxed paper pad using metal spatula
Resin-modified glass ionomer cements	Chemically bonds both to the metal and the tooth Easy to use and mix Reduced post-restorative sensitivity	Standard cements for metal and zirconia-based crowns and bridges	Glass slab or waxed paper pad using metal spatula
Zinc oxide-eugenol (ZOE)	Not as strong as some other cements Not irritant to pulp Can affect setting of some composites and may contaminate tooth surface if used prior to use of bonding agents	Cement, lining, temporary dressing (provisional restoration), impression paste	Glass slab using metal spatula or paper pad
Zinc phosphate	Strong cement Irritant to pulp Adheres only to dry surfaces Reacts with, and therefore not used with, composite restorations	Cement, lining, bridge and crown cementation	On a cool thick glass slab using metal spatula
Zinc polycarboxylate	Adheres chemically to tooth structure The most adhesive cement and cement of intermediate strength	Cement, bridge and crown cementation	On glass slab or waxed paper pad using metal spatula

- Zinc polycarboxylate
- Glass ionomer cements (GICs; polyalkenoates)
- Resins (bis-GMA or urethane acrylate)
- Resin-modified glass ionomer cements.

See also Chapter 9 for the clinical aspects of using dental cements.

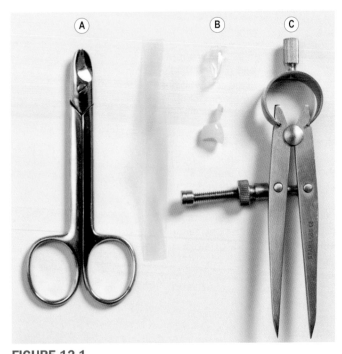

FIGURE 12.1
(A) Bee bee scissors;
(B) acrylic crowns for an incisor and premolar; (C) dividers.

294

Dental Restorative Materials

PROVISIONAL (TEMPORARY) RESTORATIONS

- Provisional fillings (temporary dressings) are made of ZOE (Cavit), resin-reinforced ZOE (Kalzinol), and self-curing acrylics or composites.
- Provisional crowns are made of aluminium or stainless steel for posterior teeth (Chapter 9) and of acrylic or composites for anterior teeth (Figure 12.1).

PERMANENT RESTORATIONS

- Common direct restorative materials (see Chapter 9) are dental amalgam, glass ionomer cement and composite resins.
- Common indirect restorative materials are gold, porcelain and zirconia.

Table 12.6 gives an overview of dental restorative materials.

TABLE 12.6 Overview of Dental Restorative Materials

	Material	Properties	Uses
Plastic (mouldable)	Amalgam	Does not adhere to tooth	Non-aesthetic fillings
	Composites (resins)	Adheres to enamel etched with phosphoric acid	Aesthetic fillings Resin-bonded bridges Veneers Fissure sealants
	Glass ionomer cements	Adheres to tooth structure via chemical (ionic) bonds	Aesthetic fillings Release fluoride
Non-plastic	Gold	Does not adhere to tooth	Non-aesthetic fillings Crowns Bridges
	Porcelain (ceramic)	Does not adhere to tooth	Aesthetic onlays Veneers Crowns or bridges
	Zirconia	Does not adhere to tooth	Aesthetic fillings Veneers Crowns Bridges

DIRECT RESTORATIVE MATERIALS

Dental Amalgam

Dental amalgam is an inexpensive, widely available restorative material that has been used in dentistry for over 150 years. It is also relatively easy to use and manipulate during placement. Other advantages are that it is strong, has a long shelf-life and it lasts longer (about 10–12 years) than other direct restorative materials, such as composite resins (5–6 years).

Dental amalgam is a mixture of *metallic mercury* with an alloy of mainly silver and tin, copper and zinc. Such a mixture of metals is called an alloy. When mercury is mixed with metals it forms an amalgam. Hence the name 'dental amalgam'. Metallic mercury can be an occupational hazard if, for example it is spilt and it vaporises. Since mercury vapour is highly fat-soluble, it is absorbed through the skin and lungs, and accumulates in the brain, liver, kidneys, spleen, muscle and glands (e.g. thyroid gland, salivary glands and testes). Mercury is **neurotoxic.**

When the tooth is first filled with amalgam, the restoration is silver in colour but it may corrode and/or become darkened over time. Thus it is not aesthetically pleasing and is not used to restore anterior teeth in most patients. Better dental health overall coupled with increased demand for more modern cosmetic alternatives such as resin composite fillings, have resulted in a steady decline in dental amalgam use. Amalgam safety has also been a concern over many years

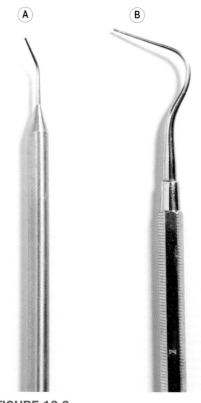

FIGURE 12.2
(A) Dycal applicator; (B) Thymozine probe.

Safety Issues Related to Dental Amalgam Use: Historical Background

In the past, before encapsulated amalgam (Figure 9.15) became available, mercury for dental use was supplied in bottles and mixed by hand to make fillings. Thus it frequently spilt in the dental surgery. Several surveys in the past showed mercury vapour in the dental surgery atmosphere (and levels of mercury in the blood, hair, nails and urine in clinicians and nurses) to be at levels above control levels. Some research has shown that the mercury from amalgams affected some clinicians, albeit mildly. Several large studies showed that clinicians' performance on many cognitive and behavioural tests was slower than the normal population. One study also found that clinicians were also more likely to have memory disturbances or kidney disorders.

> **Term to Learn**
> **Neurotoxic:** a substance that is poisonous to the nerves or nerve cells.

Safety Issues Related to Dental Amalgam Use: Current Perspectives

Modern mercury hygiene however, has substantially reduced any hazard. There is now ample evidence that, provided care is taken and only capsulated amalgam used, there is little mercury contamination in dental practices, and no hazard to staff. More recent studies of clinicians and dental nurses have *not* shown increased levels of mercury and no evidence of mercury poisoning in them.

Nevertheless, Sweden and Denmark have banned the use of amalgam, and opponents of amalgam argue that long-term exposure to mercury vapour causes **neuro-degenerative diseases**, birth defects, and mental disorders: although this may be true for metallic mercury, in amalgam, the mercury is largely bound.

Considerable research moreover, confirms that *amalgam has an established record of safety and effectiveness*. There is no scientific evidence linking dental amalgam as a cause of clinically significant toxicity, except for rare local hypersensitivity reactions. Support for amalgam safety comes from a number of findings in research and public bodies. Research findings are that:

> **Term to Learn**
> **Neuro-degenerative disease:** a disease in which there is gradual but worsening decline in the structure and functions of tissues of the brain.

- Very little free mercury is released from amalgams (except when they are placed or removed)
- The general health of people who have amalgams is no different from those who do not have amalgam fillings
- Dental staff these days do not have health problems because of amalgam/mercury exposure.

The official bodies that support the use of dental amalgam are listed below.

- The United States National Institute of Health (NIH): 'Reports that suggest mercury from amalgam causes the above-mentioned symptoms, conditions and other diseases like Alzheimer's or multiple sclerosis, are not backed up by current scientific evidence. The evidence also suggests that the removal of amalgam has no health benefits'. Also, 'Children whose cavities are filled with dental amalgam have no harmful health effects. The findings include no detectable loss of intellect, memory, co-ordination, focus, nerve conduction, or kidney function during the 5 to 7 years the children were followed' (http://www.cdc.gov/oralHealth/publications/factsheets/amalgam.htm).
- The European Commission Scientific Committee on Emerging and Newly Identified Health Risks (SCENIHR): 'All the materials are considered safe to use and they are all associated with very low rates of local adverse effects with no evidence of systemic disease. There is, obviously, a greater level of aesthetic appeal with those alternatives that are tooth coloured compared to the metallic amalgam. Furthermore, these alternatives allow the use of minimally interventional adhesive techniques. These clinical trends themselves ensure that there will continue to be a sustained reduction in the use of dental amalgams in clinical practice across the European Union' (http://ec.europa.eu/health/ph_risk/committees/04_scenihr/docs/scenihr_o_016.pdf).
- The European Commission Scientific Committee on Health and Environmental Risks (SCHER) (http://pr.euractiv.com/node/3052):
  - 'Both dental amalgams and alternative tooth filling materials are effective and safe to use.
  - 'The main exposure of patients to mercury from dental amalgam happens when fillings are placed or removed. To limit exposure, it is best to leave amalgam fillings in place unless there is a medical reason to remove them, for example if patients are allergic to one of the metals in the amalgam.
  - 'Wastewater released by dental clinics could increase the concentration of inorganic mercury in water bodies, but the added risk for aquatic organisms is considered low. In addition, the cremation of individuals with dental amalgam fillings also leads to releases into air and deposition on soil. The main environmental concern relates to the fraction of elemental mercury that is converted to methylmercury, an organic form of mercury which can accumulate in organisms and along the food chain. It is not possible to say what proportion of the risk associated with methylmercury present in the environment is due to releases from amalgams.'
- The Medicines and Healthcare Regulatory Agency (UK) (MHRA): 'there are no plans to further restrict the addition of mercury to dental amalgam' and 'the safety of dental amalgam has been reviewed nationally and internationally over last 10 years – concluding that it is safe to use'. MHRA suggests that it may be wise not to remove or place fillings during pregnancy where clinically reasonable (although there is no evidence to suggest that this is harmful) and advises that alternatives should be used in cases of allergy and hypersensitivity (http://www.mhra.gov.uk/Safetyinformation/Generalsafetyinformationandadvice/Product-specificinformationandadvice/Mercuryinmedicaldevices/CON019599).

FIND OUT MORE

What is the view of the British Dental Association (BDA) on dental amalgams? Visit the BDA website and read the Amalgam Fact File (http://www.bda.org/dentists/policy-research/bda-policies/public-health/fact-files/amalgam.aspx).

See Subchapter 1.2 for what you should do in the event of a mercury spillage and how to safely dispose of mercury.

Mercury is also released into the environment from industrial uses, waste disposal and pollution from fossil fuels. It enters the rivers, lakes and seas and is taken up by fish. The highest levels therefore are found in tuna, swordfish and shark and, in the UK, in skate and dogfish. People who eat a lot of these fish have the highest levels of mercury in their bodies.

AMALGAM BONDING

Although conventional amalgam does not bond to the tooth, if enamel and dentine are conditioned with 10% phosphoric acid, and 2-hydroxyethyl methacrylate (HEMA) is applied to the dentine for dentinal bonding, and then a layer of very *loose-filled* composite resin is applied, amalgam condensed into the tooth while the resin is unset will cause tags of amalgam and filled resin to intermingle so that when both materials set, they are locked together, and bonded to the tooth.

Composite Resins

Composite resin fillings (also called white or tooth-coloured fillings) can be made to resemble the appearance of the natural tooth. They are strong, durable and cosmetically far superior to amalgams. However, they are also much more expensive than amalgam, allergies sometimes occur and there has been concern about the potential health effects from leaching of various chemicals from the resins (see below).

Besides their aesthetic advantage, the tooth preparation for composite fillings requires less tooth structure removal because resins bond (adhere) to enamel (and dentine too, although not as well) via a micro-mechanical bond. Composites bond to the tooth surface after the enamel has been etched with a special acid (phosphoric acid), and are usually light cured (some are chemically cured).

Modern dental composite materials are a blend of glass or ceramic particles in a photo-polymerisable, synthetic, organic resin matrix. Composites are all combinations of silane-coated inorganic filler particles (commonly based on barium, quartz or strontium glass particles) with a dimethacrylate resin, either bis-GMA or urethane dimethacrylate (UDEMA). The silane agent holds the filler and resin together. An initiator package begins the polymerisation reaction of the composite when external energy (light/heat etc.) is applied to 'cure' the filling.

In summary, composite resins contain:

- Bis-GMA or urethane dimethacrylate
- Other chemicals, especially: acrylated expoxides or acrylated urethanes; **aliphatic** acrylates
- Initiator (e.g. benzoyl peroxide)
- Activators (e.g. tertiary **aromatic** amines)
- Inhibitors (e.g. hydroquinone).

'Conventional' composites have been superseded by the others with smaller particles (small particle, hybrid and microfine). But even the small-particle composites are disappearing from the scene. The commonest types used today are the hybrids, which have particles graded in size to achieve the maximum packing – enhancing the mechanical properties and also giving better aesthetics as they can be highly polished.

Composite resin fillings are less durable than amalgam with much lower wear-resistance. They also undergo some shrinkage on curing, causing the material to pull away from the cavity walls. This makes the tooth vulnerable to microleakage and recurrent decay.

297

Terms to Learn
Aliphatics and aromatics: the two classes of hydrocarbon compounds.

Safety Issues Related to Composites

Composite resin fillings often contain the chemical bis-GMA (also called BPA), which *theoretically* might contribute to the development of breast cancer. However, there is no scientific evidence of this. Bisphenol A is widely used in the manufacture of many consumer plastic products such as hard polycarbonate water bottles, some baby bottles, and the lining of food cans and bottle tops. The American Dental Association states that: 'any concern about potential BPA exposure from dental sealants or composites is unwarranted [at the time of writing] …. When compared with other sources of BPA, these dental materials pose significantly lower exposure concerns'.

Pex (cross-linked polyethylene)-based composite materials do not contain bis-GMA.

Glass Ionomer Cements (GICs)

Conventional GICs are applied directly to unconditioned enamel and dentine, where they dissolve some of the hydroxyapatite. Then the metallic polyalkenoate salts in the GIC combine with hydroxyapatite to chemically adhere the GIC to the tooth.

GICs are almost as expensive as composite resins but less aesthetic. They also do not wear as well. However, they are generally considered good materials to use for root caries and for fissure sealants, not least because they release fluoride. There seem to be no significant safety concerns.

Several faster-setting, high-viscosity conventional GICs are available, developed for use with the **atraumatic restorative technique (ART)** used in developing countries.

The term compomer, a combination of COMPosite and ionOMER, was intended to suggest the combination of composite and glass-ionomer technology. Resin-modified (RM)-GIC is the current term for the combination of GIC and composite resin that hardens when light cured. It lasts longer and can achieve a better aesthetic result than GIC but not as well as composite. RM-GICs are not recommended for occlusal restorations, and the cost is similar to composites.

Other developments of GICs include metal-reinforced GICs. These either contain silver amalgam alloy powder or silver particles, which are **sintered** onto the glass to increase the physical strength and provide radiopacity (e.g. cermet (ceramic-metal)). However, the clinical performance of cermets is inferior to other restorative materials, so their use is not encouraged.

INDIRECT RESTORATIVE MATERIALS

Gold

Gold fillings (inlays or onlays) have excellent durability and wear well. They do not cause excessive wear of the opposing teeth, but they are unaesthetic. They are also expensive and conduct heat and cold.

Ceramics

Porcelain restorations have excellent aesthetics, but are brittle and hard. Thus they can cause wear of the opposing teeth. Porcelain veneers are good for anterior teeth but porcelain is rarely recommended for posterior fillings.

Yttria-stabilised zirconia is as aesthetic as porcelain. But it has high mechanical resistance, is highly biocompatible and is stronger than porcelain.

Endodontic Materials

Endodontic materials include:

- Devitalising agents (relatively rarely used – they 'kill' the tissue).
- Sterilising agents (decontaminating).
- Irrigation agents (used throughout canal preparation and beyond).

Term to Learn
Atraumatic restorative technique (ART): a technique of treating teeth with caries in which the carious tissue is removed using only hand instruments; the cavity is then filled with a GIC. ART is not suitable for all teeth with caries.

Term to Learn
Sintered: the process by which the powder particles are 'welded' together using heat.

Term to Learn
Biocompatible: a material that will not harm living tissues when inserted into the body.

298

- *Gutta-percha*: most root canal fillings are done with gutta-percha. Some gutta-percha brands contain 0.6–0.7% cadmium, probably due to cadmium-based pigment. Cadmium-pigments are prohibited in some countries but may be permitted for dental materials.
- *Chloroform*: may be used both as an ingredient in a so-called sealer and as a solvent for the gutta-percha itself but is banned in some countries due to its carcinogenic potential.
- *AH26*: an epoxy-based sealer which contains bis-GMA. It may release formaldehyde and has a potential effect like oestrogens.

> **KEY POINT** Hypochlorite can cause burns if spilt on soft tissues and will bleach clothes.

HISTORICAL NOTES

A wide range of materials has been used in the past in endodontics, including asphalt, benzene, lead oxide, phenol, phenylmercury, formaldehyde, cadmium, creosote, sulphuric acid and others. For devitalising, materials such as arsenic, phenol and cocaine were used. Many ingredients in root canal filling materials have also been regarded as environmental hazards. A few, such as N2 (a lead-containing root filling material) have been declared by some authorities not to conform to acceptable treatment standards.

Main Hazards from Other Dental Materials

The main dangers to dental nurses from other dental materials include burns, allergies or irritant dermatitis (see also Subchapter 1.1).

BURNS
Corrosives

Acids such as phosphoric acid, chromic acid and trichloroacetic acid, and corrosives such as para-mono-chlorphenol, and sometimes even glutaraldehyde, can cause burns to clinical dental staff.

Inflammable Liquids

Many alcohols, acetone and solvents and thinners are toxic and may be flammable. They can also cause dermatitis. Many are irritant to the eyes and respiratory tract and some are suspected carcinogens.

Chronic exposure to high levels of solvents may cause renal or liver damage and some, such as toluene, may be teratogenic.

BERYLLIUM

Beryllium is found in some metal alloys used in dental appliances; the dust from it can be a hazard in the dental laboratory. About 1–15% of all people occupationally exposed to beryllium in air become sensitive to beryllium and may develop chronic beryllium disease. This is an irreversible and sometimes fatal scarring of the lungs.

X-RAY SOLUTIONS

Developers for radiographs contain hydroquinone; fixatives contain acetic acid and sodium thiosulphate. These solutions should be handled carefully and with rubber gloves, avoiding contact with the eyes (it is best to wear protective eyewear) and avoiding excessive inhalation. This is because they may cause dermatitis, conjunctivitis or bronchitis. Never let skin come into contact with processing fluids. Wash off any spillages immediately in running water. Spilt chemicals should be mopped up immediately.

> ### BOX 12.2 DENTAL MATERIALS AND ALLERGIES
>
> Dental materials and healthcare products that may occasionally cause allergic reactions are:
>
> - Denture fixatives
> - Essential oils (e.g. eugenol)
> - Iodides
> - Latex
> - Metals (amalgam, gold and other alloys, wires)
> - Methyl methacrylate (acrylic)
> - Oral healthcare products: mouthwashes, toothpastes
> - Periodontal dressings
> - Resins (colophony, composite and epoxy)
> - Rubber base impression materials.

ALLERGIES

A number of dental materials may cause allergies (Box 12.2), but latex allergy is the most common.

Latex Allergy

Latex allergy is an important occupational problem, especially with abrasive handwashing, which increases the risk of sensitisation. Allergic reactions have become increasingly common since the widespread use of protective medical/dental gloves. (This is in response to the advent of HIV/AIDS.) Latex exposure may occur via the skin, mucous membranes, or the lungs with inhalation of latex glove powder. (Allergens may attach to lubricating powder, and become aerosolised, causing sensitisation or, in those who are allergic, respiratory, ocular or nasal symptoms.) Many items used in dental practice can contain latex (Box 12.3).

> **IDENTIFY AND LEARN**
>
> Find 10 items in your workplace that may contain latex.

People with latex allergy may also have allergen cross-reactivity and react to foods such as avocado, banana, chestnut and kiwi.

Latex antigens must be avoided by people who are allergic. 'Low-allergen' latex gloves are available but there is little certainty that these offer any real benefit. Alternative choices in gloves, medical or dental or other products for persons with latex allergy include:

- Butadiene
- Nitrile (acrylonitrile butadiene),
- Polychloroprene (Neolon)
- Polystyrene-poly(ethylene-butylene)-polystyrene (Tactylon)
- Polyurethane
- Styrene
- Vinyl (polyvinyl chloride)
- Vitrile (a blend of vinyl and nitrile).

DENTAL TREATMENT OF PATIENTS WITH PROVEN OR POSSIBLE LATEX ALLERGY

All patients claiming to be sensitive to latex should have their claims taken seriously. Non-latex (Vinyl, Neoprene, Neolon, nitrile-based or polymer) gloves should be used and an alternative (rubber) dam can be fashioned from vinyl sheet or a vinyl glove. There is only a single report of a supposed allergic reaction to gutta-percha in the literature, but no definitive proof that the patient had a true allergic reaction to it. Gutta-percha does not cross-react with latex, but some gutta-percha products include gutta-balata, which can cross-react. Occasionally, healthcare workers have reacted to gutta-percha.

However, in patients with a true immediate hypersensitivity to natural rubber latex, the patient's doctor should be consulted prior to initiating the obturation phase of treatment.

BOX 12.3 LATEX IN DENTAL ITEMS

The following may have latex:

- Equipment and laboratory work previously handled with latex gloves
- Adhesive dressings and their packaging
- Amalgam carrier tips
- Bandages and tapes
- Chip syringes
- Dappen dishes
- Endodontic stops
- Gloves
- Gutta-percha and gutta-balata
- Headgear and head positioners
- Induction masks
- Latex ties on face masks
- Local anaesthetic cartridges*
- Mixing bowls
- Needle guards
- Orthodontic elastics
- Prophylaxis cups and polishing wheels and points
- Protective eyewear
- Rubber dam
- Rubber (latex) gloves
- Rubber sleeves on props, and bite blocks
- Spatula
- Suction tips
- Surgical face masks and other protective items of clothing, for example gowns, overshoes
- Tourniquets and blood pressure cuffs
- Wedges.

* Latex is present in some rubber dental local anaesthetic cartridges, stoppers or plungers – where either the harpoon penetrates or where the flat piston end of a self-aspirating syringe rests. At the other end of the cartridge is the diaphragm, which the needle penetrates. Any of these components may contain latex. Although there are no documented reports of allergy due to the latex component of cartridges of dental LA, the UK preparation of prilocaine (Citanest) contains no latex.

Essential Oils

Essential oils (eugenol, cinnamon, peppermint, aniseed, spearmint, eucalyptol, menthol and thymol) and related substances (such as balsam of Peru, benzoin, rosin, vanilla and perfumes) in soaps, cleansers and some dental materials may occasionally induce contact dermatitis.

SKIN EXPOSURE TO MATERIALS, CHEMICALS AND DRUGS

Direct skin contact with materials, chemicals and drugs should be minimised. Always wear gloves wherever possible. Wash areas of skin exposed to chemicals liberally in tap water or a suitable neutralising agent.

In the dental laboratory, attempts to reduce exposure to acrylic monomer include the use of a protective monoglyceride skin ointment, of changing to an injection moulding technique for denture flask packing, or of using a no-touch technique.

Disposable latex and vinyl gloves are most commonly used for clinical work, and polymer (especially polyethylene) gloves for some laboratory work. Latex gloves protect against many physical, chemical and microbial agents but they will not, of course, prevent puncture injuries. They also do not completely prevent penetration of some organic solvents such as methyl methacrylate monomer. It is likely that there is little monomer penetration of polyethylene gloves during the short period of mixing acrylic, and, for clinical work, butyl rubber gloves seem more impervious. Wear heavy duty rubber gloves at other times – except when fire-resistant gloves are more appropriate.

SAFE USE OF MATERIALS, CHEMICALS, AND DRUGS

- Never use domestic bottles or containers to hold toxic materials.
- Toxic agents and poisons must be stored in appropriate leak-proof containers with correct labelling containing:
  - The identity of the substance
  - Appropriate hazard warnings
  - Information on how to handle accidental exposure to the substance.
- Drugs must be kept in a locked receptacle (the Medicines Act 1968). Any drug and material safety datasheets should be retained for information about the agent and good work practices.
- Any unmarked materials or drugs should be disposed safely: never re-label bottles incorrectly
- Spills should be readily cleaned up.

USING DENTAL EQUIPMENT

When selecting new equipment for the workplace, as a dental nurse you can think about:

- What you want the equipment to do – will the equipment selected be fit for this purpose? Is there any evidence? Is it compatible with other equipment in the surgery?
- How easy it will be to use and maintain – is it CE marked (to demonstrate it conforms to European Standards)?
- How easy it is to decontaminate – what are the manufacturer's recommendations? When selecting new hand instruments avoid difficult-to-clean serrated handles and check that hinges are easy to clean.
- Can the material covering the dental chair and work surfaces be cleaned and disinfected regularly without deterioration? Check with the manufacturer.
- Select foot-controlled equipment whenever possible.
- Training – is it required? Will the manufacturer provide it?

Care and Maintenance of Dental Instruments and Equipment

KEY POINT Dental equipment is often precision equipment and usually very expensive, so take care neither to damage or lose any of it. It must be cleaned and maintained carefully.

Decontamination of dental instruments and equipment is discussed in Subchapter 1.2 and has three stages:

1. Pre-sterilisation cleaning
2. Sterilisation
3. Storage

Pre-sterilisation Cleaning

Instruments must be cleaned or the sterilisation process will not be effective. Cleaning can be done either manually or by using an ultrasonic bath or thermal washer. It is good practice to use an automated washing process with a thermal washer-disinfector whenever practical for the following reasons:

- It is a more controlled process than manual washing
- It reduces the risk in handling contaminated instruments
- It increases productivity by allowing more clinical time.

The cycle time may vary so additional instruments may be required.

The approximate cycle for a thermal washer-disinfector or sterilisation in a vacuum steriliser takes two hours.

MANUAL CLEANING

Before you manually clean instruments, make yourself familiar with the written local policy for staff for manual cleaning. You will also be given appropriate training. Damaged instruments are more difficult to clean and corrosion may reduce the life of an instrument.

1. Place the instruments in a dedicated deep sink and not the basin used for hand washing (see Figures 1.2.2 and 1.2.3).
2. Take care when handling sharp instruments.
3. Put on protective clothing:
   - Disposable apron
   - Visor or face mask
   - Heavy duty gloves.
4. Use a non-foaming detergent.
5. Use a nylon brush (which can be sterilised) or a disposable brush.
6. Fill the sink with lukewarm water.
7. Immerse instruments and clean below the water line.
8. Some instruments may require dis-assembling first.
9. Inspect instruments after cleaning and repeat cleaning if required.
10. Dry instruments with a disposable paper towel – wet instruments inhibit the sterilisation process.
11. Place in the receptacle for sterilisation.

> **KEY POINT** Instruments should be cleared away immediately after use. If you cannot clean instruments immediately, soak them in a non-ionic solution.

MECHANICAL CLEANING

Ultrasonic baths are effective for removing blood and debris from intricate, serrated and jointed instruments. They are also effective for removing cement.

1. In the deep sink rinse off blood and debris below the water line using lukewarm water.
2. Open jointed instruments and/or dismantle instruments and place in the basket. Use warm water according to the manufacturer's instructions, for example, 40 °C for three minutes.
3. Use the detergent as per manufacturer's instructions, for example, low temperature and low foaming.
4. Rinse thoroughly below the water line in clean water to remove detergent if the machine does not have a rinse cycle.
5. Drain and dry instruments.
6. Inspect instruments and repeat if necessary.
7. Always operate with the lid on.

GOOD PRACTICE WHEN USING ULTRASONIC BATHS
- Empty the bath every four hours or sooner if the solution is contaminated.
- Empty, clean and dry at the end of the day.
- Test weekly by placing a foil strip in forceps in the centre of the bath for three minutes. Inspect the foil: the edges should be serrated and pitted or the centre should be perforated. The manufacturer should provide a test kit.
- A qualified designated person should regularly maintain and test the bath.

303

Thermal Washer-Disinfectors

Bench-top thermal washer-disinfectors are suitable for the dental surgery. The type, size and model depends on the workload, time requirements and space.

Cycle
- Pre-wash below 45 °C
- Main wash
- Thermal disinfection 80–90 °C
- Post disinfection.

Cleaning of Handpieces

Pre -sterilisation dental handpiece cleaning machines are recommended by the BDA. Many handpieces are thermal/disinfectant safe, but always refer to the manufacturer's instructions.

> **KEY POINT** Handpieces should be lubricated with service oil after the thermal disinfector stage.

Manual Cleaning of Handpieces
1. Flush handpiece with water from the water line for 20 seconds.
2. Remove the bur.
3. Do not immerse in disinfectant or place in ultrasonic bath.
4. Wipe outer surface with an alcohol wipe (isopropyl alcohol).
5. Dry water channel with compressed air.

Internal Cleaning of Handpiece
1. Check oil canister has the correct attachment.
2. Shake the oil can.
3. Lay on a flat surface and hold the handpiece head with a paper towel.
4. Insert nozzle into the end of the handpiece.
5. Spray oil for approximately one second.
6. Place handpiece downwards to drain off excess oil.
7. Clean off any excess.
8. Steam sterilise at 134–137 °C for three minutes.
9. Lubricate after sterilisation if manufacturer recommends.

Pain and Anxiety Control

CHAPTER POINTS

- This chapter covers the requirements of the NEBDN syllabus Section 13: Pain and anxiety control in dentistry. The chapter is highly relevant in the day-to-day situation you will face in a dental surgery or other dental environment.

INTRODUCTION

Any patient can become anxious or experience pain in a dental environment. They are managed accordingly by using different methods of anxiety and pain control. Patients who are very anxious may need sedation. As a dental nurse student, you are not permitted to assist in conscious sedation (CS) but, once you have qualified, you may consider doing a post-qualification course in dental sedation nursing. This will involve completing a record of experience in the workplace and sitting an examination.

The mental state can significantly influence our level of anxiety and pain perception. Most patients are able to accept non-invasive dental treatments with simply sympathetic management. However, operative treatments, especially those involving cutting or removing soft or hard tissue (surgery, implantology, endodontics, much conservative dentistry and some periodontology) can cause significant discomfort. In these situations, drugs may be needed for analgesia, sedation or anaesthesia. Orofacial pain is discussed in Chapter 5. Analgesic medications are discussed in Chapter 12.

> **KEY POINT** The most important aspect of pain and anxiety control is a calm, confident and reassuring manner by the dental staff including the dental nurse.

Some practitioners use hypnosis or other techniques in an effort to help. Physical interventions (restraint, holding still or containing) must only be considered if alternative approaches have been considered and are not possible.

PRECAUTIONS IN USE OF DRUGS FOR ANXIETY AND PAIN CONTROL

It is important always to take a full medical and drug history, since the medical status or medications a person may already be taking can influence the choice of drugs (see Chapters 2 and 6). Certain drugs may need to be avoided or doses reduced in specific conditions. It is particularly important to ensure there is no history of allergy or untoward effect from the drug being considered.

The clinician can check drug doses, contraindications, interactions and adverse reactions in the *British National Formulary* (BNF) or the special dental version called the *Dental Practitioners' Formulary* (DPF).

If aspirin or paracetamol is indicated, it should be given at least 30 minutes before food, since the absorption of these drugs is otherwise delayed.

Special Situations

In general, drug doses will need to be reduced in:

- Children
- Older people
- Liver disease
- Kidney disease.

PREGNANCY

In relation to pain and anxiety control drugs should be avoided where possible in pregnancy, in case they affect the fetus.

CHILDREN

The following drugs should be avoided:

> **KEY POINT** Always check: (i) that the correct drug (and solvent) is used; this is particularly important if another person makes up the drug; and (ii) that the drug expiry date has not passed.

- Aspirin – it can cause a serious liver problem (Reye syndrome; see Chapter 12)
- Diazepam (Valium) – it may have unwanted effects, causing overactivity rather than sedation
- Tetracyclines – they may discolour the teeth (see Chapter 5).

ANAESTHESIA AND SEDATION

DEFINITIONS

- *Analgesia* – the inability to feel pain while still conscious (from the Greek *an-*, 'without', plus *algesis*, 'sense of pain').
- *Anaesthesia* – loss of bodily sensation with or without loss of consciousness (from Greek *anaisthēsia*, 'lack of sensation').
- *Local anaesthesia* (LA) – loss of feeling in a part of the body such as a tooth or an area of skin without affecting consciousness.
- *Topical anaesthesia* – loss of feeling in a part of the body such as an area of mucosa or skin, produced by a locally applied drug; there is no effect on consciousness.
- *Regional anaesthesia* – numbness of a larger part of the body, also without affecting consciousness.
- *General anaesthesia* (GA) – numbness of the body, with loss of consciousness and protective reflexes (e.g. cough reflex).
- *Sedation* – depression of a patient's awareness to the environment and reduction of their responsiveness to external stimulation. Achieved by the administration of drugs. Often given to facilitate a procedure under local anaesthesia. Consciousness and protective reflexes (e.g. cough reflex) are retained.
- *Conscious sedation* (CS) – a state of sedation in which the patient remains aware of his or her person, surroundings and conditions, but without experiencing pain or anxiety. Consciousness and protective reflexes (e.g. cough reflex) are retained.
- *Relative analgesia* (RA) – the relief of pain without loss of consciousness or protective reflexes (e.g. cough reflex). This is inhalation sedation.

There are two types of anaesthetic used in medicine:

- Local – used only in a specific area
- General – has an effect on the whole body.

Local anaesthesia (or local analgesia) is required for many dental procedures. Thousands of patients are treated successfully using LA, without any problem. Some people, however, cannot accept injections and others have a pronounced gag reflex or fear of 'the drill'. In these patients LA cannot be used or will not help. Such patients may benefit from using CS.

CS can be induced through several routes:

- Oral
- Inhalational (nitrous oxide or 'laughing gas') – also called 'relative analgesia' or RA, or inhalational sedation
- Intravenous or IV (usually midazolam)
- Intra-nasal.

In extreme cases where the patient is unable to co-operate, or in major procedures such as maxillofacial surgery, GA is indicated. However, GA can be potentially dangerous and life-threatening. Therefore GA must be given in a hospital with **critical care** facilities.

> **Term to Learn**
> **Critical care:** the care provided to patients who are critically ill and who usually require very intensive monitoring, e.g. patients in an intensive care unit (ICU or ITU for short).

LOCAL ANAESTHESIA

Local anaesthesia is generally a very safe procedure. It is made safer by ensuring that:

- Any medical problems or previous untoward reactions are noted while taking the history
- The patient has eaten meals as normal
- The injection is not given intravenously by accident
- The correct dose is given
- The patient is lying back when the injection is given.

Types of Local Anaesthesia

307

SURFACE OR TOPICAL ANAESTHESIA

This is the application of LA spray, solution, gel or cream to the skin or a mucous membrane which has a short-lasting effect restricted to the area of contact. For example:

- Paste (e.g. benzocaine (Ultracare)) and spray formulations or a tablet which is sucked (lidocaine/benzocaine) can be used before giving LA injections or before taking an impression or radiograph to prevent retching
- Gel (Oraquix, which is a lidocaine plus prilocaine periodontal gel) formulations can be applied to the gingiva before scaling
- Cream (e.g. EMLA, which is lidocaine plus prilocaine), gel (e.g. Ametop, which is tetracaine) and medicated plaster (e.g. Rapydan, which has lidocaine plus tetracaine) formulations can be applied to the skin before injections.

> **Term to Learn**
> **Neo-natal tooth:** a tooth that erupts in the first month of life. Rarely, a child is born with a tooth already erupted – this is called natal tooth.

Ethyl chloride is a highly volatile liquid spray which evaporates and produces a near freezing temperature that causes numbness. This can be used before a minor procedure such as the quick incision of an abscess or extraction of a **neo-natal tooth**. It is flammable.

INJECTED LOCAL ANAESTHESIA

The preferred method of dental and oral pain control is often injected LA, since it is very safe and is adequate for most procedures. When LA is injected it blocks transmission in the nerve that is in that area. This allows patients to undergo procedures without pain. It is also used in most cases where CS or GA are used. LA is given with an aspirating syringe to prevent the accidental injection of the LA agent into a vein or artery, which could cause the patient to collapse. Disposable needles are used (and never re-used; Figure 13.1) to avoid any risk of transmitting infections. Needlestick injuries must be avoided (see Subchapter 1.2).

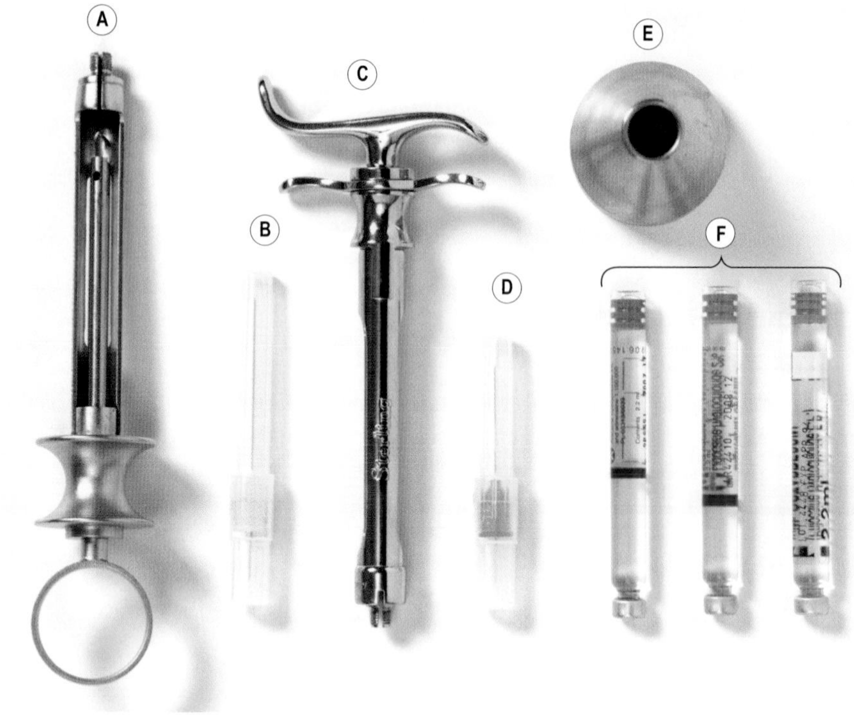

FIGURE 13.1
(A) Self-aspirating syringe;
(B) dental needle; (C) non-
aspirating syringe; (D)
dental needle; (E) Jenker
needle guard/holder; (F)
local anaesthetic cartridges.

Types of Injection

There are several ways in which LA can be given by injection. The most common techniques used in dentistry are: infiltration, regional block and intraligamentary injection. Following infiltration and regional block anaesthesia there is not much systemic absorption of the drug, that is, it does not get distributed in the entire body.

- *Infiltration anaesthesia* – this is injection of LA into the tissue alongside the tooth to be anaesthetised. It can be effective for deciduous teeth, permanent anterior teeth or maxillary premolars and molars. This is because the bone surrounding these teeth is thin enough to allow the solution to diffuse through the porous alveolar bone to the dental nerves of one or two teeth. This injection rarely works for the posterior teeth in the mandible as the bone is denser, but can be used to aid haemostasis.
- *Regional block anaesthesia* – this is injection of LA into the tissue in the vicinity of a major nerve to anaesthetize that **nerve's area of innervation**. Thus a regional block of the inferior alveolar nerve (inferior dental block or ID block) will anaesthetise the lower teeth and gingiva on that side (plus chin and lower lip). The ID block is given at the back of the oral cavity so as to deposit the LA at the site of the mandibular foramen where the inferior alveolar nerve enters the mandibular bone (see Chapter 4). The injections block the incoming impulses from all surrounding nerve branches, producing a wide area of anaesthesia. It is used during fillings, endodontics and surgical procedures in the mandible. The posterior superior alveolar nerve block will do the same in the upper jaw (anaesthetise the upper teeth and gingiva on that side).
- *Intraligamentary anaesthesia* – this is given directly into the periodontal ligament through the gingival sulcus for small fillings or extraction of a single tooth.

In addition:

- *Intra-osseous anaesthesia* – is given directly into the bone via an access hole (only rarely used).

Term to Learn
Nerve's area of innervation: the part of the body supplied by a particular nerve.

Local Anaesthetic Solutions

The main LA solution that is used in the dental workplace is lidocaine (formerly called lignocaine). It belongs to a class of drugs called amides. Other commonly used amides for dental procedures are prilocaine, articaine and mepivacaine. See also Table 13.1.

The majority of LA dental cartridges also contain a **vasoconstrictor**. The vasoconstrictor used in dental LA is either adrenaline (epinephrine) or felypressin (Table 13.1).

- Adrenaline is a naturally occurring hormone which makes the heart beat faster and harder to supply the muscles with more blood during exercise (see Chapter 4). Thus it is not used for patients with angina and high blood pressure.
- Felypressin is a hormone that constricts the blood vessels but does not make the heart beat faster, so it can then be used in place of adrenaline.

> **Term to Learn**
> **Vasoconstrictor:**
> these substances help constrict blood vessels, which reduces the bleeding in the operative field and concentrates the anaesthetic in the area (there is reduced absorption by blood), thus increasing its effect and making it last for longer.

CONTENTS OF A LOCAL ANAESTHETIC CARTRIDGE

Local anaesthetic is supplied sterile for dental use in a glass cartridge (Figure 13.1). This contains (Table 13.1):

- Local anaesthetic agent (mainly lidocaine 2% or prilocaine 3% or mepivacaine 3% or articaine 4%)
- Vasoconstrictor (adrenaline or felypressin)
- Saline solution
- Additives:
  - Buffer to control pH level (acidity)
  - Antiseptics
  - Preservatives.

Dental Local Anaesthetic Syringes

A dental syringe (Figures 13.1 and 13.2) is a hand-held device that carries the LA cartridge for injection of LA. The major problem with most syringes is that the needle has to be removed from the syringe prior to sterilisation. This puts the operator at increased risk of injury (sharps or needlestick injury) during the dismantling process. The rising awareness of infection control is also putting increased pressure on manufacturers to introduce fully disposable instruments. These issues have led to the development of dental safety syringes. The types of safety systems include:

> **KEY POINT** LAs have a limited shelf-life so you should always check before use that it has not expired.

- *Aspirating syringes* – the clinician pulls back on the thumb grip to see whether a blood vessel has been penetrated

TABLE 13.1 Commonly Used Local Anaesthetics

Name (Generic)	Trade Name Example	Working Time in Minutes	
		Infiltration	Inferior Dental Block
Lidocaine 2% with adrenaline in the concentration of 1:80 000 or 1:100 000	Xylocaine	60	90
Prilocaine 3% with felypressin in the concentration 1:200 000	Citanest	33–45	50–70
Prilocaine 4%	Citanest	15	20–30
Articaine 4% with adrenaline in the concentration of 1:100 000 or 200 000	Septanest	60	90

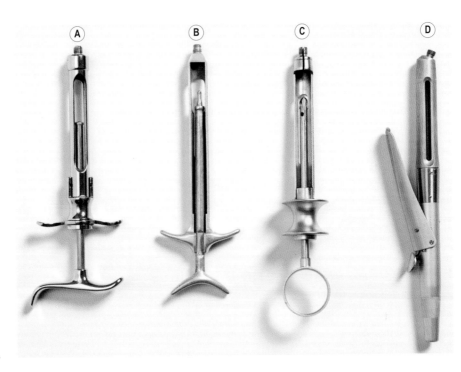

FIGURE 13.2
(A) Non-aspirating syringe;
(B) aspirating syringe;
(C) self-aspirating syringe;
(D) intraligamentary syringe.

310

- *Self-aspirating syringes* – aspiration occurs automatically after the clinician stops giving the injection; nowadays self-aspirating syringes should be used
- *Wand system* – has a 'computer-controlled local anaesthetic delivery' (C-CLAD) system for the improved and painless delivery of local anaesthetic
- *Safety system* – constructed in such a way as to avoid needlestick injuries; it is disposable.
- *SafetyWand system* – like the Safety system, it has sharps protection features to aid in the prevention of needlestick injuries and also C-CLAD.

FIND OUT MORE

Does your workplace have a Safety or SafetyWand system? If not, type 'safety wand syringe' into a search engine such as Google and check out the results.

With regard to loading a cartridge, syringes may be:

- *Breach loading* – in this the plunger is pulled against the spring so the end can be turned sideways. This opens the barrel to allow the LA cartridge to slide in.
- *Side loading* – this has a spring-loaded collar at the plunger end. This is pulled back by the plunger to allow the cartridge in.

LOADING AN LA SYRINGE

1. Always check with the clinician which LA, syringe and needle they require:
   - Sterile syringe type – self-aspirating or non-aspirating
   - Sterile needle type – short needles of size 30G (where the G stands for 'gauge') are usually used for infiltration injections for anterior teeth and all maxillary teeth. Long needles of size 27G are usually used for ID block injections, which anaesthetise a whole side of the mandible
   - Sterile cartridge type (usually lidocaine, prilocaine or articaine).
2. Check for:
   - Correct anaesthetic

- Whether the solution is discoloured
- The expiry date
- Cracks or breaks
- The correct type of bung (stopper) – with or without indentation.

3. Setting up:
- Always put the needle in the syringe first, since if the cartridge is inserted first the needle may bend
- Ensure the anaesthetic passes through the needle by gentle pressure on the syringe; you will see the solution come out in the clear sheath
- Place re-sheathed needle in a needle guard.

Patient Management during Local Anaesthetic Administration

See Box 13.1 for essential advice that needs to be given to the patient before and after the procedure.

- Ensure the patient is wearing suitable eye protection.
- Place topical anaesthetic on a cotton wool roll or pledget and pass to the clinician.
- Pass loaded syringe with the needle sheathed to the clinician.
- Never pass with needle unsheathed or over the patient's face or vision.
- The clinician may take the sheathed needle from the needle guard or ask you to pass it. The *clinician* must re-sheath the needle after use.
- Monitor patient throughout and support by holding hand or shoulder if necessary.
- Ensure re-sheathing device/needle guard is available.
- Monitor how many cartridges are used, only discard when the patient's procedure is completed. Record number used in the patient records.
- The *clinician* should discard needle into the sharps container.

> **KEY POINTS** Most dental patients can be quite satisfactorily treated using LA.
>
> Anaesthesia usually lasts for 30–60 minutes depending on type used.

Hazards and Complications Related to Local Anaesthesia

PATIENT COMPLICATIONS

Possible adverse events about which patients should be warned are:

- Fainting – especially if they are anxious or have not eaten or are hurt during the procedure

BOX 13.1 LOCAL ANAESTHESIA: PRE- AND POST-OPERATIVE INSTRUCTIONS

Pre-operatively, the patient should:

- Declare any medical history
- Declare any previous history of local anaesthesia and any reactions
- Have a light meal before the procedure
- Take their normal medications unless otherwise advised by their doctor or clinician.

Post-operatively the patient should be told that:

- The anaesthetic make take up to three hours to wear off and there may be some 'pins and needles' sensation as recovery occurs
- Take care not to bite or burn the anaesthetised area
- Not to smoke or have hot drinks for two hours after the procedure
- Report any untoward reactions to the person who treated them by contacting the surgery (details provided).

TABLE 13.2 Complications Related to Local Anaesthetic Injections

Complication	Causes
Collapse	Fainting
	Overdose
	Allergy
	Intravenous administration by mistake
Drug interactions	Adrenaline interacts with cocaine, antidepressants, beta-blockers
Failure of anaesthesia	LA given in wrong place
	LA solution out of date
	Infection
	A problem with the nerve supply
Needle complications	Needlestick injury (see text)
	Needle break
Pain	Bleeding into tissues or muscle
	Infection
Paraesthesia (tingling)	Nerve damage from needle or LA solution (usually from prilocaine or articaine)
Paralysis (temporary)	Facial or ocular palsy from misplaced injection
Trismus (restricted mouth opening)	Bleeding into tissues or muscle infection

- Prolonged anaesthesia – when they can bite or burn themselves
- Bleeding into tissues which can cause temporary bruising or difficulty in mouth opening (trismus).

Patients may also experience palpitations, cold sweat, restlessness and excitation. Table 13.2 provides an overview of possible complications. Allergic reactions to LA are very rare.

Intraligamentary injection can result in rapid absorption into the systemic circulation, but the volumes used for this technique are very small.

Intravascular Administration of Local Anaesthetic

Reports of serious interactions between LA preparations and medicines are rare. Clinicians can minimise the risk of interactions by using an aspirating syringe, which reduces the likelihood of the LA being administered directly into a blood vessel and several of the other possible complications of LA listed in Table 13.1.

OPERATOR COMPLICATIONS: NEEDLESTICK INJURY

The main danger is of a sharps (needlestick; inoculation) injury, which can cause not only local damage but could transmit a bloodborne infection. It is the clinician's rather than the dental nurse's responsibility to re-sheath and place it in a needle guard. Care must be taken while re-sheathing, in particular, to avoid needlestick injuries. One-third of all reported sharps injuries in dental practice are due to the use of non-disposable dental syringes, and most injuries occur during removal and disposal of the needle from the non-disposable syringe.

KEY POINT *Always* handle all sharps carefully, *never* re-sheath needles, and dispose all sharps and needles directly into sharps bins.

Several different types of safety syringe are now available on the market.

CONSCIOUS SEDATION

As explained at the start of this chapter, some patients require more than just an LA – they may require CS or GA to be able to have treatment (Box 13.2). Conscious sedation is a technique in which the use of a drug produces a state of depression of the central nervous

BOX 13.2 MAIN INDICATIONS FOR CONSCIOUS SEDATION (OR GA)

- Patients with dental phobia.
- Extensive procedures, major surgery.
- Patients unable to co-operate with just LA.
- Nervous children.
- Patients with a strong gag reflex.

system to enable treatment to be carried out (but LA is also given). Verbal contact with the patient is maintained throughout the period of sedation.

The level of sedation must be such that the patient:

- Remains conscious
- Retains protective reflexes
- Is able to respond to verbal commands.

> **KEY POINT** Conscious sedation is *not* general anaesthesia as the patient does not lose consciousness. Verbal contact is maintained throughout.

Sedation beyond this level of consciousness must be considered to be GA.

CS is usually given as:

- Inhalational sedation
- IV sedation.

In the dental workplace, inhalation sedation is the method of choice in most cases and it is sometimes termed relative analgesia (RA). Minimal nitrous oxide plus oxygen (usually at least 30%) is used.

The patient must have no contraindications (Box 13.3), and must have a responsible escort with them. Also, the patient's responsibilities (e.g. their job, night duty, caring for young children) must be such as to permit them to receive sedation safely.

BOX 13.3 MAIN CONTRAINDICATIONS FOR CONSCIOUS SEDATION (OR GA)

- Unavailability of:
  - ○ Necessary equipment
  - ○ Necessary staff
  - ○ Escort.
- Empty stomach (if patient has taken nothing except plain water by mouth in the previous six hours).
- Medical contraindications such as:
  - ○ Respiratory disease
  - ○ Ludwig angina (infection around throat)
  - ○ Angioedema (swelling around throat)
  - ○ Severe cardiovascular disease
  - ○ Hypertension
  - ○ Bleeding tendency
  - ○ Severe anaemia
  - ○ Metabolic or endocrine disorders, including liver disease, kidney disease; poorly controlled diabetes; hyperthyroidism (thyrotoxicosis); hypothyroidism; Addison disease (hypoadrenalism); adrenocortical suppression.
- Specific contraindications to GA drugs:
  - ○ Halothane sensitivity or recent anaesthesia with halothane
  - ○ Porphyria
  - ○ Suxamethonium sensitivity.

Continued...

> ### BOX 13.3 MAIN CONTRAINDICATIONS FOR CONSCIOUS SEDATION (OR GA)—continued
>
> - Malignant pyrexia.
> - Drug usage, particularly:
>   - Corticosteroids
>   - Anticoagulants
>   - Alcohol or narcotics
>   - Antidepressants.
> - Cervical spine pathology (e.g. trauma, Down syndrome, rheumatoid arthritis).
> - Pregnancy.
> - Myopathies.
> - Multiple sclerosis.

Requirements before Using CS

Where inhalational or IV sedation techniques are to be used it is wise to have one clinician perfom the sedation and another to carry out the dental work, but a suitably experienced practitioner may assume the responsibility of sedation of the patient, as well as operating. However, this is acceptable only provided that, as a minimum requirement, a second appropriate person is present throughout (Box 13.4). Such an 'appropriate person' might be a suitably trained dental nurse, whose experience and training enables them to be capable of monitoring the clinical condition of the patient. The second person *must* conform to the definition of a second 'appropriate person'. Should the occasion arise, the second appropriate person must also be capable of assisting the clinician in case of emergency.

Emergency procedures should be revised with that person at regular and frequent intervals. This second 'appropriate person' must be present throughout the treatment and must not leave the surgery at any time: therefore, when patients are being sedated, a third person must also be present and available to fetch, carry out administrative duties and answer the telephone or make calls.

314

> **KEY POINT** Inhalation sedation is the CS method of choice in most cases.

> ### BOX 13.4 REQUIREMENTS BEFORE AND AFTER ADMINISTERING CONSCIOUS SEDATION
>
> - Written medical history.
> - Previous dental history.
> - Written instructions to be provided pre- and post-operatively.
> - The presence of an accompanying adult.
> - The patient has complied with pre-treatment instructions.
> - The medical history has been checked and acted on.
> - Records of drugs employed, dosages and times given including site and method of administration.
> - Previous CS/GA history noted.
> - Pre-sedation assessment done.
> - Any individual specific patient requirements.
> - Suitable supervision has been arranged.
> - There is written documentation of consent for sedation (consent form).
> - Records of monitoring techniques.
> - Full details of dental treatment provided.
> - Post-sedation assessment.

> ## BOX 13.5 INHALATIONAL SEDATION: PRE- AND POST-OPERATIVE INSTRUCTIONS
>
> Pre-operatively the patient should:
>
> - Declare any medical history
> - Declare any previous history of sedation or general anaesthesia and any reactions
> - Not to drink alcohol for 24 hours before procedure
> - Eat a light meal before the procedure
> - Take their normal medications unless otherwise advised by their doctor or clinician.
>
> Post-operatively the patient should be told that:
>
> - The effects of the sedative gas normally wear off very quickly
> - They will be fit to go back to work or travel home
> - Although recovery is very rapid, they should avoid driving, particularly two-wheeled vehicles, immediately after treatment, or taking alcohol or other drugs.

Informed consent for sedation must be taken. This means that the patient must be given a full explanation of the procedure, and the nature, purpose, effects, and balance of risks. The clinician should get a consent form signed, which gives permission for a sedation technique to be used together with LA, as well as consent for the operative procedure (see also Chapter 3).

Written instructions with pre-operative advice must also always be given (Box 13.5).

Precautions during CS

- *Protect the airway* – especially in restorative dental and surgical procedures, i.e. use rubber dam, butterfly sponges, etc. The airway must be protected because protective laryngeal reflexes are impaired, especially after the administration of benzodiazepines.
- *Protect the patient's eyes* – with eye protection during operation.
- *Monitor the patient frequently before, during and after the administration of sedatives* – the patient should remain conscious and able to respond when directed. Monitoring may detect early signs of patient distress, such as changes in pulse, blood pressure, ventilatory status, cardiac electrical activity, and clinical and neurological status, before clinically significant problems arise. Standard monitoring includes recording:
  - Heart (pulse) rate
  - Blood pressure
  - Respiratory rate
  - **Oxygen saturation**.

Continuous electrocardiogram (ECG) monitoring is reasonable, especially in high-risk patients; although the necessity for such monitoring has not been proved in good quality studies, patients who may benefit from ECG monitoring include those who have a history of significant arrhythmia or cardiac dysfunction, older patients, and those for whom prolonged procedures are anticipated.

Inhalational Sedation

Inhalational sedation means breathing a combination of nitrous oxide (N_2O) and oxygen (O_2) to achieve a state of relaxation in which treatment can be carried out. Inhalational sedation is convenient both for the operator and patient, and the level of sedation can be easily controlled by withdrawing the drug as required.

Term to Learn
Oxygen saturation:
in the dental/medical context, oxygen saturation is the amount of oxygen that is bound to the haemoglobin in the blood at a particular time. It is expressed in per cent (of the maximum binding capacity of the haemoglobin (normal is 95–100%). It is commonly measured by pulse oximetry. This involves clipping or taping a small sensor on usually the tip of a finger or a toe. The sensor measures the oxygen saturation by transmitting light waves into the body.

315

INDICATIONS

- Anxiety.
- Marked gagging.

CONTRAINDICATIONS

- Fear or non-acceptance of the nasal mask.
- Inability to communicate with the patient.
- Nature of procedure warrants general anaesthesia.
- Medical contraindications such as:
  - A heavy cold (temporary contraindication) or a deviated nasal septum (permanent contraindication) or nasal obstruction
  - Cyanosis at rest due to chronic cardiac (e.g. congenital cardiac disease) or respiratory (e.g. chronic bronchitis or emphysema) disease
  - Severe psychiatric conditions in which co-operation is not possible
  - First trimester of pregnancy
  - Some neuromuscular diseases.

ADVANTAGES

- Patient remains conscious and co-operative.
- It is non-invasive.
- No strict fasting is required beforehand.
- Level of sedation is easily controlled.
- Protective reflexes are minimally impaired.
- Nitrous oxide can be easily and rapidly discontinued if required.
- Nitrous oxide is administered and excreted through the lungs; virtually total recovery takes place within the first 15 minutes of cessation of administration. The patient may, therefore, attend and leave surgery or hospital unaccompanied.
- Nitrous oxide provides a degree of analgesia (although LA is often still required).
- It also provides some degree of amnesia.
- There is no significant hypotension or respiratory depression.

DISADVANTAGES

- The level of sedation is largely dependent on psychological reassurance/back-up.
- Nitrous oxide needs to be administered continuously as long as it is required.
- The patient may have amnesia or a distorted perception of time, but this may be advantageous.
- Nitrous oxide pollution of the surgery atmosphere; this can be reduced by:
  - Use of scavenging equipment
  - Venting the suction machine outside the building
  - Minimising conversation from the patient
  - Testing the equipment weekly for leakage
  - Keeping the equipment well maintained with six-monthly servicing
  - Ventilating the surgeries with fresh air (e.g. open window and door fan, air conditioning)
  - Monitoring the air (e.g. Barnsley nitrous oxide monitor).

ESSENTIAL ADVICE TO THE PATIENT

See Box 13.5.

PROCEDURE FOR INHALATIONAL SEDATION

- *Check* – that the inhalational sedation machine is ready and working, that extra nitrous oxide and oxygen are available, and that you are completely familiar with the machine. Use a scavenging system.

- *Lie the patient* comfortably supine in the chair with legs uncrossed.
- Check that the equipment is as unobtrusive as possible.
- *Explain* the procedure to the patient.

The *signs* of inhalation sedation are positive and pleasant. The patient will:

- Feel relaxed
- Feel warm
- Have some tingling or numbness
- Have some visual or auditory changes
- Experience slurring of speech
- Have slower responses (e.g. reduced frequency of blinking, delayed response to verbal instructions or questioning).

Machine output flows of between 20% and 35% nitrous oxide in oxygen commonly allow for a state of feeling detached, as well as analgesia, without any loss of consciousness or danger of reduced reflexes. At these levels, patients are aware of operative procedures and are co-operative without being fearful.

> **KEY POINT** If the sedated patient cannot maintain an open mouth then he or she is too deeply sedated.

A possible exception may be in the case of a disabled patient, who may be unable to maintain an open mouth even without sedation. If a prop is then used, extra careful observation of the depth of sedation is essential.

If after a period of relaxation, the patient becomes restless or apprehensive, this usually means the level of nitrous oxide is too high and the percentage should be dropped to a more comfortable level. The patient can then be maintained at an appropriate level of sedation until the operative procedure (or that part of it which the patient does not usually tolerate) is complete.

- *Monitor the patient* throughout by checking the pulse and respiratory rate at frequent intervals. The patient should be conscious and able to respond when directed. Dozing is safe, but snoring indicates partial airway obstruction and must be corrected immediately. Both operator and assistant should carefully monitor the patient.

TERMINATING INHALATIONAL SEDATION

- Shut off the nitrous oxide flow, so that 100% oxygen is given for two minutes to counteract possible diffusion hypoxia.
- Remove the face mask.

TASKS AFTER INHALATIONAL SEDATION

Slowly bring the patient upright over five minutes, after which they should recover over at least another 15 minutes under the direct supervision of a member of the dental team or escort. The length of the follow-up observation is dependent upon the perceived risk to the patient. Patients may be discharged from the post-procedure recovery area once vital signs are stable, and the patient has reached an appropriate level of consciousness. See Box 13.5 for the post-operative instructions.

Intravenous Sedation (IV Sedation)

Intravenous sedation (IV sedation) involves the use of a benzodiazepine, usually midazolam. Like inhalational sedation it is convenient both for operator and patient, and the level of sedation can be controlled. However, the drug *cannot* be withdrawn once given. See Chapter 12 for more about benzodiazepines.

ADVANTAGES

- Adequate level of sedation is attained pharmacologically rather than with psychological back-up.
- Amnesia removes unpleasant memories.
- The patient may take a light meal up to two hours before treatment.

DISADVANTAGES

- Once administered, the drug cannot be 'discontinued' or 'switched off'. Flumazenil injection can, however, reverse the sedation.
- There is a short period after injection when laryngeal reflexes may be impaired. Therefore a mouth sponge/gauze or rubber dam must be used to protect against accidental inhalation of water or debris.
- Patient must be accompanied home from surgery and may not drive, ride bicycles or motor cycles of any kind, or work machinery (including domestic appliances), make important decisions or drink alcohol for 24 hours.

CONTRAINDICATIONS

- Psychological reasons: patient is frightened of needles and injections.
- Social reasons: patient will have to fulfil responsibilities after the treatment (e.g. caring for young children, shift work); inability to bring an escort.
- Medical reasons, such as:
  - History of reaction to IV agents or any benzodiazepine
  - Pregnancy (also caution during breastfeeding)
  - Severe psychiatric condition
  - Liver or kidney disease
  - **Glaucoma**
  - Alcohol or **narcotic** dependency (may render usual doses ineffective).
- Children: there is a considerable variability in reaction to benzodiazepines.

> **Terms to Learn**
> **Glaucoma:** an eye disease in which an increase in the pressure within the eye damages the optic nerve (see Subchapter 4.1), which impairs vision and can sometimes progress to blindness.
> **Narcotic:** an addictive drug, such as heroin, which reduces the feeling of pain and induces a feeling of numbness or sleep.

318

> **KEY POINT** Patients given flumazenil following IV sedation procedures must still follow the usual instructions given after sedation (i.e. no driving, operating machinery, etc.).

ESSENTIAL ADVICE TO THE PATIENT

See Box 13.6.

TASKS AFTER IV SEDATION

Following intravenous sedation, patients may have a prolonged period of amnesia (forgetfulness) and/or impaired judgement and reflexes despite appearing to recover appropriately. The patient must therefore not be discharged home until:

- At least one hour has elapsed since the drug was given
- They appear fully conscious.

In addition, patients must be discharged into the care of a responsible escort, after giving the general post-operative instructions listed in Box 13.6, together with any pertaining to the dentistry performed. The instructions should be given verbally and also written down for the patient to refer to later, after the amnesic effect of the sedative has cleared.

Other Forms of CS

INTRANASAL SEDATION

This also involves use of a benzodiazepine, usually midazolam.

BOX 13.6 IV SEDATION: PRE- AND POST-OPERATIVE INSTRUCTIONS

Pre-operatively the patient should:

- Declare any medical history
- Declare any previous history of sedation or general anaesthesia and any reactions
- Come with responsible adult to escort to and from premises
- Not drink alcohol for 24 hours before procedure
- Eat a light meal three hours before the procedure
- Take their normal medications unless otherwise advised by their doctor or clinician
- Not wear tight sleeved clothes
- Not wear nail varnish
- Wear flat shoes.

Post-operatively the patient should:

- Take private transport home
- Have an adult escort with them for the rest of the day
- Rest quietly at home for the remainder of the day.

For 24 hours, they should refrain from:

- Drinking alcohol or taking drugs that could affect the central nervous system
- Driving a vehicle or flying an aircraft
- Riding a bicycle or motor cycle of any kind
- Operating machinery
- Making important decisions.

ORAL SEDATION

Again, this is a convenient way of using a benzodiazepine (e.g. diazepam or temazepam) to sedate the patient. However, the level of sedation cannot be controlled, and there can be a delay while waiting for the drug to take effect.

Advantages

- It is easy to administer.
- Helpful for the moderately apprehensive patient.
- Relatively safe, since protective reflexes are maintained.

Disadvantages

- Variability in absorption time: the patient may become sedated too soon, possibly endangering themselves on the way to the surgery (this risk can be minimized by administering drug on arrival), or they may become sedated too late, thus delaying treatment.
- The level of sedation is unpredictable.
- Unpredictable effect of benzodiazepines in certain patients:
  - Some children become hyper-excited, some are rather resistant
  - Older patients may be very sensitive.

GENERAL ANAESTHESIA

As a dental nurse, you may be involved in pre- and post-anaesthesia care of the patient. Box 13.7 summarises the pre- and post-operative instructions for patients undergoing GA for dental procedures or oral and maxillofacial surgery.

KEY POINT GA is used only in a hospital environment where there are critical care facilities.

BOX 13.7 GA: PRE- AND POST-OPERATIVE INSTRUCTIONS

Pre-operatively the patient should:

- Declare any medical history
- Declare any previous history of sedation or general anaesthesia and any reactions
- Come with responsible adult to escort to and from the hospital
- Not drink alcohol for 24 hours before procedure
- Not eat or drink (except water) for six hours before the procedure
- Take their normal medications unless otherwise advised by their doctor or clinician
- Not wear tight sleeves or collars
- Not wear nail varnish
- Wear flat shoes.

Post-operatively the patient should:

- Take private transport home
- Have a responsible adult escort with them for the rest of the day
- Not make important decisions, drive, fly aircraft, or ride a bicycle or motorcycle of any kind, or operate machinery or electrical appliances until the following day
- Not drink alcohol for 24 hours after the procedure
- Report any untoward reactions to the person who operated on them by contacting the hospital (contact details provided).

HYPNOSIS

Hypnosis may be used to help patients relax and control their anxiety and fears or the gagging reflex. In other words, hypnotherapy can transform a scared dental patient into one who is relaxed and co-operative.

320

KEY POINT Hypnosis can be a powerful method in the treatment of anxiety states and many phobias and **psychosomatic disorders**.

Many patients are anxious about dental treatment and the anxiety can range from mild apprehension to extreme phobia. However, patients with extreme anxiety are rarely seen in general practice dentistry. When they have great pain or severe infection they will usually go to their GP.

Term to Learn
Psychosomatic disorder: a disorder in which physical symptoms or disease are thought to have (or are made worse by) a mental cause such as stress and anxiety. For example, high levels of anxiety worsening eczema or causing high blood pressure or arrhythmia.

The relaxation routines employed in the 'talking therapies' (such as cognitive behavioural therapy or CBT) are the same as those used to induce a hypnotic state. The mainstay of hypnotherapy is the post-hypnotic suggestion. This is an idea given to the patient while in the hypnotic state, which afterwards influences the patient's behaviour in a beneficial but completely unconscious way. At the same time as dealing with a specific phobia, suggestions can be made to boost the patient's confidence and overall anxiety (and improve their relaxation at the next session). Unfortunately, not all patients are able to achieve a degree of relaxation with hypnosis that is therapeutically useful.

FIND OUT MORE

To read more about CS, see the 'A Referral Guide for Dental Practitioners' (website of the Dental Sedation Teachers Group: http://www.dstg.co.uk/teaching/conc-sed/). To read more about hypnosis, see the British Society of Clinical Hypnosis (http://www.bsch.org.uk/).

Dental Imaging

INTRODUCTION

Dental imaging mainly consists of taking X-rays (radiographs) and photographs. Both of these are used routinely in the dental environment as aids to diagnosis and treatment planning. More advanced imaging, such as computed tomography (CT), magnetic resonance imaging (MRI), and ultrasound (US) are also used, especially in surgical and hospital practice.

Qualified dental nurses can process radiographs and may also mount radiographic films. Under supervision of an **IR(ME)R operator**, as a qualified dental nurse you may press the button on the X-ray machine. However, you are only allowed to place the films in the patient's mouth or position the X-ray tube, and to take radiographs, if you are suitably trained with a post-registration certificate in dental radiography. Nurses are not under any circumstances permitted to interpret radiographs.

DEFINITIONS AND BASICS OF RADIOGRAPHY

- *Radiography* – the techniques involved in producing X-ray images.
- *Radiology* – the interpretation of radiographic images.

X-rays, like light, are electromagnetic waves but they have more energy than light so can penetrate the body tissues to varying degrees (which affects the number of X-rays reaching the film). When the X-rays hit a radiographic film, they sensitise the silver crystals on the film, which then turn black when put in a developer. The image thus formed on the film enables the clinician to see different (distinct) structures because of the large differences in absorption of X-rays by hard and soft tissues. Metals and really hard tissues such as tooth enamel appear white, other hard tissues such as dentine and bone appear grey, and soft tissues appear almost black on the film.

RADIATION HAZARDS

X-rays are a type of ionising radiation. Thus, while radiography can be essential for diagnosis and treatment planning, it involves exposure of patients and, potentially, staff to ionising radiation. The problem with ionising radiation is that it can damage DNA, causing mutations that may possibly lead to cancer. Ionising radiations, particularly X-rays, are also a potential hazard to body organs and tissues where cells are proliferating rapidly (e.g. in the fetus or a young child, or in the gonads and bone marrow). Here ionising radiation has the

Term to Learn
IR(ME)R operator: a person who is trained in dental radiography, for example a dentist, therapist, hygienist or a dental nurse who has undertaken a post-registration certificate course in dental radiography. (This involves completion of a record of experience in the workplace and passing an examination.) See also p. 333.

321

capacity not only to induce malignant tumours (this is called an oncogenic effect) but also to damage reproductive tissues (teratogenic effect).

Therefore, since there is always a slight risk from excessive exposure to radiation, the benefit of it must always outweigh the risk to the patient. These advantages and disadvantages must be discussed with the patient and the patient must give informed consent. Women should always inform their clinician if there is any possibility that they are pregnant. Exposure to ionising radiation in pregnant women must be kept to the absolute minimum and X-rays taken only when absolutely essential: benefit must well exceed any possible harm.

> **KEY POINT** Since no X-ray exposure can be completely free from risk, the use of radiography is accompanied by a responsibility to ensure protection.

We are all constantly exposed to normal background ionising radiation arising from the earth (especially in areas where the rocks emit radon gas – in UK this is mainly in mountainous areas). People are also exposed to radiation when travelling by air. So diagnostic X-rays produce radiation in addition to this background radiation. As such the dose of X-rays that a person receives while undergoing basic dental radiography (intra-oral X-rays and panoramic radiography) is quite low, probably equivalent to only a few days of background radiation. However, it might still increase the risk of salivary gland and thyroid tumours. Having a CT scan means much higher exposures.

In the past, ionising radiation was also a serious occupational hazard to radiographers and clinical dental staff. Some clinicians even developed radiation-induced dermatitis or cancer of their hands from holding X-ray films in the patients' mouths during radiography. Having one's hand in the X-ray beam gives about 4000 times the exposure compared with that received 2 m away from the X-ray tube (the recommended 'safe' distance). Therefore this practice is illegal now, and there have been tremendous improvements in technology and techniques resulting in greater ionising radiation safety. Specific precautions to take in dental radiography are discussed later in this chapter.

TYPES OF DENTAL RADIOGRAPH

Dental radiographs are taken to aid:

- Detection of problems not visible on clinical examination (e.g. caries on the proximal surfaces of teeth, subgingival calculus or bony changes)
- The follow-up of disease progression
- Treatment planning (e.g. to decide implant placement)
- Assessment of prognosis.

Dental radiographs can be taken with the film held within the mouth (intra-orally) or extra-orally – when the film is outside the mouth.

Intra-oral Radiographs

For these radiographs, the X-ray films commonly used are called the periapical, bitewing and occlusal films (Figure 14.1), all of which are small enough to be partially inserted into the mouth. Intra-oral radiographs are taken to detect dental pathology including small carious lesions. They can be useful in the diagnosis of:

- Interproximal caries
- Other pathology of the tooth crown
- Pathology and assessment of the morphology of tooth roots
- Periapical pathology (abscess, granuloma, cyst, etc.)
- Pathology in the periodontium and adjacent bone.

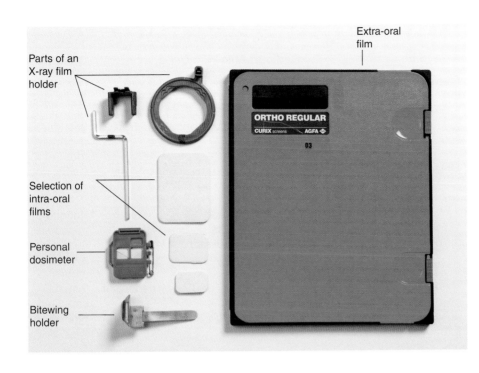

Parts of an
X-ray film
holder

Selection of
intra-oral
films

Personal
dosimeter

Bitewing
holder

Extra-oral
film

ORTHO REGULAR

CURIX screens   AGFA ◆

03

FIGURE 14.1
A selection of intra-oral films, extra-oral film in the cassette, holders and radiographic monitoring badge.

POSITIONING THE PATIENT AND THE FILM

- Precise positioning of the patient's head is important to ensure the correct area is radiographed. The tissues to be radiographed and the X-ray beam must be in proper relationship to produce an accurate radiographic image.
- As in photography, movement during exposure will result in a blurred image so, in adjusting the chair and headrest, it is important to ensure the patient is as comfortable as possible to minimise movement during exposure. (Blurring may also be greatly reduced through the use of fast-speed film.)
- Various film holding devices (Figure 14.1) should be used to secure the film in place. Most film holders will also have a beam aiming device which allows the shape of the X-ray beam to match the shape of the film, further decreasing the dose to the patient (rectangular collimation).

IDENTIFY AND LEARN
Find a couple of film holders in your workplace and ask your supervisor to explain how they help aim the X-ray beam precisely.

Extra-oral Radiographs

Extra-oral radiography means using large films to visualise the skull, jaws, temporomandibular joints and sinuses. These films are used with **intensifying screens** in a cassette (Figure 14.1).

Examples of the use of intra- and extra-oral radiographs in dentistry are given in Table 14.1.

IDENTIFY AND LEARN
Find an occipito-mental radiograph in your workplace to see how it shows the sinuses, or look it up on the internet.

CEPHALOMETRIC RADIOGRAPHS

These are a type of extra-oral radiograph often used in orthodontics (see Chapter 11 for more details).

Term to Learn
Intensifying screen:
a screen that permits a lower radiation exposure but good quality films; digital systems can also help in the same way.

323

TABLE 14.1 Examples of the More Common Dental Radiographs and Their Main Uses

Area to be Examined	Radiographic Film Used	Often Used for
Whole of the mandible and the maxilla	DPT (dental panoramic tomograph; Figure 14.2)	Presence and position of teeth; jaw fractures
A single tooth or three to four teeth plus the supporting bone	Periapical film (Figure 14.3): size varies from 35 × 22 mm to 40.5 × 30.5 mm	Assessing the periapical area, for root canal treatment and to assess root fractures
Molar/premolar region	Bitewing (horizontal) (Figure 14.4): size varies from 35 × 22 mm to 54 × 27 mm	Caries detection interproximally
	Bitewing (vertical)	Periodontitis
Maxillary incisor/canine region	Anterior occlusal (Figure 14.5): size is about 57 × 76 mm	Impacted canines; super-numerary teeth; palatal cysts; salivary duct stones
Third molars	Oblique lateral, or DPT, or periapical	Inspecting unerupted or impacted third molars
Sinuses	DPT or occipito-mental radiograph	Sinusitis, root in sinus

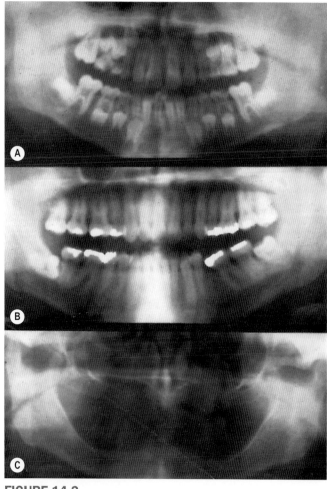

FIGURE 14.2

Examples of dental panoramic radiographs. (A) Mixed dentition period. (B) An adult with full dentition. (C) An edentulous mouth.

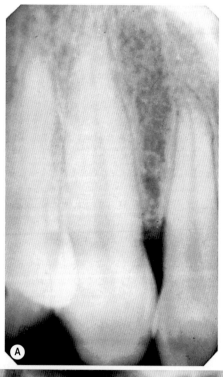

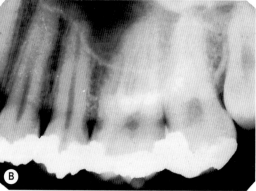

FIGURE 14.3

(A, B) Examples of periapical films.

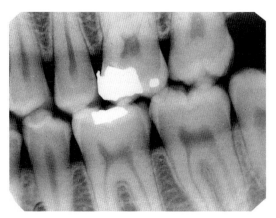

FIGURE 14.4
A bitewing film.

TOMOGRAPHS

Tomography (Greek *tomos* = slice) involves taking films of sections or slices of a part of the body. Panoramic radiography is a specialised tomographic technique that is commonly used in dentistry but the radiation dose may be higher than intra-oral films to show the same areas under examination.

Dental Panoramic Tomographs

A dental panoramic tomograph (DPT or orthopantomograph (OPG)) is used mainly to assess the lower part of the face. A DPT displays both the upper and lower teeth in a long flat film (Figure 14.2). It also gives a good overview of the maxillary sinuses, mandibular rami and the temporomandibular joints. It shows the number and position of all teeth including unerupted ones. However, it does not show fine detail of the anterior part of the jaws, as the spine gets superimposed during taking the film. DPTs are also not adequate for caries diagnosis. One panoramic film gives about the same radiation dose as 18–20 bitewings (see below).

FIND OUT MORE

How does the spine get superimposed on the front teeth when taking a DPT?

Computed Tomography (CT) Scans

Being a radiographic technique, CT scans also show the bone and teeth as 'white', and can be useful in diagnosis of hard tissue pathology. A fairly high radiation exposure is required to produce CT scans. Cone beam CT (CBCT) is a fairly recent development that has the advantage of a lower radiation dose than conventional CT; it is especially helpful in implant treatment planning.

KEY POINT When a DPT is being taken the patient needs to bite on a small plastic mouthpiece attached to the machine, to keep the arches separated, and to keep still while the arm of the machine rotates around the head (but they will not come into contact with it).

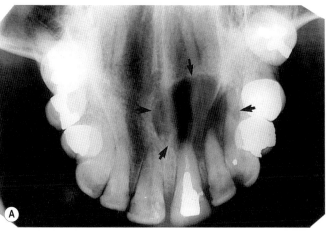

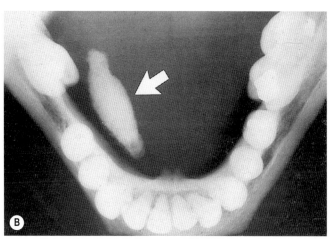

FIGURE 14.5
(A) Maxillary anterior occlusal film, showing a cyst. (B) Mandibular anterior occlusal film, showing a salivary stone.

Angiography

Angiography is an invasive technique with a relatively high radiation dose, but useful in diagnosis of blood vessel lesions and tumours.

Arthrography

Arthrography was used in the past for diagnosis of suspected temporomandibular joint problems but, in most centres, has been superseded by MRI (see below).

Sialography

Sialography can be useful in diagnosis of salivary duct obstruction.

Scintiscanning

Also known also as 'gamma scanning', this is the injection of a radio-isotope (radiopharmaceutical) such as iodine or technetium which concentrates strongly in specific parts of the body. The emitted gamma rays are collected by a gamma camera, which produces images on a computer.

- *Bone scintiscanning* is a high radiation dose technique useful in diagnosis of bone cancer and other bone disease.
- *Salivary scintiscanning* is now rarely used since ultrasound has become the imaging modality of choice for assessing salivary glands.

OTHER TYPES OF IMAGING USED IN DENTISTRY

Ultrasound Scans

Ultrasound is the non-invasive use of sound waves to produce images that can be used to help diagnosis of diseases. It is the preferred method of imaging for diagnosing soft tissue swellings (e.g. lymph nodes, thyroid or salivary glands). There are no known contraindications to ultrasound.

Magnetic Resonance Images

Magnetic resonance imaging (MRI) also does *not* use ionising radiation. On MR images, the bone shows up as black (rather than white as in X-ray films), and soft tissue lesions can be well visualised, including malignant lesions. The disadvantages of MRI are that it is expensive and liable to produce image artefacts where ferromagnetic metal objects are present (e.g. dental restorations, orthodontic appliances, metallic foreign bodies, joint prostheses, implants etc.). Contraindications to MRI include:

- Implanted electric devices (e.g. heart pacemakers and defibrillators, nerve stimulators, cochlear implants)
- Intracranial vascular clips, if these are ferromagnetic
- Prosthetic cardiac valves containing metal
- Obesity (because of the weight limit on the **gantry** and size of scanner)
- Claustrophobia (unless open scanner is available).

Term to Learn
Gantry: in radiology, a gantry is a device that helps to rotate the radiation source around the patient so that images can be taken from various angles and in various planes.

Photography

Photographs are part of the clinical record and are needed especially in orthodontics, cosmetic dentistry and after assaults including child abuse (non-accidental injury). Patient consent to all imaging is required.

PROCESSING RADIOGRAPHS

Digital X-rays need no processing (see below). Otherwise, the radiographic film has several components apart from the actual celluloid film coated with emulsion (Table 14.2).

X-ray processing can be automated or manual. X-ray film processing takes place in the dark, using an automated processor, or a locked darkroom with light for illumination compatible with the red or orange filter. The solutions must be at normal room temperature (18–22 °C)

The manual steps are as follows:

1. The correct sequence is: developing, washing, fixing, washing.
2. Wearing protective latex or other gloves, open packet and discard lead foil into special waste. Discard case into clinical waste and black paper into domestic waste.
3. Handle the film only by its edges.
4. Start the timer.
5. Immerse film in developer for one minute.
6. Remove film from developer (replace lid) and wash film in running cold water.
7. Immerse film in fixer for one minute.
8. Remove film from fixer (replace lid) and thoroughly wash film in cold running water.
9. Dry the film in warm air.
10. Mount and label radiographic film with patient's details (first and last name, date of birth and number).

Faults in Radiograph Exposure and/or Processing

Faults in radiograph exposure and/or processing are shown in Table 14.3 and the accompanying figures.

> **KEY POINT** Good developing is essential for good quality images; poor processing not only can produce a poor image but may necessitate repeating the radiography procedure – and hence unnecessary radiation exposure.

FIND OUT MORE

For a helpful summary of automated processing and quality assurance in dental radiography, and examples of faults, see the Kodak 1998 publication *Quality Assurance in Dental Radiography* (http://www.tunxis.commnet.edu/claudia-turcotte/publications/Kodak%20QA%20%20in%20Dental%20Radiography.pdf).

TABLE 14.2 Components of Radiographic Film, their Function and Disposal

Intra-oral X-ray Film Packet Component	Function	Dispose into Waste Marked
Plastic envelope	Protects the film from moisture and light	Clinical
Black paper	Protects the film from light	Domestic
Celluloid film	Produces the radiograph	Domestic
Lead foil	Prevents radiation that has not been absorbed by the film passing on into the patient	Special

327

TABLE 14.3 Radiographic Film Faults

Film Appears	Reasons	Comments
Faint or blank	Under-developed, under-exposed, not fixed	Low temperature; wrong developing time; wrong strength of developer. See Figure 14.6A
Dark	Over-developed or over-exposed	High temperature; wrong developing time; wrong strength of developer. See Figure 14.6B
Foggy	Exposed to light before developing or old film	
Fading	Under-fixed	
Black line	Bent, or finger nail marks	
Brown or green	Under-washed, so fixer not fully removed	
Cracked or crazed	Dried too quickly	
Blurred image	Patient moved while the radiograph is being taken	See Figure 14.7
Double exposure	Using the same film twice	See Figure 14.8
Poor image	Wrong side of film facing the tube	See Figure 14.9
Area of interest not on film	Poor positioning of film or patient	See Figure 14.10

DIGITAL RADIOGRAPHY

Digital radiography produces images of high diagnostic quality, at least equal to that of intra-oral radiography. It obviates the need for (toxic) processing chemicals and, with intra-oral images, significantly reduces the patient X-ray exposure.

It is vital to ensure a regular back-up of the database and not to rely on the computer's hard disk alone. From a dento-legal standpoint, it is also important to store digital radiographs securely and within a format that cannot be corrupted. The Digital Imaging and Communications in Medicine (DICOM) standard ensures security by containing the image and information about the image, such as patient name, type of image, dimensions, and changes. However, at present, relatively few dental digital systems are DICOM compatible.

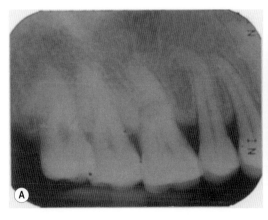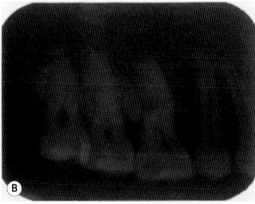

FIGURE 14.6
(A) Under-exposed and (B) over-exposed periapical films.

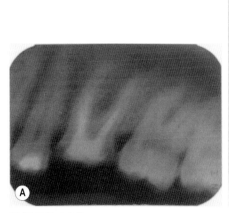

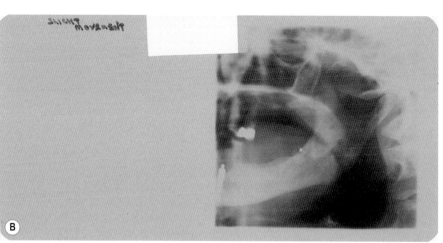

FIGURE 14.7
(A) Blurred periapical film. (B) Only half of a DPT exposed due to patient movement.

FIGURE 14.8
Double exposed film.

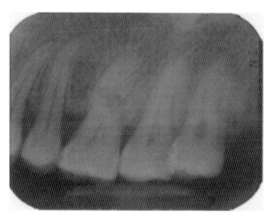

FIGURE 14.9
Back of film was facing the tube when this radiograph was taken.

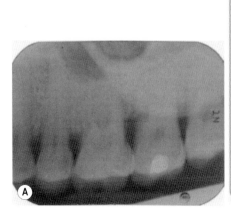

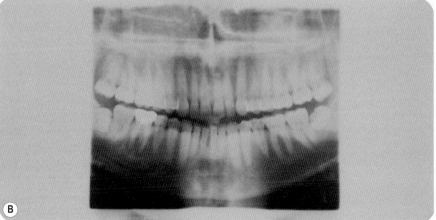

FIGURE 14.10
(A) The cone of the X-ray tube is seen in the top part of this periapical radiograph. (B) The mandibular condyles are not seen in this DPT. Compare with Figure 14.2.

RADIATION SAFETY

REDUCING RADIATION EXPOSURE

Radiation exposure of the patient can best be minimised by:
- Taking only essential radiographs
- Ensuring high quality and useful radiographs
- Reducing field size
- Using the fastest X-ray films
- Processing films properly.

Radiation precautions in practice should include the following.

Minimise Radiographs Taken and the Exposure

The government legislation lays down controls for radiation safety (see below); but the best way to reduce exposure is to take radiographs only when and where they are absolutely essential for diagnosis or treatment. Therefore no patient should undergo dental radiography without having received a clinical examination. The clinician will also take into account the efficacy, benefits and risk of available alternative techniques having the same objective but involving no or less exposure to X-rays. If radiography is deemed necessary, patient X-ray doses should be kept **as low as reasonably achievable** (ALARA principle). Exposure can be minimised by:

- Only taking radiographs when essential
- By reducing field size
- By use of fast films or digital dental imaging.

KEY POINT The need for an X-ray should be decided after weighing the total potential diagnostic benefits against the individual detriment that the exposure might cause.

Radiographs may also need to be taken to avoid medico-legal difficulties. For example, if a patient has pain following a tooth extraction but no dry socket is apparent, it is prudent to take a film to exclude, for example, a fracture of the jaw.

Take and Develop Films Correctly

It cannot be emphasised too strongly therefore that it is well worthwhile in the interests of both safety and economy to make sure that radiographic apparatus and techniques are up to the highest possible standards. Films should be taken and developed correctly. Each film should yield the maximum amount of diagnostic information possible. To achieve this, the following are required:

- Correct alignment and *collimation* (see next section) of the X-ray beam.
- Correct placing of the film and positioning of the patient.
- Choice of the fastest film compatible with image quality.
- Choice of the most effective intensifying screens compatible with image quality.
- Correct processing of the film to give optimum image quality.
- Correct film processing:
  - Processing solutions should be used at the recommended temperature and changed regularly, as advised by the manufacturer.
  - The developer should be changed at least once a month but preferably fortnightly.
  - Processing must be carried out in a light-proof environment – either an automatic film processor or a darkroom.

330

○ Panoramic films are particularly light sensitive and a special filter is required for the dark-room safelight if they are used.

○ Films once processed should be washed to remove chemicals and then dried in a dust-free atmosphere before viewing. They should be filed carefully in the patient's records afterwards.

COLLIMATION

Collimation in radiology means focusing the X-rays into a narrow beam to reduce unnecessary exposure of other parts of the body. Rectangular collimation can achieve dose reductions of around 50%. In intra-oral radiography, beam field size is constrained by using film holding devices (see Figure 14.1) with a beam alignment guide to prevent *cone cuts*. Rectangular collimation for intra-oral periapical and bitewing radiography offers levels of thyroid protection similar to those provided by lead shielding. There is no evidence to justify routine use of abdominal (gonadal) lead protection for intra-oral dental radiography.

FIND OUT MORE

Why was lead shielding considered important while taking dental radiographs? What is meant by a cone cut? Ask the person responsible for taking X-rays in your workplace to demonstrate this to you.

Maintain Radiation Equipment Carefully

All X-ray equipment leaks radiation. Modern and well-maintained apparatus must therefore be used, to keep leakage to a minimum. Collimating diaphragms must be used to restrict the useful X-ray beam to the area under study and aluminium filters to reduce skin absorption must be installed. It is also important to check that the duration of X-ray emission corresponds exactly with what is indicated on the timer switch.

Keep Well Away from the X-ray Source

The X-ray film must not be held by the operator during exposure and only the patient and operators should be in the room during the exposure. Distance is important since trebling the distance from an X-ray source reduces the radiation dose to about one-tenth (the inverse square law). The exposure switch should be so arranged that the operator can stand at least 2 m away from the X-ray tube, out of line of the direct beam, and that the switch cannot be operated accidentally. This aspect is covered in more detail in the section on the Dental radiography room (p. 337)

> **KEY POINT** It is good practice for non-essential staff to leave the room during intra-oral radiography.

Use the Fastest Films

Film speed is an important aspect in determining the amount of radiation exposure. The fastest X-ray film consistent with adequate image quality should be used: speed groups E or F are recommended because they reduce the radiation dose more than 50% compared with group D-speed films. The fastest films currently available are the group F films Kodak Ektaspeed and AGFA DM4. Ektaspeed and AGFA DM2 are available for periapical, bitewing, and occlusal films. Many now recommend that E-speed films should be used almost exclusively.

331

Use of Intensifying Screens

Extra-oral radiography uses cassettes containing intensifying screens to reduce the radiation to about one-tenth of that necessary to produce an image of the same density on wrapped packet film. Cassettes are light-tight containers for light sensitive film and contain sheets of card covered with rare earth crystals which emit light when struck by X-radiation and thereby expose the film. Unfortunately, the detail is not as good as with intra-oral film because of the very poor edge definition produced by the crystals' diffuse light emission. The larger the crystals the poorer the definition – but the shorter the exposure. Rare earth screens (e.g. Kodak Lanex or 3M Trimax or Fuji RX ranges) not only further reduce the exposure but the X-ray tube also lasts longer because of the reduced load. However, for ordinary dental use there is little if any advantage because of the relatively low kilovoltage used in dental sets, and for oblique lateral films the exposure may be made unmanageably short.

A panoramic film may reveal unsuspected disease in the jaws or elsewhere. However, the clinician needs to bear in mind the limitations of panoramic films especially in the anterior region and the lesser quality of detail of the periodontal and periapical tissues. Digital panoramic radiographs do not reduce the dose to the patient as much as digital intra-oral systems. This is because non-digital system panoramic radiography can use intensifying screens.

CONSENT AND QUALITY ASSURANCE

Informed consent should be obtained from patients prior to imaging. Quality assurance (QA) is required to ensure consistently adequate diagnostic information. A well-designed QA programme should include:

- Image quality assessment
- Practical radiographic technique assurance
- Patient dose and X-ray equipment checks
- Darkroom, film, cassettes, digital sensors and processing checks
- Staff training.

Surveys and checks should be performed according to a regular timetable, and a written log of this programme should be maintained. This ensures adherence to the programme and raises its importance among staff. A named person should be leader for the QA programme in a dental workplace.

RADIOGRAPHY AND PREGNANCY

When taking dental radiographs, the risk to the developing fetus is low as the radiation dose is low. Thus there is no contraindication to dental radiography of women who are or may be pregnant provided that it is clinically justified. There is also usually no need to use a lead protective apron; although it is required if the X-ray beam is pointed directly towards the fetus. At other times, the use of a lead apron may actually impair the quality of the radiograph produced. Lead aprons are contraindicated for DPTs.

Staff rarely receive radiation doses above 1 mSv (milli **Sievert**) per year provided the ALARA principle is applied. So special precautions for pregnant staff are not normally required – if it can be assured that the dose during pregnancy is no more than 1 mSv to the abdomen during pregnancy (which is normally the case in dental practice). However, female employees should inform the employer, in writing, as soon as they discover that they are pregnant so that the dose situation may be reviewed.

Terms to Learn
Sievert (Sv): this is the unit of radiation absorbed dose producing the same biological effect, in a specified tissue, as 1 Gray of high energy X-rays.
Gray (Gy): the unit of radiation. 1 Gy = 100 Rads (an older unit of radiation)

LEGAL ASPECTS
Legislation Applying

- European Council Directive 96/29/Euratom, of 13 May 1996 – this lays down the basic safety standards for the health protection of workers and the general public against dangers arising from ionising radiation (this ensures the protection of workers exposed to ionising radiation, including clinicians and their assistants, and of members of the public).
- European Council Directive 97/43/Euratom of 30 June 1997, on health protection of individuals against the dangers of ionising radiation in relation to medical exposure (Medical Exposures Directive) (provides a high level of health protection from ionising radiation in medical exposure).
- The Ionising Radiation Regulations 1999 (known as IRR).
- The Ionising Radiation (Medical Exposure) Regulations 2000 (known as IR(ME)R).

The EU Directives are concerned not only with avoiding unnecessary or excessive exposure to radiation but also with improving the quality and effectiveness of medical uses of radiation.

IRR and IR(ME)R 2000

In the UK, following the establishment of the Radiological Protection Act 1970, the National Radiological Protection Board (NRPB) was created as the authority primarily concerned with safety of ionising radiation. The NRPB is now part of the Health Protection Agency (HPA).

Dental radiography in the UK is subject to the IRR and the IR(ME)R, enacted under the Health and Safety at Work etc Act 1974. The IRR and IR(ME)R Regulations have implications for every dental practice and cover all aspects of radiography from equipment selection and installation through to radiographic procedures and protocols. General guidance on complying with IRR99 is given in the Approved Code of Practice (ACOP). Actions taken under the IR(ME)R 2000 come under criminal and not civil law.

333

FIND OUT MORE

The 2001 publication *Guidance Notes for Dental Practitioners on the Safe Use of X-Ray Equipment* of the Department of Health and NRPB explains the content, scope and implications of the ionising radiation regulations and the regulation of clinical practice as relevant to dental practice. You can find this document easily by searching for it on the internet, for example on the HPA website (http://www.hpa.org.uk).

The IR(ME)R regulations classify dental professionals involved in radiography as follows.

IR(ME)R REFERRER

An IR(ME)R referrer is a medically or dentally qualified person who is legally allowed to refer patients for radiographic examination for diagnostic or treatment planning purposes. They have a responsibility to ensure that the examination they request justifies the associated radiation dose. The referrer is usually a dentist.

IR(ME)R PRACTITIONER

An IR(ME)R practitioner must be dentally qualified. It is usually the clinician who authorises a radiographic examination once they are satisfied that the radiation dose is justified.

IR(ME)R OPERATOR

An IR(ME)R operator is any person carrying out any practical aspect of the exposure. Regulation 11 paragraph 1 of IR(ME)R 2000 states that 'no practitioner or operator shall carry out a medical (or dental) exposure of any practical aspect without having been adequately trained'. Radiographs can thus be taken, *provided they are trained*, by a clinician *or dental nurse*.

Schedule 2 of the regulations details the requirements for adequate training and states that: 'practitioners and operators shall have successfully completed training, including theoretical knowledge and practical experience, in a 'core of knowledge'. This includes knowledge of: radiation production and protection; the relevant statutory obligations relating to ionising radiation; and diagnostic radiology as relevant to their specific area of practice.

> **KEY POINT** The Referrer, Practitioner and Operator can be one and the same person, i.e. the clinician. Conversely several IR(ME)R operators may be involved in a single procedure.

Dental nurses who are not trained in radiography are still counted as IR(ME)R operators if they are involved in any aspect of production of the X-ray image – processing, mounting of films or QA of systems, and they need to be appropriately trained.

RADIATION PROTECTION ADVISER (RPA)

Every dental practice should have an RPA to advise about observance of the regulations and other health and safety matters connected with ionising radiation, such as:

- Direct advice to management on legal and other matters.
- Radiation measurements to assess potential hazards and to control exposure of the workforce.
- Assistance in drawing up:
  - Prior risk assessments
  - Contingency plans
  - Local rules
  - Radiation protection programmes.
- Statutory testing of radiation monitors.
- Statutory tests for leakage of radioactive material from sealed sources.
- Personal dosimetry (see below).
- Critical examinations.
- Radiochemical analysis.
- Restorative action and dose assessment following accidents or incidents.
- Radiation protection training.
- Audits of radiation protection arrangements.

LOCAL RADIATION SAFETY RULES

Every employer who undertakes work with ionising radiation must have a set of written local rules that enable staff working with ionising radiation to do so in compliance with the regulations. They also need to ensure that staff are aware of such of the rules as are relevant to them and any other persons who may be affected by them. The information in the rules should include:

- Name of the RPS (p. 335).
- Identification of controlled areas where X-rays will be used.
- Safe working instructions:
  - Switch off machines when not in use
  - Keep 2 m away from the X-ray tube head
  - Do not enter controlled areas when X-rays are operating.
- Contingency arrangements to be followed in the event of machine failure.
- The name of the 'legal person' – usually the employer.
- Name of person responsible for contacting engineer.
- Contact details of the RPA.

RADIATION PROTECTION SUPERVISOR (RPS)

All dental practices should also have an RPS, who is usually a dentally qualified member of the practice. The RPS has a supervisory role and assists the employing dentist to comply with the regulations. In a single-handed practice the RPS is usually the clinician.

The RPS must have knowledge and understanding of the requirements of the ionising radiation regulations and local rules. They should be directly involved with the work with ionising radiation and should undertake close supervision to ensure that the work is done in accordance with the local rules. They should also ensure that the necessary precautions are taken in the work which is being done and to what extent these precautions will restrict exposure. Although the RPS need not be present at all times, adequate supervision must be maintained in their absence.

> **KEY POINT** The RPS ensures that local rules are in place and followed by all members of the dental team.

The employer carries the ultimate responsibility for compliance with the regulations; this cannot be delegated to the RPS.

STAFF EXPOSURE TO X-RAYS

The European Basic Safety Standards (BSS) Directive requires designation of 'controlled areas' (areas subject to special rules to ensure staff safety). For panoramic and intra-oral units, the controlled area is defined during X-ray exposure as: within 1.5 m of the X-ray tube and patient and within the primary X-ray beam until sufficiently attenuated by distance or shielding.

To ensure staff are fully aware of the precautions to be taken it is desirable that written instructions (local rules and working procedures) are in place and displayed near the X-ray equipment. These instructions should include:

- The responsibility for exposure
- Positioning of staff
- Use of protective devices
- Any restriction on primary beam direction
- Personal monitoring arrangements (if appropriate; see below).

Personal Monitoring

In the average dental practice, exposure to radiation of any staff is highly unlikely to exceed 1 mSv, even in a whole year. The doses received by staff working with dental X-ray equipment are such that there should be no need to alter normal good working practice. For comparison, on average each person living in the UK receives more than 2 mSv every year from *natural* radiation. It is, however, good practice that even for small workloads all staff wear a personal dosimeter (Figure 14.1). This provides reassurance that safe conditions continue to prevail. There are at least three types of personal dosimeters: film 'badges', the new Luxel technology and TLDs (thermoluminescent dosimeters).

> **KEY POINT** Anyone who works with radiation and actually gets or might get 10% of the annual limit is recommended to wear a dosimeter. Dental practices generally are not *required* to provide dosimeters to staff since the exposures are low and the beam sizes small.

Dosimeters *do not* protect or shield you from radiation exposure; they merely inform how much radiation (if any) that the wearer received. The guidance for wearing personal dosimeters is:

- WEAR IT when working.
- DO NOT WEAR IT:

- When you are receiving X-rays for your personal healthcare
- Away from the workplace.
- DO NOT:
  - Share it with someone else
  - Tamper with it, or anyone else's dosimeter.
- DO:
  - TURN IT IN promptly on leaving employment
  - REPORT A LOST/DAMAGED unit immediately
  - STORE the dosimeter in a radiation-safe area and a place that is not hot.

The recorded occupational doses should be reviewed by the RPS on receipt of the dose reports, and action taken if any dose exceeds that expected, e.g. 150 exposures per week should result in a dose no greater than 0.25 mSv. A three-month wearing period is suitable.

For dentistry, personal monitoring should usually demonstrate a dose no greater than 0.2 mSv accumulated during the monitoring period. The RPS should carry out a formal investigation if the cumulative dose received by any individual member of staff in particular year exceeds 1 mSv.

When personal dosimeters are not in use they should be stored outside the radiography room, in a dry place away from heat. The HPA provides an advice and monitoring service 'The Dental Monitoring Service'.

PERSONAL DOSIMETERS

- Personal dosimeters can be obtained from the Radiological Division of the HPA at Chilton, Didcot, Oxon (tel: 0235 831600) or from RRPPS, PO Box 803, Edgbaston, Birmingham, B15 2TB (tel: 0121–627–2090/1)
- At least two companies offer electronic personal devices that give an audible and visual alarm of acute and chronic over-exposure (X-Alert, Evident Dental Co Ltd, 57 Wellington Court, Wellington Road, London NW8 9TD: GXR1 alarm, Nesor Products, Claremont Hall, Pentonville Road, London, N1 9HR).

Training

It is the responsibility of the 'legal person', that is the dental practice owner, to ensure that all staff receive adequate training. Training aims to ensure that you are aware of the dangers and potential hazards of ionising radiation and your own safety, that of your patients and members of the public.

The General Dental Council (see Chapter 3) has set out the level of training in radiography that therapists, hygienists and dental nurses should receive. As a dental nurse, your basic training should include the hazards of radiography and instruction on film processing, mounting and QA procedures. These elements are included in the National Certificate for Dental Nursing and in the current NVQ syllabus.

Specialist dental radiography courses are offered by a number of institutions. The Certificate in Dental Radiography allows the holder to undertake dental radiographic procedures under the prescription of an IR(ME)R practitioner.

Under the regulations, all practitioners and operators (clinicians or other dental care professionals) must undertake continuing education in dental radiology and radiation protection. On an average, practitioners are expected to devote 12.5 hours or 5% of their CPD to the subject of dental radiology. Attendance at formal courses would usually provide at least five hours of verifiable CPD and certified evidence of continuation training in the area.

X-RAY TUBE VOLTAGE, BEAM SIZE AND FILTRATION, AND DISTANCE CONTROL

- Dental X-ray equipment should be designed, constructed and installed in compliance with British Standards (e.g. BS 5724). It should be maintained in accordance with the recommendations of its manufacturer or the manufacturer's authorised representative.
- The *X-ray tube voltage* should not be lower than 60 kilovolts (kV) and for intra-oral radiography should be preferably 70 kV, since lower kV values necessitate higher localised patient exposure.
- Every X-ray source assembly (comprising an X-ray tube, an X-ray tube housing and a beam limiting device) should be constructed so that, at every rating specified by the manufacturer for the X-ray source assembly, the air kerma from the leakage radiation, at a distance from the focal spot of 1 m averaged over an area not exceeding 100 cm^2, does not exceed 1 mGy (milli gray) in one hour. For equipment intended for dental radiography with an intra-oral film, radiation leakage should not exceed 0.25 mGy in one hour.
- The total *filtration of the beam* (made up of the inherent filtration and any added filtration) should be equivalent to not less than the following:
  - 1.5 mm aluminium for X-ray tube voltages up to and including 70 kV
  - 2.5 mm aluminium of which 1.5 mm should be permanent for X-ray tube voltages above 70 kV.

> **Terms to Learn**
> **Kerma:** is an acronym for **k**inetic **e**nergy **r**eleased in **m**aterial.

EXPOSURE CONTROL

- *Exposure control* (timer): timers must operate accurately and reproducibly, and repeat exposures must not be possible without first fully releasing the exposure switch. Older timers are likely to need to be replaced.
- *Exposure switches* on all dental X-ray equipment should be so arranged that exposure continues only while continuous pressure is maintained on the switch and terminates immediately the pressure is released. To guard against automatic timing failure, an additional means of termination should be provided and must be independent of the normal means. Release of the exposure switch may be regarded as the additional means when this action overrides the timer. Exposure switches should also be designed to prevent inadvertent production of X-rays. If re-setting is automatic it should be ensured that pressure on the switch has to be released completely before the next exposure can be made.
- All dental equipment *control panels* should be fitted with a light which gives an indication, clearly visible (and preferably also an audible warning) to the operator, that an exposure is taking place. The light should be triggered by the flow of current directly responsible for the start and termination of the emission of radiation. For equipment fitted with an audible warning the warning should be triggered by the same conditions. The exposure should be terminated automatically when a predetermined condition, such as a pre-set time, has been attained.

The Dental Radiography Room

- Dental radiography should be carried out in a room (the X-ray room) from which all persons whose presence is unnecessary are excluded while X-rays are being produced. This room, which may be a dental surgery or a separate examination room, should not be used for other work or as a passageway while radiography is in progress.

> **KEY POINT** The X-ray room should be large enough to provide safe accommodation for those persons who have to be in the room during X-ray examinations.

- The workload in most dental surgeries is not likely to exceed 300 intra-oral films, or 50 panoramic examinations, each week. However, protective panels having a protective equivalent of not less than 0.5 mm of lead should be provided if the workload is likely to exceed this, that is:
  - ○ 150 mA minutes per week for panoramic tomography
  - ○ 30 mA minutes per week for other procedures.
- Persons in all occupied areas immediately outside the X-ray room should be adequately protected. The X-ray room should be arranged so that:
  - ○ The radiation beam is directed away from those areas
  - ○ Use is made of the natural shielding of the walls, floor, ceiling of the X-ray room where these are relatively thick or dense, e.g. of brick or concrete
  - ○ Advantage is taken of the reduction in radiation level by distance.
- If the normal structural materials do not afford sufficient shielding (e.g. a light-weight partition wall may sometimes be in the radiation beam), protective material such as lead ply should be attached to the wall concerned. The equipment should be installed so that the useful beam is directed away from any door or window, if the space immediately beyond is occupied.
- Adjacent areas, for example, those used as waiting rooms, should not be controlled or supervised areas.
- There should be a radiation warning sign, together with appropriate words, on any X-ray room door that opens directly into an area where the instantaneous dose rate is greater than 7.5 μSv/h (μSv = micro Sievert).
- When the **controlled area** extends to any entrance of the X-ray room an automatic warning signal should be given at that entrance while radiation is emitted.
- If more than one X-ray set is sited in any room, e.g. in open plan accommodation, then arrangements should be made, in consultation with the RPA, to ensure that patients and staff are adequately protected.
- Since the beam is not always fully absorbed by the patient, it should be considered to extend beyond the patient until it has been attenuated by distance or intercepted by a primary protective shielding such as a brick wall.
- If it is necessary to support a disabled patient or child, this should only be done in accordance with the local rules drawn up with the advice of the RPA.
- The tube housing should never be held by hand during an exposure. The operator should stand at least 2 m away, making use of the full length of cable to the exposure switch. A protective panel should, if possible, be provided and the operator should stand behind it.
- If the advice on avoidance of the beam and the protection afforded by distance is followed for ordinary dental radiography and for panoramic tomography, the operator should be outside the controlled area and should not therefore need to be designated as a classified person.
- Any staff who enter a controlled area should either be classified persons or do so under a written system of work, which may include the need to wear a personal dosimeter.
- As mentioned earlier, the operator should check that the equipment warning light and, where provided, any audible warning signal operates at each exposure and ceases at the end of the intended exposure time. If the warning does not operate or there is reason to think that the timer is defective or that there may be some other fault (for example, signs of damage, excessive X-ray tube temperature), the equipment should be disconnected from the supply and not used again until it has been checked and, if necessary, repaired (see below).

Term to Learn
Controlled area: in radiology, this is a designated area into which entry and exit as well as the activities carried out are controlled. The aim is to ensure only the minimal, necessary occupational exposure of staff to radiation.

338

Intra-oral Radiography

- Equipment for radiography using an intra-oral film should be provided with a field-defining spacer-cone which will ensure a minimum focal spot to skin distance of not less than 20 cm for equipment operating above 60 kV and not less than 10 cm for equipment operating at lower voltages.
- When alternative spacers are available or interchangeable spacers are provided, the one most suited to the technique to be employed should be fitted. The correct setting of the equipment is particularly important where interchangeable cones for different radiological techniques are available.
- The open end should be placed as close as possible to the patient's head to minimise the size of the incident beam: beam diameters should not exceed 6 cm and preferably should be collimated to a rectangular field. If a larger focal spot to skin distance is required, a longer spacer should be employed.
- The beam should not be directed towards the gonads. If the patient is a woman who is, or who may be, pregnant, care should be taken that the fetus is not irradiated inadvertently. Where such a beam direction cannot be avoided, the body should be covered by a protective apron having a protective equivalent of not less than 0.25 mm lead.
- The dental film should be held by the patient only when it cannot otherwise be kept in position. It should virtually never be hand-held by anyone else. Exceptionally it may be held by someone other than the patient using a pair of forceps to avoid direct irradiation of the fingers, for example, when a child or a disabled person cannot hold it themselves. In such cases protective gloves and aprons should be worn in accordance with advice obtained from the RPA.
- The exposure factors should be checked by the operator on each occasion before an examination is made. This is particularly important when a short spacer is used after a long one and when there is more than one beam size setting. The larger apertures may be quite unsuitable for use with intra-oral films.

Dental Panoramic Tomography (DPT)

- Intensifying screens should be used with all extra-oral films.
- If the rotational movement fails to start, or stops before the full arc is covered, the switch should be released immediately to avoid high localised exposure of the patient.
- A lead apron is not indicated for DPT radiography where it may interfere with the process.
- For panoramic tomography the beam size at the cassette holder should not exceed 10 mm × 150 mm. The total beam area should not exceed the area of the receiving slit of the cassette holder by more than 20%.

Panoramic Radiography with an Intra-oral X-ray Tube

- Because of the unnecessary exposure of tissues not being examined, intra-oral panoramic units still in use are required to be phased out as soon as practicable.
- In those still in use, beam applicators should be used to protect tissues such as the tongue which do not have to be irradiated for the production of a satisfactory radiograph.
- Care should be taken in positioning the X-ray tube in order to get satisfactory and consistent results.

FIND OUT MORE

For more information on dental radiography, see *Radiography and Radiology for Dental Nurses* (Whaites E, Wincott D, 2005, published by Elsevier).

The British Dental Association (BDA) advice sheet 'Radiation in Dentistry' also includes advice on radiation protection.

339

Communication

WORKING WITH PATIENTS

As a dental nurse you need to have, and be able to demonstrate, an interest in people: the dental nurse works with, rather than on, patients. You will need to listen to and to explore, with the patient, the beliefs and practices that are important to them and their situation, their feelings and their concerns about healthcare. Patients vary, for example in how they wish to be addressed, and so need to be asked. Remember, as mentioned in Chapter 6, not everyone is happy to be addressed by their first name. Some may also wish to involve in discussions and/or decisions people who are close to them. Check!

KEY POINT 'Patients know if you care well before they care if you know' (John Maxwell, American author and motivational speaker)

Communication

Greetings can 'make' or 'break' the professional relationship with a patient. So do greet patients with a smile. Always strive also to communicate in such a way that the person can understand what is being told them. This includes your facial expression and body language as well as what you say.

GOOD PRACTICE POINTS IN COMMUNICATION

- Smile.
- Speak clearly and directly to the patient, making eye contact as appropriate.
- Greet by saying 'good morning' or 'good afternoon', or the greeting appropriate to the culture concerned. For many people, especially people of African, American (North or South), European and other Western descent, the customary greeting is a gesture or a handshake but some patients may be uncomfortable shaking hands with a person of the opposite gender. Unless you are certain of their culture or religion, it is better to greet a patient with a handshake, seeing first if a woman offers her hand, and then say 'Good morning/afternoon' and use their title (Mr, Mrs, Dr, Professor) followed by their last name. Different cultures and religions have different traditions in greetings (Box 15.1).
- Never use the first name alone, except for children and when requested. Ask the patient for their family name and their most used personal name, and if they prefer, use their title and surname, confirming pronunciation if uncertain.
- Be very careful about touching anywhere but especially the upper arm or leg or chest (see Box 15.1 and below).

- Explain who you are and what you do, what is happening and what will happen.
- Sensitively enquire as to whether the patient understands the conversation.
- If possible, say something to put the patient at ease or say a few words in the person's language.
- Encourage the patient to establish a relationship.
- Do not cut across conversations between the operating clinician and patient.
- A carer, family member, partner or companion may be present as an advocate to provide any information that the patient cannot perhaps provide. They may also help address any questions, but the essential rule in communicating is to address the patient directly.
- One of the most obvious ways to assist communication is to have clinic and other signs and material easily visible, in large enough font, readable and understood and available in relevant different languages.

FIND OUT MORE

What methods are used in your workplace to assist communication?

Communicating across a language and/or cultural barrier can be time-consuming, difficult and frustrating. It is important to:

- Ask patients about their preferred language
- Recognise those situations in which use of an interpreter will minimise or eliminate barriers in communication
- Remember that even those with a good grasp of the language may not understand medical or dental terminology
- Explain as you go along
- Remember that head-nodding and smiles do not necessarily indicate understanding or agreement. And silence can have many meanings and sometimes indicates lack of agreement
- Never assume agreement or fluency until you are sure from the feedback from the patient.
- Remember oral fluency in a language often exceeds skills in reading and writing.
- Do not get disturbed if a bi-lingual patient reverts to their native tongue to speak with family or friends, as they are almost certainly *not* gossiping.

Notions of Modesty

Virtually all patients can be embarrassed by feeling exposed, particularly to the gaze of strangers or people of the opposite gender. Particular cultures may have specific rules or concepts about:

- What areas of the body can be exposed
- Touching
- Personal space
- Clothing to be worn.

Establish the patient's wishes about opposite gender healthcare professionals and try to comply. If it is not possible, a chaperone of the same gender as the patient should be available. As a dental nurse, you may well have to act as the chaperone (see Chapter 6).

Do not remove from patients any clothing, head coverings, amulets or jewellery unnecessarily and, if they really must be removed, place them carefully in a clean receptacle and never directly on the floor. Ensure appropriate facilities for washing are available if working in a hospital.

BOX 15.1 GREETINGS IN DIFFERENT CULTURES AND RELIGIONS

Arabs: Greet with 'As Salamu Alaikum'. Use title (Mr, Mrs, Dr, Professor) followed by last name.

To avoid any offence, wait to see if person wishes to shake hands.

Asians: Unless you are aware they are Hindu or Muslim (see below), bowing is a common practice in Asia, as a way of expressing respect as well as a form of greeting. Greet with a slight bow and a handshake. Shake hands with a woman only if she offers hers.

Buddhists: Greet with 'Good morning/afternoon' and use title (Mr, Mrs, Dr, Professor) followed by the last name.

Bowing is a common practice in Asia, a way of expressing respect and reverence, as well as a form of greeting. Greet Buddhist monks/nuns with a small bow with hands together in front of the chest and avoid hand shaking.

Chinese: Greet with 'Good morning/afternoon' and use title (Mr, Mrs, Dr, Professor) followed by the last name.

Christians: Greet with 'Good morning/afternoon' and use title (Mr, Mrs, Dr, Professor) followed by the last name.

Handshake, or, in some cultures such as those of southern European origin, if the person is known, by a touch of the cheek on the cheek of the other person.

Hindus: Greet with 'Namaste' and their title (Mr, Mrs, Dr, Professor) followed by their last name.

Handshake. When a Hindu meets a Hindu, they greet each other with the hands folded together at chin level.

Jains: Use their title (Mr, Mrs, Dr, Professor) followed by their last name and say 'Jai Jinendra'.

Greet only men with a handshake. Whenever a Jain meets a Jain, they place hands together at chin level, and bow.

Jews: Greet with 'Good morning/afternoon' and use title (Mr, Mrs, Dr, Professor) followed by the last name.

To avoid any offence, wait to see if person wishes to shake hands.

Muslims: Greet with 'As Salamu Alaikum' (May peace be with you). Use title (Mr, Mrs, Dr, Professor) followed by the first and last names. The naming system used depends on the area from which the person comes.

To avoid any offence, wait to see if the person wishes to shake hands.

Roma: Use their title (Mr, Mrs, Dr, Professor) followed by their last name and say 'Good morning/ afternoon' or the words in Roma for luck and health ('baxt hai sastimos').

Handshake. When a Roma meets a Roma, they greet each other with a raised palm.

Sikhs: Use their title (Mr, Mrs, Dr, Professor) followed by their first and last names and say 'Waheguru Ji Ka Khalsa, Waheguru Ji Ki Fateh' or less formally by saying 'Sat Sri Akal'.

Greet men with a handshake. When a Sikh meets another Sikh, they greet each other with folded hands.

Touching Patients

Males should:

- Volunteer the right hand to shake the right hand with a male
- Not shake hands with a female unless she offers her hand first.

Females should:

- Volunteer the right hand to shake the right hand with a female
- Not shake hands with a male unless he offers his hand first.

Give things with your right hand only, even if you are left handed. In some cultures, both hands are used.

Keep a respectful distance and touch within gender only; take care to touch only hands or upper limbs, not the head or legs and never anywhere near the breasts or genitals.

Interpreting

Interpretation requires time, patience and expertise. Try not to use family members, or interpreters/advocates of different sects, since there could be:

- Role conflicts
- Lack of medical vocabulary or understanding
- Confused perceptions or misunderstandings
- Withholding or distorting of information
- Differences in health beliefs
- Danger of conflict.

Translation services are available but, in some cultures and with some individuals, there can be concern and mistrust if the patient believes the interpreter may not accurately convey their messages to the dental care professional (DCP). In these circumstances, the patient may prefer a different professional interpreter. Where indicated, use interpreters of the same gender as the patient, preferably no younger than the patient – always ensuring first that the patient is comfortable with the interpreter. They should therefore meet, before the interview, which allows the interpreter also to assess the patient.

It is crucial before proceeding to take the history, for the clinician to check the interpreter's understanding and to:

- Tell the interpreter what they want to achieve
- Ask the interpreter not to omit or to insert information
- Allocate adequate time.

344

Term to Learn
Placebo effect: this is the well-known scientific fact that, for example, if someone believes that they have been given a medication or treatment to help them feel better they will feel better even if the medication or treatment was a dummy pill or tablet or sham treatment.

DEVELOPING A GOOD DCP–PATIENT RELATIONSHIP

The relationship of a patient with their DCP can have a powerful therapeutic effect on them. In fact, it can be thought of like having a **placebo effect**. Failure to develop a satisfactory relationship means that this therapeutic effect will not be obtained. That's why the communication with patients should include:

'CLASS':

- Context or setting
- Listening skills
- Acknowledge emotions and explore them
- Strategy for management
- Summary and closure.

Any bad news, e.g. telling a patient they have cancer, must be thought through carefully, and the 'SPIKES' protocol used for breaking the news:

- Setting and listening skills
- Perception by patient of condition and seriousness
- Invitation from patient to give information
- Knowledge – giving medical facts
- Explore emotions and empathise as patient responds
- Strategy and summary.

TEAMWORKING

The dental team includes as a minimum a dentist and dental nurse but, much more commonly, a number of dental professionals as well as receptionists and secretaries. Technological advancements in clinical practice dictate that as a dental nurse, you should be a skilled professional with a broad range of knowledge of current techniques, materials and, most importantly, patient care.

The scope of practice of the dental nurse is outlined in Chapter 3, and is summarised here:

- Providing clinical and other support to other General Dental Council (GDC) registrants and patients
- Undertaking clinical tasks in relation to the scope of work of the clinician
- Providing patient care including post-operatively, for the patient undergoing treatment.

As mentioned previously, typical roles of a dental nurse may involve both clerical and clinical work. The clerical duties may include:

- Working at reception
- Greeting and reassuring patients
- Booking appointments
- Taking payments.

Clinical duties typically include:

- Preparing the dental surgery
- Maintaining sterile and safe conditions, following health and safety guidelines, including infection control
- Patient care including acting as chaperone
- Helping ensure that the patient is and remains relaxed and comfortable
- Helping the clinician (DCP) record information about patients
- Passing instruments to the clinician
- Aspirating water and saliva from the patient's mouth during treatment
- Preparing and manipulating dental materials, for example, fillings and impressions
- Cleaning the surgery after treatment, and decontaminating and sterilising instruments
- Carrying out stock control.

The roles of the various other dental professionals, as stipulated by GDC, are outlined below together with additional roles available after more training, and guidance as to what certain professionals are by law *not* permitted to do.

The GDC's Definition of Roles of the Various UK Professionals in the Dental Care Team

The General Dental Council (Illegal Practice, 2005) states:

> The Dentists Act 1984 makes it an offence for a person who is not a registered dentist or a registered dental care professional to practise dentistry, or hold themselves out – whether directly or by implication – as practising or as being prepared to practise dentistry.
>
> By law, the following groups of professionals have to be registered with the GDC to work in the UK:
>
> - Dentists
> - Clinical dental technicians
> - Dental hygienists
> - Dental nurses

- Dental technicians
- Dental therapists
- Orthodontic therapists.

All registrants are individually accountable to the GDC, and dentists are additionally accountable as leaders of the team.

The scope of practice of various members below is taken from the GDC 2009 document *Scope of Practice*.

Dental nurses

'Dental nurses' are registered dental professionals who provide clinical and other support to other registrants and patients.

Dental nurses:

- Prepare and maintain the clinical environment, including the equipment
- Carry out infection-control procedures to prevent physical, chemical and microbiological contamination in the surgery or laboratory
- Record dental charting carried out by other appropriate registrants
- Prepare, mix and handle dental materials
- Provide chairside support to the operator during treatment
- Keep full and accurate patient records
- Prepare equipment, materials and patients for dental radiography
- Process dental radiographs
- Monitor, support and reassure patients
- Give appropriate advice to patients
- Support the patient and their colleagues if there is a medical emergency
- Make appropriate referrals to other health professionals.

Additional skills dental nurses could develop during their careers include:

- Further skills in oral health education and oral health promotion
- Assisting in the treatment of patients who are under conscious sedation
- Further skills in assisting in the treatment of patients with special needs
- Intra-oral photography
- Shade taking
- Placing rubber dam
- Measuring and recording plaque indices
- Pouring, casting and trimming study models
- Removing sutures after the wound has been checked by a dentist
- Applying fluoride varnish as part of a programme which is overseen by a consultant in dental public health or a registered specialist in dental public health
- Constructing occlusal registration rims and special trays
- Repairing the acrylic component of removable appliances
- Tracing cephalographs.

Additional skills on prescription:

- Taking radiographs to the prescription of a dentist
- Applying topical anaesthetic to the prescription of a dentist
- Constructing mouthguards and bleaching trays to the prescription of a dentist
- Contstructing vacuum formed retainers to the prescription of a dentist
- Taking impressions to the prescription of a dentist or a CDT (where appropriate).

Dental nurses do not diagnose disease or treatment plan. All other skills are reserved to one or more of the other registrant group (GDC 2009).

Dentists

The scope of practice covers the areas listed below under DCPs, plus:

- Diagnose disease
- Prepare comprehensive treatment plans (this is a 'strategic' role, as a treatment plan can be taken to any appropriate dental care professional for delivery. The 'tactical' planning of delivery of care is not unique to clinicians; overall long-term responsibility for treatment planning is)
- Prescribe and provide endodontic treatment on adult teeth
- Prescribe and provide fixed orthodontic treatment
- Prescribe and provide fixed and removable prostheses
- Carry out oral surgery
- Carry out periodontal surgery
- Extract permanent teeth
- Prescribe and provide crowns and bridges
- Carry out treatment on patients under general anaesthesia
- Administer inhalational and intravenous conscious sedation
- Prescribe drugs as part of dental treatment
- Prescribe and interpret radiographs.

Additional skills that a dentist could develop during their career:

- Provision of implants (GDC 2009).

REGISTERED DENTISTS AND DENTAL SPECIALISTS

According to the GDC, all *registered dentists* are legally entitled to practise any clinical aspect of dentistry, such as cosmetic surgery, provided they undertake only procedures within their competence and do not use the title of 'specialist' unless entitled to do so.

Specialist dentists are those who fulfil certain criteria and thus have a right to call themselves specialists in particular areas of dentistry. As of 2010, the GDC maintains 13 *Specialist Lists in Distinctive Branches of Dentistry* (Box 15.2) to enable patients to identify specialist dentists. Not all areas in dentistry that may be thought of as specialties are recognised as such by the GDC.

Clinical Dental Technicians

Clinical dental technology builds on dental technology. Thus CDTs are registered dental professionals who provide complete dentures directly to patients and other dental devices on prescription from a clinician. They are also qualified dental technicians. 'A CDT may set up an independent practice but must have the correct protocols in place to enable referral to an appropriately qualified and registered dental professional, should they be faced with a patient whose needs are outside their scope of practice. They specialise in the manufacture and fitting of removable dental appliances directly to patients. Working independently they can provide patients who have no natural teeth with full dentures. They can also provide removable appliances in the form of partial dentures, mouth guards and anti snoring devices under the prescription of a dentist' (NHS Education for Scotland, *A Career in Clinical Dental Technology*; http://www.nes.scot.nhs.uk/documents/publications/classa/clinicaldentaltech.pdf).

Patients with natural teeth or implants must see a clinician before the CDT can begin treatment. CDTs refer patients to a clinician if they need a treatment plan or if the CDT is concerned about the patient's oral health.

347

Clinical dental technicians *can*:

- Take detailed dental history and relevant medical history
- Perform technical and clinical procedures related to providing removable dental appliances
- Carry out clinical examinations
- Take and process radiographs and other images related to providing removable dental appliances
- Distinguish between normal and abnormal consequences of ageing
- Recognise abnormal oral mucosa and related underlying structures and make appropriate referrals
- Fit removable appliances
- Provide appropriate advice to patients (GDC 2009).

Clinical dental technicians *cannot* provide treatment for patients as described under the sections for hygienists, therapists, orthodontic therapists or dentists. The skills set out in each section are meant for those relevant groups.

Additional skills that a CDT could develop during their career:

- Oral health education
- Providing sports mouth guards
- Re-cementing crowns with temporary cement
- Providing anti-snoring devices on prescription of a dentist
- Removing sutures after the wound has been checked by a dentist (GDC 2009).

Dental Hygienists

These are registered dental professionals who 'help patients maintain their oral health by preventing and treating gingival disease and promoting good oral health practice' (GDC 2009).

Dental hygienists *can*:

- Provide dental hygiene care to a wide range of patients
- Plan the delivery of patient care to improve and maintain periodontal health
- Obtain a detailed dental history and evaluate medical history
- Complete periodontal examination and charting and use indices to screen and monitor periodontal disease
- Provide preventive oral care to patients and liaise with dentists over the treatment of caries, periodontal disease and tooth wear
- Undertake supragingival and subgingival scaling and root debridement, using manual and powered instruments
- Prescribe appropriate anti-microbial therapy in the management of plaque-related diseases
- Adjust restored surfaces in relation to periodontal treatment
- Apply topical treatments and fissure sealants
- Give patients advice on how to stop smoking
- Take, process and interpret various film views used in general dental practice
- Give infiltration and inferior dental block analgesia (see Chapter 13)
- Place temporary dressings and re-cement crowns with temporary cement
- Take impressions
- Identify anatomical features, recognise abnormalities and interpret common pathology, carry out oral cancer screening
- If necessary, refer patients to other healthcare professionals
- Place rubber dam (GDC 2009).

348

Dental hygienists *cannot*:

- Diagnose disease
- Restore teeth
- Carry out pulp treatments
- Adjust unrestored surfaces
- Extract teeth (GDC 2009).

These skills are reserved for dental therapists and clinicians. Dental hygienists also do not undertake any of the skill areas that the GDC describes as being those for dental technicians, CDTs or dentists.

Additional skills that a dental hygienist might develop during their career:

- Tooth whitening to the prescription of a clinician
- Prescribing radiographs
- Administering inhalational sedation (see Chapter 13)
- Suture removal after the wound has been checked by a clinician.

Dental Technicians

These are registered dental professionals who 'make dental devices including dentures and crowns and bridges to prescription from a dentist or clinical dental technician' (GDC 2009).

Dental technicians *can*:

- Review cases coming into the laboratory to decide how they should be progressed
- Work with the dentist or clinical dental technician on treatment planning and outline design
- Design, plan and make a range of custom-made dental devices according to a prescription
- Repair and modify dental devices
- Carry out shade taking
- Carry out infection control procedures to prevent physical, chemical and microbiological contamination in the laboratory
- Keep full and accurate laboratory records
- Verify and take responsibility for the quality and safety of devices leaving a laboratory
- Make appropriate referrals to other healthcare professionals (GDC 2009).

Dental technicians *cannot*:

- Work independently in the clinic
- Perform clinical procedures related to providing removable dental appliances
- Undertake independent clinical examinations
- Identify abnormal oral mucosa and related underlying structures
- Fit removable appliances (GDC 2009).

Dental technicians do not provide treatment or advice for patients as described by the GDC for hygienists, therapists, orthodontic therapists or dentists.

Additional skills which dental technicians could develop during their career:

- Working with a dentist in the clinic assisting with treatment by:
  - Taking impressions
  - Recording facebows
  - Carrying out intra-oral and extra-oral tracings
  - Carrying out implant frame assessments
  - Recording occlusal registrations

    ○ Carrying out intra-oral scanning for CAD/CAM
    ○ Helping dentists to fit attachments at the chairside
- Working with a clinical dental technician in the clinic assisting with treatment by:
    ○ Taking impressions
    ○ Recording facebows
    ○ Carrying out intra-oral and extra-oral tracings
    ○ Recording occlusal registrations
    ○ Tracing cephalographs
    ○ Taking intra-oral photographs (GDC 2009).

Dental Therapists

These are registered dental professionals who 'carry out certain items of dental treatment under prescription from a dentist' (GDC 2009). Dental therapy covers the same areas as dental hygiene.

Dental therapists *can also*:

- Carry out direct restorations on permanent and primary teeth
- Carry out pulpotomies on primary teeth
- Extract primary teeth
- Place pre-formed crowns on primary teeth
- Plan the delivery of a patient's care (GDC 2009).

Dental therapists *cannot*:

- Make the initial diagnosis
- Take overall responsibility for planning a patient's treatment.

They do not undertake any of the skill areas described by the GDC within the roles of the dental technician, clinical dental technician or dentist.

Additional skills that dental therapists could develop during their career:

- Administering inhalational sedation
- Varying the detail of a prescription but not the direction of a prescription
- Prescribing radiographs
- Carrying out tooth whitening to the prescription of a dentist
- Removing sutures after the wound has been checked by a dentist (GDC 2009).

Orthodontic Therapists

These are registered dental professionals who 'carry out certain parts of orthodontic treatment under prescription from a dentist' (GDC 2009).

Orthodontic therapists *can*:

- Clean and prepare tooth surfaces ready for orthodontic treatment
- Identify, select, use and maintain appropriate instruments
- Insert passive removable orthodontic appliances
- Insert active removable appliances adjusted by a dentist
- Remove fixed appliances, orthodontic adhesives and cement
- Take impressions
- Pour, cast and trim study models
- Make a patient's orthodontic appliance safe in the absence of a clinician
- Fit orthodontic headgear
- Fit orthodontic facebows which have been adjusted by a clinician
- Take occlusal records including orthognathic facebow readings
- Place brackets and bands

- Prepare, insert, adjust and remove archwires
- Give advice on appliance care and oral health instruction
- Fit tooth separators
- Fit bonded retainers
- Make appropriate referrals to other healthcare professionals (GDC 2009).

Orthodontic therapists *cannot*:

- Remove subgingival deposits
- Give local analgesia
- Re-cement crowns
- Place temporary dressings
- Place active medicaments (GDC 2009).

These tasks are reserved for dental hygienists, dental therapists and clinicians. In additions, orthodontic therapists do not carry out laboratory work other than that listed above as according to the GDC, these skills are reserved for dental technicians and CDTs. They cannot diagnose disease, treatment plan or adjust orthodontic wires as these areas are carried out by the dentist.

Additional skills that orthodontic therapists could develop during their career:

- Applying fluoride varnish to the prescription of a dentist
- Repairing the acrylic component part of orthodontic appliances
- Measuring and recording plaque indices and gingival indices
- Removing sutures after the wound has been checked by a dentist (GDC 2009).

At the time of going to press, the GDC is finalising a consultation on learning outcomes: readers should consult the GDC website for further information on roles of dental professionals.

BOX 15.2 THE GDC SPECIALIST LISTS IN DISTINCTIVE BRANCHES OF DENTISTRY

Dental and Maxillofacial Radiology

Involves all aspects of medical imaging which provide information about anatomy, function and diseased states of the teeth and jaws.

Dental Public Health

This is a non-clinical specialty involving the science and art of preventing oral diseases, promoting oral health to the population rather than the individual. It involves the assessment of dental health needs and ensuring dental services meet those needs.

Endodontics

Concerned with the cause, diagnosis, prevention and treatment of diseases and injuries of the tooth root, dental pulp, and surrounding tissue. [Endodontics is part of Restorative Dentistry.]

Oral Medicine

Concerned with the oral health care of patients with chronic recurrent and medically related disorders of the mouth and with their diagnosis and non-surgical management.

[Oral Medicine is the specialty of dentistry that sits at the interface between dentistry and medicine. Many Oral Medicine specialists have dental and medical qualifications, and both are now requirements for entry to training that leads to appointment as a Consultant in Oral Medicine. This reflects that the specialty had its origins in dentistry, but has evolved to formally encompass medical aspects of care.]

Continued...

BOX 15.2 THE GDC SPECIALIST LISTS IN DISTINCTIVE BRANCHES OF DENTISTRY—continued

Oral Microbiology

Diagnosis and assessment of facial infection – typically bacterial and fungal disease. This is a clinical specialty undertaken by laboratory-based staff, who provide reports and advice based on interpretation of microbiological samples.

Oral and Maxillofacial Pathology

Diagnosis and assessment made from tissue changes characteristic of disease of the oral cavity, jaws and salivary glands. This is a clinical specialty undertaken by laboratory based personnel. [It includes the scientific study of the causes and effects of disease in the oral and maxillo-facial complex, an understanding of which is essential for diagnosis and for the development of appropriate treatments and preventative programmes.]

Oral Surgery

Deals with the treatment and ongoing management of irregularities and pathology of the jaw and mouth that require surgical intervention. This includes the specialty previously called Surgical Dentistry.

[Oral and Maxillofacial Surgery is a specialty of medicine concerned with the diagnosis and treatment of diseases affecting the mouth, jaws, face and neck, that sits at the interface between dentistry and medicine. Oral and Maxillofacial Surgery specialists are registered on the Register of the General Medical Council but usually have dental and medical qualifications. This reflects that the specialty had its origins in dentistry, but has evolved to formally encompass surgical aspects of care.]

Orthodontics

The development, prevention, and correction of irregularities of the teeth, bite and jaw.

Paediatric Dentistry

Concerned with comprehensive therapeutic oral health care for children from birth through adolescence, including care for those who demonstrate intellectual, medical, physical, psychological and/or emotional problems.

Periodontics

Diagnosis, treatment and prevention of diseases and disorders (infections and inflammatory) of the gums and other structures around the teeth. [Periodontics is part of Restorative Dentistry.]

Prosthodontics

Replacement of missing teeth and the associated soft and hard tissues by prostheses (crowns, bridges, dentures) which may be fixed or removable, or may be supported and retained by implants. [Prosthodontics is part of Restorative Dentistry.]

Restorative Dentistry

Deals with the restoration of diseased, injured, or abnormal teeth to normal function. Includes all aspects of Endodontics, Periodontics and Prosthodontics. [At the time of going to print, the GDC is seeking views on how it regulates the practice of Implant Dentistry.]

Special Care Dentistry

Special Care Dentistry is concerned with the improvement of the oral health of individuals and groups in society who have a physical, sensory, intellectual, mental, medical, emotional or social impairment or disability or, more often, a combination of these factors. It pertains to adolescents and adults.

CHAPTER 16

Dental Emergencies

CHAPTER POINTS

In the context of dental emergencies, for the purpose of the dental nurse qualification, the NEBDN syllabus specifically mentions having an understanding of:

- Dental haemorrhage
- Aetiology and progression of dental caries.

However, we believe it will be helpful for you and others to have background knowledge of the commonplace dental emergencies covered in this chapter. This will help you care better for the patients who present with these conditions. Therefore, we recommend that you read this chapter to learn about the diagnosis and management of commonplace dental emergencies.

INTRODUCTION

Most dental emergencies relate to trauma or pain from a tooth affecting a person at home, work, while studying, or while doing leisure activities. The conditions that commonly cause dental pain are listed in Table 16.1 and these appear to be increasing.

Other dental emergencies such as bleeding are usually related to operative procedures (pp. 46, 61). These are also discussed in this chapter. Allergies are discussed in Chapter 2 (see p. 56).

KEY POINT With all emergencies, it is essential to keep clear and accurate records, including records of the time of events and procedures; not least because medico-legal proceedings are increasingly common.

TRAUMA

- Trauma is especially common in young males, particularly those who have been using alcohol or other recreational drugs. The face, mouth and teeth are often involved.
- Avoiding alcohol and drugs, and routinely using safety measures such as seat belts and child safety harnesses, can reduce the risk of trauma as a result of road traffic accidents.
- Many other injuries occur in contact sports or recreational activities and could be prevented through the use of protective safety equipment such as helmets.
- Mouth guards made of soft plastic adapted to fit the shape of the upper teeth, protect both the lips and teeth. Pre-formed guards are available, or a clinician can create a custom-fit guard.

General Management of a Patient with Trauma

In all cases of trauma, the medical team should assess the patient if there has been any serious injury. First the clinician will:

- Ensure that the patient is breathing freely
- Exclude head injury (particularly assessing any change of consciousness) or other serious injuries.

Mosby's Textbook of Dental Nursing

TABLE 16.1 Overview of Common Dental Emergencies

Emergency	Definition	Clinical Features and Diagnosis	Potential Complications	Management
Abscess	Localised bacterial infection	Localised pain and swelling. Tooth tender to touch or biting. Tenderness on palpation in adjacent buccal sulcus	Cellulitis	Incision and drainage with root canal treatment (RCT) or tooth extraction, analgesics, possibly antibiotics
Cellulitis	Diffuse soft tissue bacterial infection	Pain, erythema, and swelling	Regional spread	Analgesics, antibiotics and RCT or extraction
Pericoronitis	Inflamed gingiva over partially erupted tooth	Pain, erythema (redness), swelling and trismus	Cellulitis	Irrigation under operculum, antibiotics if cellulitis or fever also present
Pulpitis: irreversible	Pulpal inflammation	Spontaneous, and poorly localised pain	Periapical abscess, cellulitis	RCT or extraction
Pulpitis: reversible	Pulpal inflammation	Pain with hot, cold, or sweet stimuli	Periapical abscess, cellulitis	Dress cavity with zinc oxide eugenol
Tooth avulsion	Tooth knocked out by trauma	Clinical examination	Ankylosis, external resorption	Re-implantation and splinting
Tooth fracture	Broken tooth	Pain, clinical examination and radiography	Pulpitis and sequelae	Restore, with or without RCT, or extraction
Tooth luxation	Loose tooth	Clinical examination and radiography	Aspiration of tooth, pulpitis, and sequelae	Splinting, with or without RCT, or extraction

It is also important to exclude **non-accidental injury** (NAI, e.g. child abuse); images (X-ray and photographic) can help enormously when the aftermath is being resolved.

Examination then focuses on signs of jaw injury (displacement or fracture), soft tissue injuries, and the dentition. The teeth are examined for any loosening, displacement, fracture or complete loss. In addition, the location of any lost tooth or other fragments should be noted.

A proper diagnosis invariably requires at least one dental radiograph and may also require tooth vitality testing. Photographs may also be needed. A soft diet may have to be recommended.

Maxillofacial Injuries

Term to Learn
Non-accidental injury: an injury that is not consistent with the account given about how it occurred. It is usually seen as part of physical abuse in children.

KEY POINTS Keeping the patient alive is the main priority, especially ensuring they can breathe.

Basic life support (BLS) can be provided by dental nurses (see Chapter 2).

General Examination

Immediate life-threatening problems in a patient with a jaw injury include:

- Airway (breathing) difficulties – ensure the airway is clear.

354

- Damage to the neck (cervical spine) – take care not to extend the head or the patient may become paralysed or die.
- Severe blood loss – medical attention would be urgently needed.
- Bleeding into the brain (intracranial bleeding) – medical attention would be urgently needed.

All traumatised patients should also be assessed by the clinician following the advanced trauma life support (ATLS) scheme:

A Airway
B Breathing
C Cardiovascular circulation and control of haemorrhage
D Disability and neurological assessment including pupils
E Environmental control and exposure.

Records taken immediately, and every 15 minutes, include:

- State of consciousness
- Blood pressure
- Pulse rate
- Respiration
- Temperature.

Management of Maxillo-Facial Injuries

JAW FRACTURES

Jaw fractures can be severely disfiguring and can cause the patient a lot of anxiety. However, management of injuries such as these is only undertaken after the patient's general condition has been assessed and stabilised by a clinician.

Jaw fractures include:

- Fractures of the mandible – these are among the commonest jaw fractures after trauma. Patients with fractures of the mandible rarely have serious injuries to other parts of their body; however, alcohol or other drugs may be involved.
- Fractures of the middle or upper third of facial skeleton – these are more common after severe trauma (particularly road accidents or war injuries). They are more likely to be associated with life-threatening problems because of:
  - ○ Airway obstruction
  - ○ Head injury
  - ○ Serious trauma to other body parts, particularly chest injuries, ruptured organs (e.g. liver or spleen), eye injuries, fractured cervical or lumbar spine, and fractured long bones with serious internal bleeding.
  - ○ Alcohol or other drug use.

Jaw fractures are usually managed by open reduction and internal fixation (**ORIF**).

SOFT TISSUE INJURIES

Any lacerations in or around the mouth and face usually bleed heavily because of the rich supply of blood to the area. However, the injuries may not be as severe as they seem at first sight. Cleaning the area with weak aqueous chlorhexidine or hydrogen peroxide solution (one part hydrogen peroxide and one part water) often reassures the patient, relatives, and healthcare staff.

If there is bleeding, apply pressure with a clean gauze for at least five minutes under supervision. If the lip is swollen or bruised, apply a cold compress to limit swelling, bleeding, and discomfort. To do this, wrap crushed ice in a clean gauze or a clean piece of cloth, and hold it inside the cheek or lip.

Term to Learn
ORIF: this is a surgical procedure to set and fix a fractured bone in certain situations (not all fractures require ORIF). First, the site of fracture is opened by making an incision in the skin and tissues overlying the bone (open surgery) and the displaced segments of a fractured bone are set in place. Second, the segments are rigidly fixed in place with screws and/or plates to prevent any movement and allow healing to occur.

355

It is particularly important that an experienced surgeon closes (usually with stitches) cuts that cross the vermilion border, or the patient may be left with a very obvious cosmetic problem.

INJURIES TO TEETH

Teeth, usually the maxillary anterior teeth, can readily be injured in violence or play, especially in young males. Care, and the use of mouthguards, can help prevent or minimise damage.

Tooth injuries are classified as:

- Avulsion (complete displacement of the tooth from its socket)
- Luxation (lateral or extrusive)
- Subluxation (loosening and displacement of the tooth)
- Intrusion (the tooth is pushed vertically into the alveolar bone)
- Fracture.

Avulsed Tooth

- Avulsed primary teeth should not be replanted.
- Avulsed permanent anterior teeth may be replanted successfully in a child, particularly if the root apex is not completely formed (under 16 years); It is best to replant immediately. Teeth replanted within 15 minutes stand a 98% chance of being retained after further dental attention. The younger the child and the sooner the replantation is done, the better the success.

> ## WHAT TO TELL A PATIENT (OR PARENT) WHO HAS AN AVULSED TOOTH
> - Hold tooth by the crown (do not handle root as that could damage the periodontal ligament).
> - If tooth is contaminated, rinse with sterile saline or cold running tap water – but never scrub the tooth.
> - Place the tooth in an isotonic fluid (cool, fresh, pasteurised or long-life milk, sterile saline, or contact lens fluid). Otherwise, if the child is old enough and co-operative, the tooth should be placed in the buccal sulcus. (Note: Unsuitable and slightly damaging fluids are water (due to isotonic damage as a result of prolonged exposure), disinfectants, bleach, or fruit juice.)
> - Reach the dental surgery as soon as possible for care by the clinician, ideally within 30 minutes.

Term to Learn
Tissue adhesive: a glue-like material that is used instead of sutures to hold the edges of a wound together to help the wound heal.

The clinician will, if the socket contains clot, remove it with saline irrigation, replant and then splint tooth for 7–10 days to stabilise it; 'finger crimping' with a metal foil is another temporary measure, as is use of a **tissue adhesive**.

Luxated Tooth: Partially Dislodged (or Extruded) Tooth As long as the nerve and blood vessels remain intact, an extruded tooth may be saved without root canal treatment. This will depend, though, on how displaced it is.

The clinician will guide the tooth back into the right position and apply a plastic splint or orthodontic brackets and a wire to keep the tooth stable.

Intruded Tooth As long as the nerve and blood vessels remain intact, teeth that have been intruded into the alveolar bone may be saved without root canal treatment.

Fractured Teeth

- Injuries to the primary teeth may appear to be of little consequence (as regards emergency care), but even seemingly 'mild' injuries can damage the permanent teeth. However, injuries to permanent teeth are much more immediately important.

- Minor cracks, also called 'craze lines', are superficial fractures affecting the enamel only and rarely need treatment.
- Chips can be smoothed or cosmetically corrected. Other options include veneers, crowns and composite or other tooth-coloured restorations.
- Cusp fractures rarely affect the pulp and are unlikely to cause significant pain. But they may interfere with chewing, and if so they are repaired with composites, an onlay or a crown. Emergency care consists of placing a suitable dentine-bonding agent onto the fractured dentine (see Chapter 9).
- Serious fractures (those involving dentine and pulp) should be treated as urgent since pulpal infection might follow. If the pulp is damaged, the broken part of the tooth will usually bleed and there will be pain. Root canal treatment is usually required and a crown often needed to restore the tooth. So prompt treatment within the same working day or at least by the following morning is required.
- A tooth that has split vertically into two separate parts will often have to be extracted.

Bites
- Bites are painful and, in some instances can result in significant loss of tissue or damage, or infections – both local and sometimes systemic.
- Wound irrigation with sterile saline helps assessment and may reduce the risk of infection.
- In penetrating wounds surgical debridement and closure will be needed.
- Specimens should be obtained from wounds for bacteriological culture. Appropriate antibiotics and analgesics (pain-killers) will need to be prescribed.
- Except for the most superficial wounds, whether by animals or humans, tetanus prophylaxis is recommended unless immunisations are up to date. This is so despite the infrequency of contamination of human bites with the bacterium *Clostridium tetani* since tetanus can be a lethal infection. Tetanus immune globulin is the product of choice for prophylaxis.
- In animal bites, if rabies is a risk, vaccination will also be required.
- In human bites, the person who has caused the bite may need to be assessed for risk status regarding blood-borne viruses (see Subchapter 1.2). If they are a known carrier of hepatitis B virus or HIV, the wound should be thoroughly irrigated (washed). The victim may need to be immunised against HBV and receive anti-retroviral (anti-HIV) prophylaxis (post-exposure prophylaxis or PEP, see Chapter 1). They will also be followed up to monitor any risk of HIV infection. If the person who has caused the bite is HIV positive, a blood specimen of the victim should be drawn immediately to determine their HIV status at that time. It will need to be re-tested after three and six months. If the wounded person remains negative at six months it is highly unlikely that HIV has been transmitted.

> **KEY POINT** All patients with bite injuries should be followed up to ensure healing has occurred and there are no infective sequelae.

PAIN
Pulpitis

Pulpal pain is:

- Spontaneous
- Severe
- Often throbbing
- Exacerbated by temperature
- Likely to outlast the stimulus.

It is often difficult for the patient to say exactly where the pain originates. In other words, the pain is poorly localised. The pain tends to radiate to the ear, temple or cheek *on the same side* and it may stop spontaneously. As the pulp has probably died (necrosed), an acute

357

periapical periodontitis (dental abscess) is likely to follow. Endodontic treatment (root canal treatment), or tooth extraction, will be required.

Periapical Periodontitis

Periapical periodontitis pain is:

- Spontaneous
- Severe
- Persists for hours
- Well localised
- Usually exacerbated by biting.

A dental abscess may form ('gum boil'). The tooth is tender to percussion (periostitic) and the adjacent gingiva is often tender to touch (palpation). Sometimes there is also facial swelling, fever and malaise. Deeper (fascial space) infections are fortunately rare but can be serious as the associated neck swelling can compress the airway and choke and kill the patient.

MANAGEMENT OF A DENTAL ABSCESS

A dental abscess should be drained to release the pus. Analgesics such as paracetamol are given, and antibiotics are prescribed if there is facial swelling, fever, malaise or any threat to the airway. In the latter instance, urgent specialist care is required.

The clinician will drain the tooth either by incising the abscess or opening the tooth to allow it to drain through the root canal/pulp. If infection extends deeply, the patient should be hospitalised and intravenous antibiotic treatment started immediately.

Acute Periodontal Abscess

This may be seen in a patient who has periodontal disease. Symptoms include:

- Throbbing pain with erythema and swelling
- Tooth tender to percussion.

If left untreated, the abscess may rupture or, less commonly, progress to cellulitis. Drainage and debridement of the infected periodontal area are indicated. Antibiotics are not usually indicated.

Acute Pericoronitis

Acute pericoronitis is seen where there is an impacted or partially erupted tooth and is recognised by:

- Swelling of the flap (operculum) over a partially erupted lower third molar (wisdom tooth)
- Pain
- Tenderness
- Halitosis
- Bad taste.

Swollen lymph nodes are common, and trismus (restricted mouth opening) and fever can occur. Pericoronitis may be caused by plaque build-up, and by trauma to the gingiva from the opposing upper tooth. The area should be cleaned by irrigation under the flap with aqueous chlorhexidine, and any opposing tooth ground down or removed. Hot salt mouthwashes can help resolve symptoms. Penicillin and appropriate analgesia may be necessary. Eventually, the impacted tooth may need to be removed.

FIND OUT MORE
How can an upper tooth cause pericoronitis around a lower wisdom tooth?

MEDICAL AND SURGICAL COMPLICATIONS

Medical emergencies, which are generally much more serious, are described in Chapter 2. Surgical complications are described below.

Antral Complications

TOOTH/ROOT IN THE MAXILLARY ANTRUM

- The location of the tooth/root is checked on X-rays
- Antibiotics and a nasal decongestant are prescribed
- Further operation is required to retrieve the tooth/root

ORO-ANTRAL FISTULA (OAF)

This is often recognised when, on drinking fluids, the liquid appears in the nose!

- Patients should not blow their nose
- Antibiotics and a nasal decongestant may help
- If detected early, primary closure is possible
- Some OAFs may need flap closure

Bleeding

Most post-operative bleeding is a result of:

- Excessive trauma during the operation
- Inflamed mucosa
- Poor post-operative compliance (too much exercise or hot drinks)
- Post-extraction interference with the extraction socket
- Uncontrolled hypertension
- Use of aspirin or non-steroidal anti-inflammatory drugs (NSAIDs; see Chapter 12).

Oral bleeding is more likely if the patient:

- Rinses
- Disturbs the clot
- Chews hard
- Consumes hot drinks, alcohol, or does exercise.

Box 16.1 lists the instructions regarding post-operative bleeding that should be given to the patient.

If the socket bleeds continuously and the patient reports back, Surgicel (oxidised regenerated cellulose) or another haemostatic agent (collagen: synthetic (Instat); microcrystalline (Avitene); or porcine) or tissue adhesives are placed in the socket by the clinician. If the bleeding continues, the socket will most likely require sutures or the doctor will need to exclude a bleeding tendency.

Inhaled or Swallowed Foreign Body

Items that can be aspirated (or swallowed) can include restorations, restorative materials, instruments, implant parts, rubber dam clamps and

KEY POINT Care and the use of rubber dam can prevent many accidents. Rubber dam should always be used for conservative and endodontic dentistry.

359

> ### BOX 16.1 PATIENT INFORMATION AFTER TOOTH EXTRACTION
>
> After a tooth has been extracted, the socket will usually bleed for a short time, but then the bleeding stops because a healthy clot of blood forms in the tooth socket. These clots are easily disturbed and, if this happens, more bleeding will occur. To avoid disturbing the clot, DO NOT:
>
> - Rinse the mouth for 24 hours
> - Disturb the clot with the tongue or fingers
> - Eat food which requires chewing (for the rest of the day)
> - Chew on the affected side for at least three days (if both sides of the mouth are involved, have a soft diet for three days)
> - Take hot drinks, hot baths, alcohol, exercise, talk too much or get excited or too hot.
>
> If the tooth socket continues to bleed after leaving the hospital, do not be alarmed; much of the liquid which appears to be blood will be saliva. Make a small pad from a clean handkerchief or cotton wool, or a teabag. Sit down and place it directly over the socket and close the teeth firmly on it. Keep up the pressure for 15–30 minutes.
>
> If the bleeding still does not stop seek advice from the practice (or the hospital or resident dental surgeon).

impression materials. Swallowed items usually pass naturally out of the gastro-intestinal tract, unless they are sharp and penetrate the gut wall.

Inhalation of a foreign body is exceedingly dangerous as it may:

- Block the airway and cause hypoxia and death
- Cause lung collapse (atelectasis) or lung infection, such as lung abscess or pneumonia.

The main problem is to know whether the item has been swallowed or inhaled, and therefore medical attention is required urgently for all patients. Each dental surgery must have a documented protocol for the follow-up of such incidents.

Pain

Any operation involving soft tissues may cause some discomfort and most operations involving bone will cause some post-operative pain. Minimising operative trauma will reduce pain.

Pain should be controlled with analgesics (see Chapter 12) given regularly.

- Paracetamol usually provides adequate post-operative analgesia and should be given prophylactically as some discomfort is inevitable.
- Aspirin is best avoided as it can be dangerous to children and, at any age, can cause a bleeding tendency (see Chapter 12). Other NSAIDs can also cause a bleeding tendency.

Post-operative pain is usually present for the 24 hours or so after operation. At first it is constant, but eventually it is evident just on moving or touching the area.

If pain persists longer than 48 hours, or increases, some pathological process may be present, such as wound infection (e.g. dry socket; see p. 361). The patient should then contact the surgery and may have to be seen again by the clinician to exclude pathology (e.g. dry socket or fracture).

Wound Infection

- Wound infection is usually obvious if the area is inflamed, swollen and tender, discharging pus and there is fever (pyrexia).

- If the wound infection is only trivial, with no obvious pus formation (suppuration), antibiotics may alone suffice.
- If pus is draining, there may be no need to give antibiotics, as the infection may settle spontaneously within a few days. However, the clinician or dental nurse under supervision may take a sample of the pus on a swab to send for culture to identify the organism and test sensitivity to antibiotics.
- If the wound is not draining but is **fluctuant**, the clinician may remove one or more sutures from the most inflamed area to allow drainage of pus.
- Infection under neck flaps used in cancer surgery is particularly dangerous as the carotid artery may be eroded and burst, which is then usually fatal. Any suspicion of this is an emergency and the clinician must be urgently contacted.

**Term to Learn
Fluctuant:**
compressible.

Dry Socket

A dry socket is an empty and infected and inflamed extraction socket (localised osteitis). This occasionally follows an extraction, typically a difficult lower molar extraction, especially in a smoker and after extraction under LA.

If a patient develops a dry socket, they usually get the following symptoms after two to four days of the extraction:

- Increasing pain
- Halitosis
- Unpleasant taste
- Empty socket
- Marked tenderness to touch.

The clinician may take an X-ray to exclude other possible causes of the pain such as retained roots, foreign bodies, or jaw fracture.

MANAGEMENT
Dry socket is treated by:

- Irrigating the socket with warm (50 °C) saline or aqueous 0.2% chlorhexidine (Corsodyl)
- Dressing the socket with a sedative dressing, e.g. Alvogel
- Giving analgesics and/or antimicrobials, e.g. metronidazole (Flagyl).

Surgical Emphysema

Surgical emphysema is air blown into the soft tissues, It usually occurs when 3-in-1 syringes or high-speed dental handpieces are being used and the dental bur lacerates the mucosa.

Serious complications are rare but antibiotics may be prescribed.

Swelling

The amount of swelling (usually caused by inflammatory oedema and/or a haematoma) that occurs post-operatively:

- Depends largely on the extent of trauma
- Varies between individual patients.

It can be reduced by:

- Minimising the trauma and duration of operation
- Using corticosteroids or ice packs.

Trismus

- Trismus is when there is difficulty in opening the mouth.
- It may occur post-operatively because of bleeding or inflammation around the muscles of mastication.
- The chances of trismus happening can be minimised by being careful about the same factors as for swelling above, and also by minimising the stripping of muscle off the bone.
- Rest is indicated and possibly NSAIDs or, sometimes, antibiotics.

FIND OUT MORE

To read more about dental emergencies and their management see the Merck Manuals website section on Dental Emergencies (http://www.merck.com/mmpe/sec08/ch096/ch096a.html).

CHAPTER 17

Human Diseases and Health Promotion

CHAPTER POINTS

- For the purpose of the dental nurse qualification, as outlined in the NEBDN syllabus, an understanding of human diseases is *not* a requirement. However, at some time during your career you will come across patients, colleagues or friends with many of these diseases. Since it is important for all healthcare professions to promote good health, it is helpful to have background knowledge of some common human diseases and general health promotion. This is also recognised by the GDC in its document *Learning Outcomes* (see p. 351).

  17.1: Common Human Diseases

  17.2: General Health Promotion

363

17.1 COMMON HUMAN DISEASES

There are several reasons why diseases occur. These can be divided into (Box 17.1.1):

- Congenital (these are diseases that are present at birth, in the newborn)
- Acquired (these diseases develop at or after birth):
  - Environmental: chemical; inflammatory; irradiation; trauma
  - Lifestyle: diet; habits (use of tobacco, betel nut, alcohol, other recreational drugs); lack of exercise.

Many diseases result from an interaction of several of these factors (Figure 17.1.1).

THE SEVERITY OF AN ILLNESS

The severity of an illness can influence the type of operation or other medical care given, since in very ill patients such interference can cause the patient to deteriorate.

A commonly used system to classify the severity of illnesses is the American Society of Anesthesiologists' (ASA) system, shown in Table 17.1.1.

ORAL HEALTHCARE IN ILL PATIENTS

- It is generally accepted that the least operative work done should be aimed for.
- All patients with medical conditions benefit from preventive dental care:
  - Practising good oral hygiene
  - Regular dental examinations
  - Dietary counselling
  - Use of fluorides to minimise the risk of developing caries.

BOX 17.1.1 CAUSES OF HUMAN DISEASES

- *Congenital diseases* – may be genetic (due to gene abnormalities) in origin or acquired by the fetus while in the mother's uterus (from infections, or toxins such as alcohol, tobacco or drugs).
- *Acquired diseases* – may be inflammatory, neoplastic, metabolic or trauma-related.
- *Inflammatory and autoimmune diseases* – may be caused by various infections (bacteria, viruses, fungi or parasites) or by the person's own white blood cells attacking their tissues (autoimmune disease; rheumatoid arthritis is the best example).
- *Infectious diseases* – these can occur when the micro-organisms cross the skin or mucosal barrier due to, for example, a needlestick (sharps) injury, ingestion of infected food or water, inhalation of aerosol; and sexual contact (genital, anal or oral mucosae).
- *Immunocompromise* – some people develop disease because their white blood cells fail to protect them against infections, for example human immunodeficiency virus (HIV) damages CD4 white cells. These people are said to be immunocompromised.
- *Neoplastic diseases (cancer)* – these are caused due to **mutations** in the DNA. Mutations themselves are caused by certain factors, particularly tobacco and alcohol, but other chemicals, radiation (e.g. sunlight, X-rays) and some micro-organisms (e.g. human papillomavirus) can also be responsible. All of this results in uncontrolled growth of some cells. Some cancers are more serious and the growth invades the underlying tissues. The cancer may also metastasise, that is, spread via lymphatics and blood mainly to lymph nodes, bone, brain and liver. Cancer can damage vital organs and cause organ dysfunction, pain and other symptoms. In many instances, it ultimately leads to death.
- *Metabolic disorders* – these, as the name suggests, are disorders of metabolism, that is, the body's ability to produce, transport, store and distribute energy, mostly because of malfunctioning enzymes. Diabetes can be caused by malfunctioning of endocrine glands or may be due to lifestyle factors.

Term to Learn
Mutation: alteration in the DNA sequence of a cell's genome (the full DNA sequence of an organism), which can have several causes such as exposure to radiation, certain viruses and chemicals.

FIGURE 17.1.1
Interplay of factors in disease causation.

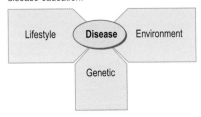

364

ALCOHOLISM

Alcohol is the most commonly misused drug. It affects the functioning of the central nervous system (CNS) as follows:

- Interfering with the cerebral cortex to **release inhibitions**
- Impairing the capacity to reason
- Interfering with the functioning of the cerebellum (see Chapter 4) to cause unsteadiness of gait (ataxia) and inco-ordination of movements.

Eventually alcoholism interferes with the working of the brain centres (e.g. respiratory) and can cause unconsciousness or even death (Table 17.1.2). The high rate of deaths among people with alcoholism is mainly as a result of road traffic accidents and assaults. Alcoholics can also drown in their own vomit.

KEY POINT People, particularly those who are ill, often have concerns about privacy, and about the social implications of their condition. You must therefore strictly adhere to data protection and patient confidentiality principles. Reassure the patient that none of their details will be discussed, even with partners, unless permission is gained from them.

Term to Learn
Release of inhibitions: when people start acting in ways or saying things they would not normally do (thus serious people start giggling, etc.).

TABLE 17.1.1 ASA Classification of State of Health

Class I	Normal healthy individual
Class II	Patient with mild systemic disease (not interfering with daily life)
Class III	Severe systemic disease (interferes with daily life)
Class IV	Incapacitating systemic disease (constant threat to life)
Class V	Moribund (very seriously ill) patient with life expectancy <24 hours

TABLE 17.1.2 Acute Effects of Alcohol

Blood Alcohol Level in mg/dl					
<100	100–200	200–300	300–400	400–500	>500
Dry and decent	Delighted and devilish	Delinquent and disgusting	Dizzy and delirious	Dazed and dejected	Dead drunk

ALCOHOL AND THE SIX Ls

Social difficulties from alcohol misuse are common and can affect the six 'Ls':

- Law – breach of the criminal, civil and/or professional codes
- Learning – intellectual difficulties
- Livelihood – job problems
- Living – housing problems
- Lover – relationship difficulties of all kinds: husband/wife; partner, employer/employee, etc.
- Lucre – (Latin *lucrum* = wealth) money problems.

Many other diseases can be caused or aggravated by alcohol including:

- Bleeding tendency
- Brain damage and epilepsy
- Cancers
- Gastro-intestinal disease
- Heart disease
- Impaired wound healing
- Infections, especially pneumonia and tuberculosis
- Injuries (including maxillo-facial), from accidents or assaults
- Liver disease
- Malnutrition
- Muscle disease
- Pancreatic disease.

Management

Alcoholic people need help in the way of admission to a rehabilitation unit. Management includes ensuring abstinence, adequate nutrition and medication to reduce dependence.

ALLERGY

Allergy is an abnormal response to an allergen (protein). Potential allergens in dentistry are:

- Latex – the most common cause (see Chapter 12 for more details)
- Anti-microbial drugs (e.g. penicillin).

Rare allergic reactions in dentistry occur in relation to:

- Local anaesthetics (LAs)
- Oral healthcare products (antiseptics, mouthwashes, oils such as eugenol)
- Dental materials (impression materials, cements, adhesives, resins, metals)
- Disinfectants.

Common allergens are listed in Table 17.1.3.

Allergies are responsible for some types of the following diseases and conditions:

TABLE 17.1.3 Common Allergens

Allergen Source	Examples
Dental materials	Amalgam, gold, mercury, resins, plasters (e.g. Elastoplast)
Drugs	Aspirin, penicillins
Environment	Animal hair, dust mites, pollens
Foods	Milk, nuts (especially peanuts), eggs, shellfish
Latex	Gloves, dressings, elastic bands, condoms

- Asthma
- Eczema
- Rhinitis (hayfever)
- Anaphylaxis (collapse, with low blood pressure and breathing difficulties) – this can be fatal (Chapter 2).

> **KEY POINTS** People at risk of anaphylaxis should carry an Epipen (syringe containing adrenaline) for self-administration.
>
> As a dental professional, you must be familiar with the medical management of anaphylaxis within a dental setting (see Chapter 2).

Early Symptoms and Signs of an Allergic Reaction

These include:

- Breathlessness and itchy rash (hives or urticaria), which typically occur within a few minutes to an hour
- Wheezing (bronchospasm).
- Fall in blood pressure (hypotension)
- Swelling of the face and lips (angio-oedema; Figure 17.1.2) and laryngopharynx. This may be followed by life-threatening anaphylactic shock.

Management

All allergies are best managed by allergen avoidance:

- Drugs – accurate documentation of drug allergies in medical notes. Use of MedicAlert bracelets.
- Food products – following an elimination diet.
- House dust mites – use of mite-proof bed linen and wooden floors.
- Pets – avoid keeping pets.
- Pollen – keeping windows kept shut and avoiding grassy spaces.

FIGURE 17.1.2
Angio-oedema.

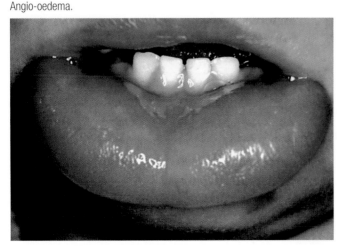

Commonly used drugs for treatment are:

- Anti-histamines
- Bronchodilators
- Corticosteroids
- Adrenaline (also called epinephrine).

ANAEMIA

A person is said to have anaemia when their haemoglobin (Hb) level is below the normal for their age, gender and ethnic background. Haemoglobin is required to carry oxygen to the brain and tissues (see Chapter 4). Anaemia has many causes as shown in Table 17.1.4.

TABLE 17.1.4 Causes of Anaemia

Nature of Anaemia	Cause
Increased loss of red blood cells (RBCs)	Menstrual blood loss Gastro-intestinal blood loss Haemolysis (breakdown of the RBCs), such as in malaria or sickle disease
Reduced RBC production	Dietary deficiency Bone marrow disease, such as in leukaemia
Increased tissue requirements	Puberty Pregnancy
Decreased tissue requirements	Hypothyroidism

Anaemia may not cause any symptoms early on. But, as it worsens and the oxygen-carrying capacity of the blood falls, symptoms and signs develop (e.g. breathlessness, palpitations).

> **KEY POINT** Pallor of the oral mucosa, conjunctiva or palmar creases suggests severe anaemia.

Management

Management includes treatment of the underlying cause. Deficiency states must be corrected with iron, folic acid, and vitamin B12 supplements. Blood transfusion may be indicated if the onset of anaemia has been rapid.

ANTI-COAGULANT-RELATED PROBLEMS

Anti-coagulants are drugs used to slow blood clotting. This is required to control and prevent clotting in people who have deep vein thromboses (**thrombo-embolic disorders**) or after heart surgery. The dose of the drug needs to be controlled or the patient will bleed too easily. Warfarin is the most frequently prescribed anti-coagulant. The dose is controlled by doing a blood test called the international normalised ratio (INR). An INR above 1 indicates that clotting will take longer than normal.

Surgery is the main hazard for the patient on warfarin. Thus alternative treatments, e.g. endodontic treatment, are always considered.

Term to Learn
Thrombo-embolic disorder: a disorder related to the formation of blood clots (thrombi) in one part of the body, of which either small portions or the whole clot can then become loose (emboli) and travel to other parts of the body in the blood stream, causing e.g. pulmonary thrombosis.

367

Dental Considerations

LA regional block injections, or those given in the floor of the mouth, may be a hazard since bleeding into the tissues of the neck can block the airway and suffocate the patient. If surgery is to be more than simple or minor, or the INR is above 3.5, the patient is usually treated in hospital or another specialist centre.

> **KEY POINT** Anti-coagulant doses should not be altered without consulting the doctor in charge. Stopping the drug before surgery is dangerous as there can be fatal thromboses (blood clots).

Aspirin and non-steroidal anti-inflammatory agents (NSAIDs) inhibit platelet aggregation and cause bleeding. Thus they should be avoided in these patients. Paracetamol is the analgesic of choice for these patients.

ANXIETY AND STRESS

Anxiety is an unpleasant emotional state characterised by fear and a variety of physical symptoms. Stress raises blood levels of the adrenal hormones: cortisol, adrenaline (epinephrine) and noradrenaline (norepinephrine). These 'stress hormones' influence many physiological functions, causing:

- Apprehension
- Fast pulse rate (tachycardia)
- Over-breathing (hyperventilation)
- Raised blood pressure (hypertension)
- Sweating
- Tremor
- Dilated pupils
- Involuntary defecation
- Urinary incontinence.

TYPES OF ANXIETY DISORDERS

- Panic disorder: the person panics apparently spontaneously
- Phobia: the anxiety is provoked by discrete stimuli, e.g. phobia of flying or dental treatment.
- Generalised anxiety disorder: such people worry all the time.

Management

- Appropriate management of any underlying organic disease.
- Lifestyle changes to reduce stressors and avoid precipitating factors.
- Behavioural therapies that aim to change anxiety-provoking behaviours (e.g. talking treatments such as cognitive behaviour therapy (CBT)).
- Drugs (anxiolytics such as diazepam or beta-blockers).
- Psychotherapy.

ARTHRITIS

Osteoarthritis (OA)

This is the most common type of arthritis, and consists of progressively worsening joint deformity. Risk factors for OA include:

- Age over 45 years
- Gender: females are more commonly affected
- Genetic predisposition
- Obesity
- Malformed joints (hereditary or acquired)
- Trauma
- Occupation (athletes).

Osteoarthritis may affect any joint, but frequently used, weight-bearing or traumatised joints such as those in the fingers, hips, knees, lower back and feet are more often affected.

SYMPTOMS AND SIGNS

Joint pain, stiffness, deformity, loss of flexibility and reduced function.

MANAGEMENT

This includes:

- Pain relief
- Information and advice, including how to access community support
- Weight reduction if appropriate
- Appropriate footwear and chiropody
- Exercise and walking aids to encourage mobility and improve muscle strength
- Heat and cold application

- Drug treatment
- Surgical treatment:
  - ○ Arthroscopy (this allows removal of diseased joint fragments)
  - ○ Joint replacement (e.g. artificial hip).

Rheumatoid Arthritis (RA)

RA affects women most frequently. It mainly affects the wrists, hands and feet (Figure 17.1.3). Patients may also have a dry mouth (Sjögren syndrome, see Chapter 5 and Figure 17.1.4).

MANAGEMENT

- General supportive measures such as splints and appliances to facilitate mobility.
- Pain relief.
- Preservation of function of affected joints.
- Use of various drugs to try to control the disease.

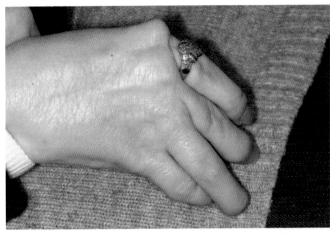

FIGURE 17.1.3
Rheumatoid arthritis.

ASTHMA

Asthma is a common condition in which there is difficulty breathing because of narrowing of the airways. This can happen because of:

- Excessive tone of the muscles in the walls of the bronchi (bronchospasm)
- Oedema
- Hypersecretion of mucus.

During an asthmatic attack a person may have difficulty breathing, cough and wheeziness.

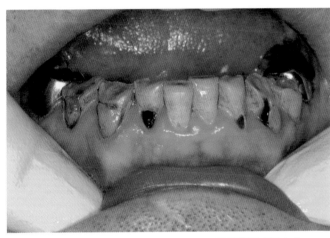

FIGURE 17.1.4
Sjögren syndrome: widespread (rampant) caries due to dry mouth.

There are two types of asthma (Table 17.1.5): extrinsic and intrinsic. Extrinsic asthma is more common and is caused by exposure to allergens. Intrinsic asthma is much less common and is often not related to exposure to allergens.

Management

This includes drug treatment, smoking cessation and avoidance of precipitants.

A prolonged asthmatic attack which is resistant to treatment may lead to life-threatening *status asthmaticus*.

TABLE 17.1.5 **Types of Asthma**

	Extrinsic	Intrinsic
Frequency	Common	Less common
Associations	Allergic disease (hay fever, eczema, allergic rhinitis)	None
Main precipitating factors	Animal hairs	Air pollutants
	House dust mite	Cold air
	Pollen and moulds	Drugs (NSAIDs)
		Stress
		Exercise

369

ATHEROMA (ATHEROSCLEROSIS)

Atheroma is the accumulation of fats (cholesterol and lipids) in the artery walls. The accumulation occurs in the form of plaques. These can cause narrowing of the arteries and reduce the blood supply to the tissues supplied by that artery.

Signs and Symptoms

These depend on the location:

- Pain in the legs (intermittent claudication)
- Pain in the chest (because of coronary artery disease (CAD) – the pain is termed angina, see Chapter 2 and coronary (ischaemic) heart disease, p. 373)
- The plaque may rupture or a clot may form (thrombo-embolism), blocking an artery. This can have potentially life-threatening consequences depending on where the artery is blocked:
  - Heart attack or myocardial infarction (due to blocked coronary artery) – see Chapter 2
  - Stroke or cerebrovascular accident (due to blocked brain artery) – see Chapter 2.

AUTISM

Autism is a developmental disorder that usually begins in the first 30 months of life. It is characterised by:

- Poor social skills – inability to get along with people
- Lack of developing interpersonal relationships – people with autism appear indifferent and remote. They are unable to form emotional bonds with others, or understand other people's thoughts, feelings, and needs. They seem to prefer being alone, and may resist attention and affection or passively accept hugs and cuddling.
- Abnormal speech and language – specialised educational help is required.
- Ritualistic or compulsive behaviour with repetitive stereotyped activities – most autistic people have an obsessional desire for maintaining an unchanging environment and rigidly following familiar patterns in their everyday routines. Asperger's is a related syndrome.

FIGURE 17.1.5
Bell's palsy. When the patient attempts to smile the mouth droops on the side of the paralysis (his right side).

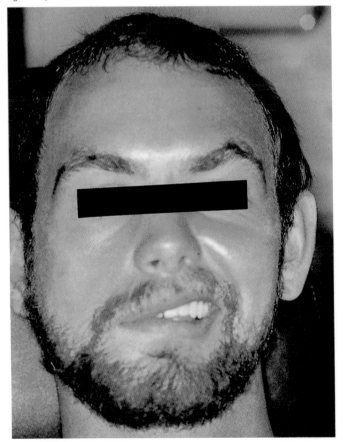

BELL'S PALSY

Bell's palsy (Figure 17.1.5) is a type of facial paralysis that usually occurs on one side. It occurs mainly due to infection with herpes simplex virus (HSV). Most patients recover totally and spontaneously within a few weeks. Treatment includes:

- Anti-inflammatory medication
- Antiviral medication.

BLOOD-BORNE VIRAL INFECTIONS

Blood-borne virus infections (e. g. hepatitis B virus (HBV), hepatitis C virus (HCV), or HIV) are transmitted mainly by sharps injuries, but also via unscreened blood and sexual contact. Occasionally they are transmitted through the mucosa of the eye or mouth (see p. 379).

BREAST CANCER

After skin cancer, breast cancer is the most common cancer among women. It is usually seen in women over the age of 50.

Risk Factors

- Personal history of breast cancer
- Family history of breast cancer
- Other factors:
  - Increased oestrogen levels
  - Late childbearing
  - Alcohol use
  - Fatty diet.

Signs and Symptoms

- Early breast cancer usually does not cause pain
- Later breast cancer can cause:
  - A lump or thickening in or near the breast or axilla
  - A change in breast size or shape
  - Nipple discharge, tenderness or inversion
  - Breast ridging or pitting.

Management

There are many treatments, and which one is offered varies from patient to patient:

- Surgery
- Radiation
- Chemotherapy
- Hormones (tamoxifen)
- Antibodies.

CANNABIS (MARIJUANA) USE

Cannabis is usually smoked as a cigarette (joint, spliff or nail) or in a pipe (bong). The main active chemical THC (delta-9-tetrahydrocannabinol), works by binding to the brain. This affects the person's:

- Sense of pleasure
- Memory
- Thoughts
- Concentration
- Sensory and time perception
- Co-ordination of movements.

KEY POINT People high on marijuana may become silly and giggly, seem dizzy and have trouble walking and have a hard time remembering things that have just happened – they thus appear drunk.

Within a few minutes of inhaling marijuana smoke, the user will often feel their heart beat increase, have a dry mouth, and red eyes. In some people, marijuana can double the normal heart rate and raise the blood pressure. Because of the effects of cannabis on perceptions and reaction times – which last for up to 24 hours – users can be involved in risky sexual behaviour, violence or in road traffic accidents. Some users may also have acute anxiety and paranoid thoughts; rarely, a user can have severe **psychotic symptoms** and need emergency medical treatment.

Term to Learn
Psychotic symptoms:
psychosis is a serious mental disorder in which a person loses touch with reality or their perception of reality is highly distorted. The classic symptoms are: hallucinations and delusions and other confused thoughts. There may also be a lack of self-awareness.

371

The long-term effects of using cannabis are not yet clear, but it may affect the lungs, heart, and immune system and mental health. Marijuana smokers may develop many of the breathing problems that tobacco smokers have, hypertension and increased heart rate and lowered oxygen-carrying capacity of blood. Because of this the risk of a heart attack is increased four-fold in the first hour after smoking marijuana. Long-term use of marijuana can trigger or worsen schizophrenia (see p. 389).

CARDIAC DISEASE

See also Coronary heart disease (p. 373).

Electrosurgery can cause heart pacemakers and implantable cardiac defibrillators to malfunction. Some older electrically operated dental equipment may also be a risk but most *modern* dental equipment is safe in this respect.

Dental Implications

In the past, patients thought to be at risk from infective endocarditis were routinely given anti-microbial prophylaxis ('cover') before dental surgery and some other procedures. But that is no longer the case (see p. 383). Some 'cardiac' drugs can cause gingival swelling.

FIND OUT MORE

Some drugs used in cardiac disease can cause the gingivae to swell up. Can you name any?

CEREBRAL PALSY

Cerebral palsy (CP) is the most common congenital physical disability. In cerebral palsy, muscle control is abnormal because of damage to a child's brain early in the course of development. The brain damage is caused mainly by lack of oxygen (hypoxia), trauma or infection. Physiotherapy is an important part of management.

CHRONIC OBSTRUCTIVE PULMONARY DISEASE

Chronic obstructive pulmonary disease (COPD), also called chronic obstructive airway disease (COAD), is a progressive, irreversible lung disease, most frequently a combination of:

- Chronic bronchitis – excessive production of mucus and persistent cough with sputum production
- Emphysema – the pathological dilatation of air spaces in the lungs with destruction of the alveoli.

Risk Factors

The most important causes of COPD are cigarette smoking and environmental pollution.

Management

Management consists of lifestyle changes and drug treatment:

- Smoking cessation
- Exercise
- Weight loss
- Drug treatment – bronchodilators, corticosteroids or antibiotics
- Oxygen therapy – long-term oxygen therapy
- Vaccination – pneumococcal and influenza vaccine.

COELIAC DISEASE

Coeliac disease (also called gluten-sensitive enteropathy; coeliac sprue, non-tropical sprue) is an allergic reaction of the small intestine mucosa to **gluten**.

Signs and Symptoms

Many affected people are asymptomatic. However, malabsorption of proteins can cause growth retardation, abdominal pain, fatty faeces (steatorrhoea) and behavioural changes.

Management

- Gluten-free diet: plain meat, fish, fruits, and vegetables do not contain gluten.
- Correction of nutritional deficiencies.

CORONARY (ISCHAEMIC) HEART DISEASE

Coronary artery disease (CAD) is the leading cause of death in the UK.

It is caused by atherosclerosis of the coronary arteries.

Risk Factors

These include:

- Increasing age
- Gender – men are at greater risk than premenopausal women
- Family history
- Cigarette smoking
- High blood cholesterol level
- Hypertension
- Diabetes mellitus
- Obesity
- Lack of exercise.

Signs and Symptoms (see also Box 17.1.2)

- Dizziness
- Shortness of breath
- Decreased exercise tolerance
- Chest pain (angina pectoris)
- Sudden death due to a myocardial infarction (irreversible damage to heart muscle).

> **Term to Learn**
> **Gluten:** a group of proteins found in all forms of wheat, and related grains (especially rye and barley).

> **KEY POINT** Myocardial infarction commonly presents with central chest pain similar to that of angina. However, the pain of myocardial infarction is not relieved by rest or with GTN.

Management

A person with myocardial infarction requires immediate aspirin and hospital admission (see Chapter 2). Up to 50% of patients die within the first hour; but early treatment halves the death rate.

BOX 17.1.2 CONDITIONS RELATED TO CAD

- *Angina pectoris* – This is the name given to episodes of chest pain caused by CAD. Angina is precipitated by exercise, particularly in cold weather, and is relieved by rest or use of glyceryl trinitrate (GTN).
- *Myocardial infarction* (heart attack) – this results from the complete blockage of one or more arteries to the heart (coronary arteries). Fewer than 50% of patients with myocardial infarction have any preceding symptoms, but angina may progress to myocardial infarction.

Lifestyle changes play a major role:

- Reduced intake of cholesterol and saturated fats
- Daily exercise
- Weight loss
- Smoking cessation.

Medications include anti-coagulant drugs (e.g. aspirin) and cholesterol-lowering drugs such as statins.

When symptoms are worsening despite this management, surgery (cardiac revascularisation techniques) may be considered such as:

- Coronary angioplasty (**stents**)
- Coronary artery bypass grafting (CABG).

CHEMOTHERAPY-RELATED PROBLEMS

Cytotoxic chemotherapy is used to treat many cancers and other malignant conditions such as leukaemia. The drugs often cause hair loss (alopecia), nausea and vomiting, and pins and needles (paraesthesia) but one of the biggest problems for the patient is a sore mouth (mucositis). Analgesics are needed, as well as a soft diet. Sucking ice cubes may help ease the pain, and many other concoctions are available to help the patient. Oral hygiene must be maintained.

CORTICOSTEROID-RELATED PROBLEMS

The adrenal hormone cortisol is released in the response to stresses such as trauma, infection, general anaesthesia or surgery. Secretion of cortisol is regulated via a **biological feedback** system that includes another hormone called adrenocorticotropic hormone (ACTH). In patients given systemic corticosteroid drugs (steroids), this feedback response may not occur. As a result, the adrenal gland is unable to produce the necessary steroid response to stress. The patient may then have a fall in blood pressure and collapse.

KEY POINT Steroid supplementation (steroid cover) may need to be considered before stressful procedures such as surgery in patients taking corticosteroids. The blood pressure must be carefully monitored during the operation and recovery.

CREUTZFELDT–JAKOB DISEASE

Creutzfeldt–Jakob disease (CJD) is a rare, progressive brain disease. It is a type of transmissible spongiform encephalopathy (TSE). Some TSEs are transmissible from animal to man; bovine spongiform encephalopathy (BSE; also known as 'mad cow disease') in cattle appears to be responsible for variant CJD (vCJD) in humans.

TSEs are caused by prions – which are abnormal cellular proteins. Prions are very resistant to normal disinfectants and sterilisation. TSEs have prolonged **incubation periods** of months to years. Persons with vCJD develop psychiatric symptoms (severe depression and behavioural disorders), followed by dementia, and finally death.

There is no effective treatment yet for vCJD and there have been few patients (172 dead and alive cases reported in UK by 2010).

Term to Learn
Stent: these are miniature wire coils put inside an artery to keep it open.

Term to Learn
Biological feedback: the system by which the body feeds back information to the various regulating organs, which then respond by either increasing or decreasing the formation of regulators, for example, hormones.

374

Term to Learn
Incubation period: this is the time period between catching an infection and displaying the symptoms of that disease.

PRIONS AND DENTISTRY

Prions are proteinaceous infectious particles. They are found in brain and are transmitted by brain surgery or use of brain products or even by transfusions of whole blood.

A unique feature of prions is their remarkable capacity to bind to steel. They resist inactivation by conventional methods: heat, most disinfectants, and by ionising, ultraviolet and microwave radiations. This presents significant infection control problems when patients with CJD undergo medical or dental interventions. Disposable equipment is the best answer.

Prions are also a rare hazard from exposure-prone (invasive) procedures. Dental interest in prion disease (CJD) and the related conditions centres on the risk of their transmission from patient to patient in the course of dental treatment through contaminated instruments. There is no known case of this happening and appropriate dental infection control precautions will reduce the scope of the theoretical risk. It is not yet known whether CJD can be transmitted via blood or other tissues encountered during dental surgery.

FIND OUT MORE

To read more about prion disease and health and safety, see HTM 01-05 (Section 1; see Chapter 1) and *Transmissible Spongiform Encephalopathy Agents: safe working and the prevention of infection* produced by the Advisory Committee on Dangerous Pathogens (http://www.dh.gov.uk/ab/ACDP/TSEguidance/DH_098253).

> **KEY POINT** CJD and related conditions raise new infection control questions because prions are much more difficult to destroy than conventional micro-organisms. So single-use instruments are recommended. All other instruments should be decontaminated.

DEMENTIA AND ALZHEIMER DISEASE

375

Dementia is a progressive loss of intellect, memory and social abilities without clouding of consciousness. The prevalence increases with age; it is rare in people younger than 60 years. Alzheimer disease is the most common form of dementia – a neurodegenerative disease in which neurones in the brain die and plaques form.

Signs and Symptoms

Early symptoms are loss of short-term memory and an inability to perform previously simple tasks.

In advanced dementia, individuals may be disoriented in time, place and person.

Management

This includes:

- Support
- Possibly drug treatment.

Long-term residential or nursing home care may become necessary.

DEPRESSION
Signs and Symptoms

Depression is characterised by:

- Persistent lowering of mood
- Negative thinking

- Feelings of hopelessness, worthlessness, helplessness and guilt
- Impaired concentration.

Biological functioning is also altered, so patients may:

- Lack energy
- Have insomnia, or early-morning awakening, or oversleep
- Lose appetite and weight
- Have chronic pains of 'unknown cause'.

Depression can be triggered by adverse life events such as a bereavement or divorce and onset is typically in the third decade of life.

Management

This includes:

- Appropriate risk assessment for suicide and self-neglect
- Anti-depressant drugs
- Psychological therapies (CBT and supportive therapy).

DIABETES

Diabetes mellitus is a common condition caused by a decreased production of the hormone insulin from the pancreas or because of insulin resistance. Insulin normally controls blood sugar by facilitating its entry into cells for use as energy. In diabetes, glucose (sugar) accumulates in the blood (hyperglycaemia) and the urine (glucosuria) leading to the production of large volumes of urine (polyuria) and to thirst (polydipsia). Fat and protein stores are metabolised to glucose with weight loss, muscle wasting and the production of ketone bodies, which may be detected on the breath (in particular acetone). Diabetes also causes damage to kidneys, nerves and eyes. Complications of diabetes can affect almost every part of the body and include:

- Cerebrovascular disease
- Coronary artery disease
- Hypertension
- **Peripheral vascular disease.**

> **Term to Learn**
> **Peripheral vascular disease:** when the blood vessels that carry blood to the extremities, such as the arms and legs, become narrowed so that blood flow is compromised. This affects the health of the local tissues.

376

HAVING A 'HYPO'

If the blood sugar level falls too much (hypoglycaemia; or 'hypo'), the brain becomes starved of energy and the patient may collapse and even die.

Hypoglycaemia is avoidable by appropriate planning, such as operating mid-morning to allow the patient to have their breakfast. Furthermore, particularly before surgical procedures, the patient's blood glucose level may be tested. More protracted procedures such as multiple extractions should only be carried out in hospital.

DOWN SYNDROME

Down syndrome (previously called mongolism or trisomy 21) is the most frequent genetic cause of learning disability. The other characteristic features include:

- Short stature
- Characteristic facial features with spaced eyes and **epicanthic folds.**

> **Term to Learn**
> **Epicanthic fold:** a fold of the skin of the upper eyelid. It typically runs from the nose to the inner side of the eyebrow.

Down syndrome also affects many, if not most, organs including the mouth. Fissured lips, periodontitis and hypoplastic teeth are common.

Management

- Long-term care is inevitably required, with protection from infection.

DRUG ABUSE (SUBSTANCE DEPENDENCE)

Drug abuse is self-administration of certain drugs without any medical indication for them, despite adverse medical and social consequences (Table 17.1.6). The use of some drugs is illegal and people found in possession of these or, particularly, if there is any intention of dealing (supplying), can be charged.

There is intense dependence on the drug and severe physical or psychological effects if the drug is stopped (**withdrawal syndrome**). Alcohol is the main drug abused.

Club Drugs

Used in nightclubs, bars, rave or trance scenes, these include LSD (acid), MDMA (Ecstasy), mephedrone, (M-Kat; MEOW), GHB, GBL, ketamine (Special-K), Fentanyl, Rohypnol, amphetamines and methamphetamine. In high doses, these drugs can cause a sharp rise in body temperature (malignant hyperthermia) leading to muscle breakdown and kidney and heart failure, and death.

> **Term to Learn**
> **Withdrawal syndrome:** when a person stops taking a drug after having being used to regular and possibly large amounts of the drug. This can cause typical symptoms in the body.

> **KEY POINT** Intravenous injection, and sharing of needles or syringes carries the risk of blood-borne infections (viral hepatitis and HIV), **septicaemia**, liver and heart damage, and eventually death.

EATING DISORDERS

Dieting to maintain a body weight lower than needed for adequate health is increasingly common, particularly in adolescent girls and young women. It is also heavily promoted in some activities (e.g. modelling) and by fashion trends and sales campaigns.

Eating disorders such as *anorexia nervosa* (self-imposed starvation) and *bulimia nervosa* (binge eating and dieting) can be life-threatening. Frequently the person also has depression or anxiety disorders or is using substances.

> **Term to Learn**
> **Septicaemia:** sepsis in the blood.

Complications

These include:

- Anaemia
- Hormone (endocrine) and metabolic disturbances; infrequent or absent menstrual periods are common

TABLE 17.1.6 Main Groups of Substances Abused

Group	Stimulants (uppers)	Depressants (hypnotic/sedatives /downers)	Hallucinogens (psychedelics)	Analgesics	Anabolic steroids
Actions	Speed brain activity	Slow brain activity	Distort brain activity	Decrease pain	Promote growth and muscle
Examples	Caffeine, Cocaine, Crack, Nicotine	Benzodiazepines, barbiturates, ethanol (alcohol), inhalants (various)	Lysergic acid (LSD), amphetamines Ecstasy, PCP, marijuana, mephedrone	Codeine, heroin, morphine	Deca-durabolin, Sustanon 250

377

- Depression
- Suicide.

Management

This includes:

- Medical care and monitoring
- Psychosocial interventions (CBT or interpersonal psychotherapy)
- Nutritional counselling.

EPILEPSY

Epilepsy is a predisposition for recurrent seizures (fits or convulsions). A seizure (fit) is a convulsion or transient disturbance in consciousness caused by abnormal brain electrical activity. An electroencephalogram (EEG) measures brain electrical activity.

Epilepsy may be the result of underlying brain pathology (injury, tumours or infections). The clinical presentation is variable (see Table 17.1.7).

Epileptic seizures may be precipitated by sleep deprivation, concurrent illness, sensory stimuli (flashing lights) and drugs.

Management

- Anti-epileptic therapy is commonly required (e.g. phenytoin) and may cause gingival swelling. See Chapter 2 for management of an epileptic fit in the dental workplace.

FIND OUT MORE

Which common anti-epileptic drug can cause gingival swelling?

GONORRHOEA

Gonorrhoea is a bacterial, sexually transmitted infection (STI). It is caused by *Neisseria gonorrhoeae.*

Signs and Symptoms

- Gonorrhoea in all sites is frequently asymptomatic – which increases the chances of transmission.
- Pain on urinating (dysuria) and urethral or vaginal discharge are common symptoms.

Management

- Treatment is with antibiotics. It also includes **contact tracing** of sexual partners.

Term to Learn
Contact tracing: the formal method of finding out the persons who may have come into contact with an infected person.

TABLE 17.1.7 **Classification and Clinical Features of Epilepsy**

Sub-type	Clinical Features
Tonic-clonic (Grand mal)	Loss of consciousness Tonic phase Clonic phase Tongue biting Incontinence Seizure lasts <5 minutes
Absence seizure (Petit mal)	Brief period of unresponsiveness Duration of absences <30 seconds

HAEMOPHILIA

Haemophilia A and B are hereditary bleeding disorders that only affect males (but females can carry the defective gene). Haemophilia A (classic haemophilia) and B (Christmas disease) are deficiencies in blood clotting factors (see Chapter 4). They cause bleeding that can be dangerous because of either blood loss or bleeding into the brain, larynx, pharynx, joints and muscles.

Haemophiliac patients should be under the care of a recognised haemophilia reference centre.

> **KEY POINT** Bleeding after dental extractions may be the presenting feature of haemophilia.

Management

The missing factors must be replaced to adequate levels during episodes of bleeding and before treatment. In the past, blood transfusions were used, but this sometimes transmitted hepatitis or HIV or even prions.

'Gene therapy' and 'gene-delivery systems' may be potential cures for haemophilia in the future.

HEALTHCARE-ASSOCIATED INFECTIONS

Meticillin-resistant *Staphylococcus aureus* (MRSA) is an important bacterium that is resistant to common antibiotics. It is widely found in healthcare facilities. *Clostridium difficile (C. diff.)* is another serious cause of healthcare-associated infections (HCAIs). There are also many others!

MRSA is not more pathogenic than other **strains** of *S. aureus* but it does not colonise normal skin. It colonises the nose, axillae and perineum, and wounds, ulcers and eczematous skin. MRSA may be found in patients who are hospitalised or who have been discharged from hospital into the community. It is not usually found in the oral cavity but may occasionally be isolated from oral infections.

> **Term to Learn**
> **Strain:** a special variety of a particular species, for example a bacterium or a domesticated animal.

379

Dental Implications

- No special precautions above standard infection control are necessary for the dental treatment of patients colonised with MRSA.
- However, dentists or ancillary staff colonised with MRSA should not undertake or assist with invasive procedures.
- A microbiologist or communicable disease physician can provide treatment to end MRSA colonisation.

HEPATITIS

'Hepatitis' means liver inflammation. The most common causes are viral – hepatitis viruses A, B (HBV), C (HCV) and D are the most important.

SPREAD OF THE HEPATITIS VIRUSES

HBV and HCV are of special significance, since they are blood-borne and transmissible, especially by needlestick injuries.

Hepatitis viruses spread also via:

- Intravenous drug abuse
- Unscreened blood
- Blood product transfusions
- Tattooing/ear-piercing
- Sexual contact (especially among individuals who do not practise safer sex).

HBV and HCV can also cause chronic hepatitis – in which the infection is prolonged, sometimes lifelong. HCV in particular can lead to liver **cirrhosis** and liver cancer.

Prevention

Prevention of hepatitis is best achieved by avoiding contact with the viruses by:

- Never sharing needles, syringes, water or 'works'
- Never sharing personal care items that might have blood on them (razors, toothbrushes)
- Being vaccinated against hepatitis A and B
- Using condoms.

> **Term to Learn**
> **Cirrhosis:** when the normal liver tissue is replaced by fibrous scar tissue, for example after exposure to toxins such as long-term alcohol and hepatitis viral infections.

> **KEY POINT** Healthcare workers should always follow standard precautions and safely handle needles and other sharps, and be vaccinated against hepatitis B.

The risks from getting hepatitis via tattoos or body-piercing should be considered.

Management

This includes:

- Bed rest
- Specific drugs
- Avoiding things such as alcohol that damage the liver
- Vaccination. Hepatitis B vaccine protects against HBV, but there is no vaccine yet against HCV.

HERPESVIRUS INFECTIONS

Herpesvirus infections are common. However, the viruses often remain dormant, commonly living in neurones (see Chapter 4). Reactivation may lead to **viral shedding** and disease, and spread through saliva and other body fluids.

> **Terms to Learn**
> **Ganglia:** Plural of ganglion, which is a collection of nerve cells.
> **Viral shedding:** The process of excretion of a virus that is present in a particular area of the body. The virus can be excreted or shed via sweating or the saliva or even via faeces.

> ### IMPORTANT HERPESVIRUSES
>
> - The most important herpesviruses are:
> - Herpes simplex viruses (HSV)
> - Varicella zoster virus (VZV)
> - Epstein-Barr virus (EBV)
> - Cytomegalovirus (CMV)
> - Kaposi sarcoma herpesvirus (KSHV).

HSV typically first causes oral infection with acute gingivo-stomatitis (see Chapter 5 and Figure 17.1.6) or ano-genital infection. It thereafter remains dormant in the sensory nerve ganglia. If reactivated it may cause lesions. Recurrent infections are often precipitated by systemic infections, sunlight, trauma, stress, menstruation or immunocompromise.

VZV causes varicella (chickenpox), a highly contagious disease spread by droplets. VZV also remains dormant within nerve **ganglia**. If reactivated, as can happen in the elderly or immunocompromised, it can lead to shingles (zoster), a painful unilateral rash.

EBV causes glandular fever (infectious mononucleosis), which consists of lymph node swelling, sore throat and fever. CMV causes similar illnesses. KSHV causes Kaposi sarcoma – most common in HIV/AIDS.

FIGURE 17.1.6
Acute herpes infection (the fingers are those of the patient, not healthcare worker–who would always wear gloves).

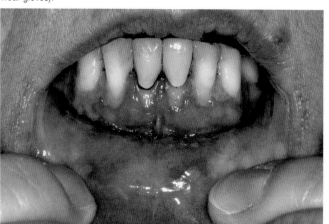

Management

- Anti-viral drugs may be used.

HIV/AIDS

The human immunodeficiency virus (HIV) is mainly sexually transmitted. Infection rates are particularly high in men having sex with men, and in intravenous drug users. HIV infection leads to acquired immune deficiency syndrome (AIDS) and has spread worldwide to create a global pandemic. The number infected increases daily, especially in Africa, Asia, Russia and other eastern European countries.

HIV TRANSMISSION

This occurs through:

- Sexual intercourse – saliva, semen and blood may contain HIV. Rectal intercourse is a particularly high-risk activity
- Contaminated blood, blood products and donated organs
- Contaminated needles – intravenous drug users and needlestick injuries in healthcare workers
- Vertical transmission (mother to child) transmission may occur in the womb (in utero), during childbirth and via breast milk.

However, there is no reliable evidence for transmission of HIV by non-sexual social contact or by insect vectors such as mosquitoes or bed bugs.

Development of the Disease (Figure 17.1.7)

- HIV infects and damages white blood cells (the lymphocytes) that protect against infection with viruses, fungi and a few bacteria (such as *Mycobacterium*).
- The cells mainly damaged are known as CD4+ helper T-lymphocytes, and so the number of these in the blood ('the CD4 count') falls.
- After infection with HIV, antibodies to HIV develop and appear in the blood within six weeks to six months of infection (called seroconversion) and the blood test for HIV becomes positive.
- Some individuals develop a clinical illness resembling glandular fever.
- An asymptomatic period of variable length usually follows seroconversion; this may last many years – even as long as five to 15 years.
- HIV-infected (HIV-positive) patients carry the virus (and many are unaware they are infected) and gradually develop low immunity. Thus other infections (especially viral, fungal, parasitic and TB) may begin to appear.
- When immunity falls to a very low level, the HIV-infected patient is said to have AIDS.
- HIV/AIDS may be complicated not only by other infections, but by cancers and brain damage. Early death is inevitable.

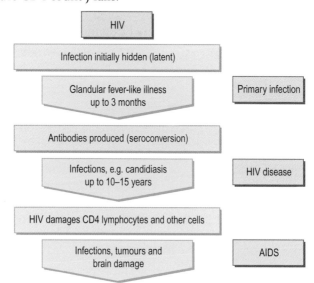

FIGURE 17.1.7
Stages in HIV infection.

MOUTH LESIONS IN HIV/AIDS

- Fungal infections (candidosis/candidiasis – see Chapter 5 and Figure 17.1.8).
- Viral infections (warts, hairy leukoplakia, herpes, and zoster).
- Tumours (Kaposi sarcoma and lymphomas).

There is also a predisposition to necrotising gingivitis and to periodontitis, and to mouth ulcers and salivary gland disease (see Chapter 5).

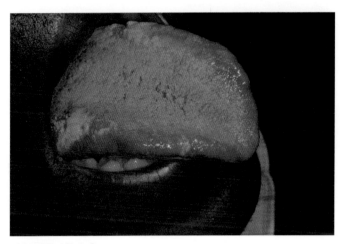

FIGURE 17.1.8
Candidosis in HIV/AIDS.

Management

There is as yet no effective treatment to eliminate HIV infection. However, several anti-retroviral drugs are available. They are used as part of the so-called anti-retroviral therapy (ART) and highly active anti-retroviral therapy (HAART). These treatments have helped to significantly increase the quality of life and the survival of infected people.

Dental Implications

HIV-infected individuals often have particular concerns about privacy and the stigma and social implications of their infection. It is therefore critical to ensure strict adherence to data protection and patient confidentiality – the patient should be reassured that none of their details will be discussed, even with their doctor, without their permission.

Caution is particularly advised to avoid needle-stick injuries – which might transmit infection.

Standard infection control procedures are sufficient.

HUMAN PAPILLOMAVIRUS INFECTIONS

There are more than 100 human papillomaviruses (HPV). They are spread by close or sexual contact and usually cause skin or mucosal warty lesions but some, such as HPV-16, can cause ano-genital or mouth cancers.

HYPERTENSION

Hypertension means a persistently raised blood pressure. Blood pressure is measured in units of millimetres of mercury (mmHg), and hypertension may be defined as a blood pressure of at least 140/90 mmHg. Blood pressure tends to increase with age, but in most people with hypertension the cause is unknown. It is, however, often related to:

- Genetic predisposition
- High alcohol intake
- High salt intake
- Smoking.

Long-standing hypertension accelerates atherosclerosis and so predisposes to damage to:

- Heart (coronary artery disease)
- Brain (cerebrovascular disease, particularly stroke)
- Kidneys (chronic renal failure)
- Hands and feet (peripheral vascular disease)
- Eyes (hypertensive retinopathy) leading to blindness.

Management

General measures to lower blood pressure include:

- Relaxation
- Smoking cessation
- Restricting alcohol intake
- No-added-salt diet
- High-fibre diet
- Weight reduction
- Regular exercise
- Anti-hypertensive drugs.

INFECTIVE ENDOCARDITIS

Infective endocarditis is a rare, but dangerous, heart infection that occasionally can follow surgery. It happens if bacteria enter the bloodstream (bacteraemia) and the patient's heart is defective, for example, with a heart valve problem. For this reason, antibiotic cover used to be recommended for patients with a heart condition that predisposed to infective endocarditis, who were undergoing a dental procedure causing a significant bacteraemia. However, concerns about the use of antibiotic prophylaxis have grown, and in 2008 the National Institute of Health and Clinical Excellence (NICE) issued a guideline that:

- Antibiotic prophylaxis against endocarditis is not recommended for patients undergoing dental procedures
- Patients should achieve and maintain high standards of oral health.

INFLAMMATORY BOWEL DISEASE

Inflammatory bowel disease (IBD) is a term which includes Crohn disease and ulcerative colitis – both chronic diseases of unknown cause:

- Crohn disease usually presents with an alteration of bowel habit as well as features of malabsorption. Diarrhoea, bleeding and painful defecation are typical.
- Ulcerative colitis frequently causes diarrhoea with stools containing intermixed mucus, blood and pus. There is a risk of colorectal carcinoma.

Management

- Medical therapy of IBD includes conservative measures (nutritional support) and drug therapy.
- Surgery in IBD is indicated if medical therapy fails, or to treat complications.

IRRITABLE BOWEL SYNDROME

Irritable bowel syndrome (IBS or spastic colon) may affect up to 30% of the population. It is characterised by recurrent abdominal pain with abnormal bowel habit. The cause of IBS is unclear but there is often a positive family history, anxious personality type and history of migraine.

Management

Symptoms of IBS usually respond to:

- Stress reduction
- High-fibre diet
- Anti-spasmodic drugs
- CBT.

LEUKAEMIAS

Leukaemias are cancers of bone marrow stem cells. Causes may include a genetic predisposition and exposure to radiation, viruses or chemicals.

Leukaemias are classified by:

- Cell of origin (lymphoblast or non-lymphoblast)
- Cell maturity – immature (acute) versus mature (chronic).

Large numbers of white blood cells (leucocytes) are seen under a microscope on a blood film and on bone marrow biopsy. These cells lack the normal protective capacity of healthy leucocytes, so the patient becomes vulnerable to infections. The malignant expansion of white

TABLE 17.1.8 Signs and Symptoms of Leukaemia

Site of Disease	Clinical Manifestation
Bone Marrow Failure	
Anaemia	Pallor, lethargy, breathlessness
Neutropenia	Recurrent infection
Thrombocytopenia	Mucosal bleeding and bruising
Tissue Infiltration	
Lymphatics	Lymph node swelling
Liver and spleen	Swollen liver and spleen
Bone	Bone pain and fractures

cells into the reticulo-endothelial system causes enlarged lymph nodes, liver and spleen. When they crowd out other bone marrow cells, the patient develops anaemia (lack of red blood cells) and a bleeding tendency (because of low blood platelet numbers).

Acute leukaemias account for nearly 50% of malignant disease in children. Chronic leukaemias are diseases of late adult life and fairly benign.

Signs and Symptoms

The clinical features broadly reflect the degree of spread of the leukaemic cells in other tissues and the extent of bone marrow failure (Table 17.1.8).

Management

Chemotherapy is usually used. But the drugs damage not only proliferating leucocytes but also other cells including hair, mucosae, bone marrow and reproductive tissues. So there are many unpleasant adverse effects such as hair loss, mucositis, infections and sterility.

LICHEN PLANUS

Lichen planus is a common skin and mucosal disease causing an itchy rash on the wrists. The mouth, genitals, nails or hair may be affected.

Management is usually with corticosteroids.

LIVER DISEASE

Liver disease or cirrhosis may be caused by excessive alcohol intake, and viral hepatitis. Jaundice, bruising, haemorrhage and infection are common.

Management

The management of patients with chronic liver disease is complicated. It includes:

- Dietary modification including reduction or cessation of alcohol use
- Careful drug prescribing in view of impaired drug handling and an increased risk of drug toxicity
- Treatment of underlying viral disease (e.g. hepatitis B or C).
- Prevention of and aggressive treatment of infection.

FIND OUT MORE

Why do people with liver disease have impaired drug handling and increased risk of drug toxicity?

LUNG CANCER

Lung cancer is the most common cancer in developed countries in males, and most frequently affects urban, adult cigarette smokers.

Signs and Symptoms

The main features are:

- Recurrent cough
- Blood in sputum (haemoptysis)
- Dyspnoea (breathlessness)
- Chest pain
- Chest infections.

Management

Management is mainly by radiotherapy.

MIGRAINE

Migraine is a recurrent headache due to the brain blood vessels becoming dilated and inflamed. It affects mainly women. It is a unilateral, throbbing headache (hemicrania) lasting for hours or days. Photophobia (wanting to be in a dark place), nausea and vomiting may also occur. Classic migraine is preceded by an aura of visual disturbances (fortification spectra), sensory abnormalities (paraesthesia), motor and speech disturbances. Episodes may be precipitated by alcohol, tyramine-containing foods (e.g. chocolate, cheese, red wine, bananas), menstrual disturbances, stress and drugs.

385

Management

This includes:

- Reassurance
- Avoidance of precipitating factors
- Suitable environment (a quiet dark room) during an attack
- Drugs – analgesics, antiemetics (for the relief of nausea) and triptans. For individuals with recurrent episodes of migraine, prophylactic drug treatment is indicated.

MULTIPLE SCLEROSIS

Multiple sclerosis (MS or disseminated sclerosis) is the most common chronic neurological disease. It is thought to be due to damage to nerve myelin sheaths (demyelination) with the development of 'plaques' throughout the CNS. The cause remains unknown but the diagnostic hallmark is a series of neurological deficits distributed in time and space. For example, there may be visual disturbances, followed by paralyses and/or patches of skin numbness.

Signs and Symptoms

Symptoms and signs depend on the area of the nervous system affected:

- Numbness, weakness or paralysis in a limb
- Brief pain, tingling or electric-shock sensations
- Tremor, lack of co-ordination or unsteady gait
- Visual disturbances and pain on eye movement (optic neuritis)
- Urinary incontinence, constipation and sexual dysfunction
- Memory loss and impaired concentration.

Management

Multiple sclerosis can be disabling and even fatal. Care may include:

- Physical and occupational therapy
- Counselling
- Drug treatment.

OBESITY

Obesity is the main nutritional problem in the developed countries. Almost 25% of adults are now clinically obese (Box 17.1.3) and more than 60% aged 20 years and older are overweight. Obesity is also increasing among children.

A certain amount of body fat is needed for, for example, stored energy, heat insulation and shock absorption. As a rule, women have more body fat than men.

Obesity results from eating more than the body needs. What causes this imbalance between calories in and calories out differs from one person to another and other factors may also play a part, including:

- Lifestyle – such as what a person eats and their level of physical activity
- Psychology – some people eat in response to negative emotions such as boredom, sadness, or anger. Some anti-depressants and other drugs can cause weight gain
- Genetic factors
- Hormonal causes rarely – although many fat people believe that they have a glandular or hormonal disorder, this is rarely the case.

Associated Problems

These include:

- It is unaesthetic and disabling
- Predisposes to or aggravates several disorders:
  - Chronic diseases (heart disease, diabetes, hypertension, stroke)
  - Some cancers.

Management

The best way to avoid obesity is to increase exercise and reduce calorie intake. Eat smaller portions!

OSTEOPOROSIS

Osteoporosis (bone-thinning or brittle bone disease) is a very common cause of fragile bones, usually in older people. The difference between how much healthy bone is formed and the rate at which it is remodelled and removed later, determines how much osteoporosis (see below) results. From age 30 years, about 1% bone is lost per year, rising to about 5% after menopause.

Risk factors for osteoporosis are shown in Box 17.1.4.

BOX 17.1.3 DEFINING OBESITY

- Men with more than 25% body fat and women with more than 30% body fat are termed obese.
- Because measuring body fat is difficult, healthcare providers often rely on weight-for-height tables – a range of acceptable weights for a person of a given height. However, these tables do not distinguish between muscle and excess fat.
- Body mass index (BMI – weight in kilograms divided by height in metres squared), is now the standard.
- A BMI of 25–29.9 indicates a person is overweight, a BMI of 30 (males) or 28.6 (females) or higher indicates obesity.

> **BOX 17.1.4 RISK FACTORS FOR OSTEOPOROSIS**
>
> - Advanced age – over the age of 60 years, nearly one-third of the population has osteoporosis – at least 1 in 3 women and 1 in 12 men.
> - Female gender and early menopause.
> - Positive family history.
> - Lifestyle factors:
>   - Lack of exercise
>   - Diet low in calcium or vitamin D
>   - Excess alcohol intake
>   - Smoking.
> - Drugs and disease:
>   - Drugs such as corticosteroids, heparin, ciclosporin, and anti-convulsants
>   - Malignant disease
>   - Chronic inflammatory states such as rheumatoid arthritis
>   - Endocrine disorders.

Complications

The main complications are fractures of the hip (neck of the femur), or wrist, or of the spine (hence the shrinking size of some older women). Low back pain is common.

Management

- The best management is to avoid falls and injuries.
- Exercise has a positive effect: walking, running, jogging, and dancing are recommended.
- Additional calcium and vitamin D may also be helpful. The main sources of calcium are dairy products and green vegetables. The main source of vitamin D is sun-exposure.
- Drug treatment – bisphosphonates are drugs commonly used to prevent osteoporosis. These drugs are also given intravenously for patients who have cancers affecting bone.

> **KEY POINT** Bisphosphonates remain in the bone for many years and have an extremely long-lasting effect, causing susceptibility to jaw **osteonecrosis** – mainly in people having intravenous bisphosphonates. Patients taking bisphosphonates (especially intravenous) must therefore be counselled about risks before they have any surgery of the jaws, including implant placement.

387

Term to Learn
Osteonecrosis: death of bone tissue.

PARKINSON DISEASE

Parkinson disease is a common but serious brain disorder. The risk of developing Parkinson disease increases with age. Mostly it is **idiopathic** but injuries (particularly boxing), drugs and toxins may be responsible.

Signs and Symptoms

These include:

- Trembling
- Muscle rigidity
- Difficulty walking
- Problems with balance and co-ordination.

Management

There is a decrease in the level of the brain **neurotransmitter** dopamine. So management is with levodopa (L-dopa), which is converted in the brain into dopamine.

Terms to Learn
Idiopathic: a disease whose cause is unknown.
Neurotransmitter: a chemical that helps to transmit electrical impulses at nerve synapses (see Subchapter 4.1).

PEPTIC ULCER

Peptic ulcer disease (PUD) develops in acid-secreting areas in the stomach (gastric ulcer) or duodenum (duodenal ulcer). Infection with *Helicobacter pylori*, a bacterium, is a key cause of PUD. Other factors include use of NSAIDs and corticosteroids, and smoking, alcohol and stress are also responsible.

Management

This includes:

- Antibiotics – if there is *H. pylori* infection
- Dietary modification (frequent small meals with no fried foods)
- Smoking cessation
- Alcohol moderation.

Surgery is usually reserved for patients with complications.

RADIOTHERAPY-RELATED DISORDERS

Radiotherapy is one of the main treatments for head and neck cancers. It kills cancer cells but also inevitably damages normal tissues in the line of the beam, such as the:

- Oral mucosa (when it causes soreness from mucositis)
- Salivary glands (when it causes hyposalivation)
- Bone (osteoradionecrosis).

Osteoradionecrosis (ORN) is particularly liable to occur after trauma/dental extractions in the irradiated area. This may be prevented by removing teeth no less than 10 days *before* the start of radiotherapy. Antibiotics and hyperbaric oxygen therapy (HBOT) may help in treatment.

RENAL (KIDNEY) DISEASE

Term to Learn
GFR: a measure of kidney function.

388

Chronic renal failure or chronic kidney disease (CKD) is defined as a low glomerular filtration rate (**GFR**). It results from progressive, irreversible kidney damage due to some other disease – diabetes is the single most common cause. Hypertension and drug effects are others.

Signs and Symptoms

CKD may be asymptomatic until kidney function has fallen to less than 25% of normal. Then hypertension, anaemia, bruising and bone disease may be seen.

Management

Initial management aims to lower the blood pressure and urea levels. Dietary modification may include salt restriction. Waste metabolites may eventually need to be removed by:

- Continuous ambulatory peritoneal dialysis (CAPD) and intermittent peritoneal dialysis – placement of a catheter into the abdominal peritoneal cavity.
- Haemodialysis – via a 'kidney machine'. Infection control to prevent cross-infection of hepatitis viruses, HIV and other blood-borne agents is of paramount importance.
- Haemofiltration – using a highly permeable membrane.

Renal transplantation may become necessary.

RESPIRATORY INFECTIONS

Viral upper respiratory infections are commonplace. Tuberculosis (see below) and *Legionella* infections are also important respiratory infections.

Prevention

The most important preventive measures are:

- Avoid treating or being in close proximity to persons with acute respiratory infections
- Minimise production of aerosols, splatter, and dusts. In clinical work use rubber dam and high vacuum aspiration. In the laboratory use guards and suction

- Avoid inhaling aerosols, dusts, vapours, smoke, or fumes by provision of masks
- Ventilate the working area adequately.

Face masks filter a great deal of debris but vary in their filtering efficiency and should preferably be changed every hour. Face protectors have the advantage of giving a flow of filtered cool air to the operator and protecting eyes and respiratory system simultaneously.

> **KEY POINT** Use of high volume aspiration and rubber dam during restorative procedures will significantly reduce the amount of infected aerosol and splatter.

SCHIZOPHRENIA

Schizophrenia is a chronic, disabling mental condition. Mood, thoughts and behaviour are disorganised and appear irrational and exaggerated. The person also has hallucinations, delusions and thought disorder and they lack insight. Concern is initially raised by a friend or relative. Treatment includes long-term psychotherapy and drug therapy.

SEXUALLY TRANSMITTED INFECTIONS

Sexually transmitted infections (STIs) are passed from person to person through unsafe sexual practices. The important STIs are syphilis, herpes and HIV, ano-genital warts, and gonorrhoea (Table 17.1.9).

Having several STIs at one time (including viral hepatitis) is not uncommon, especially in intravenous drug users. This is because of unhygienic practices and drug users often offer sex to get money to fund their habit.

Contact tracing can identify who a person was infected by, or whom they have infected.

Prevention

Risk of STI can be reduced by avoiding casual and unprotected sexual intercourse by ABC:

- Abstinence
- Being monogamous (having only one partner)
- Condom use at all times.

389

TABLE 17.1.9 The Most Important Sexually Transmitted Infections

Agents	Diseases	Caused by
Bacteria	Chancroid	*Haemophilus ducreyi*
	Chlamydia infections (including lymphogranuloma venereum)	*Chlamydia trachomatis*
	Gonorrhoea	*Neisseria gonorrhoeae*
	Syphilis	*Treponema pallidum*
	Trichomoniasis	*Trichomoniasis vaginalis*
Viruses	Herpes	Herpes simplex virus (human (alpha) herpesvirus)
	Hepatitis	Hepatitis A, B, C or D viruses
	HIV/AIDS	Human immunodeficiency virus
	Warts	Human papillomavirus (HPV)
Fungi	Thrush	*Candida albicans*
Parasites	Fleas	*Siphonaptera*
	Lice (crabs)	*Phthirus pubis*
	Scabies	*Sarcoptes scabiei*

High-risk Groups

Certain groups of people and their sexual partners who may be at especially high risk of contracting STIs are:

- Promiscuous heterosexuals or men who have sex with men (MSM)
- Prostitutes – male or female
- Drug addicts and alcoholics
- Armed forces personnel
- Merchant navy personnel
- Aircrew
- Frequent business travellers
- Learning-impaired people.

SICKLE CELL DISEASE

Sickling disorders are inherited conditions mainly affecting people of African descent. An abnormal haemoglobin (called HbS) distorts the shape of the red blood cells, causing them to block arteries.

- Sickle cell *trait* is at least ten times as common as sickle disease, but it is often asymptomatic.
- Sickle cell *disease* is a serious disease with widespread complications – sickle crises can be caused by low oxygen tension (as in general anaesthesia, at high altitudes or in unpressurised aircraft).

Painful **infarcts** form, mainly in the spleen, bones and joints, brain, kidneys, lungs, retinae and skin. Breakdown of erythrocytes (haemolysis) causes anaemia and jaundice and infections. Patients may eventually die from heart failure, kidney failure, overwhelming infection or stroke.

Management

Management of sickle cell *disease* is to prevent sickle crises. Factors that can precipitate a crisis include:

- Trauma
- Infection
- Hypoxia
- Acidosis
- Dehydration.

SJÖGREN SYNDROME

Sjögren syndrome is an autoimmune disease which affects tear (lacrimal), salivary and other glands. This leads to dry eyes and dry mouth, and sometimes gland swelling.

Management

- Sipping water or sugar-free drinks
- Sucking ice
- Using salivary substitutes.

Occasionally, salivary stimulant drugs are used but chewing gum is often more helpful.

STROKE

A stroke or cerebrovascular accident (CVA) is a common cause of death and disability worldwide, mainly in older people. The most common cause is atherosclerosis: plaque

Term to Learn
Infarct: local area of dead tissue, the cause of which is a lack of blood supply, e.g. due to obstruction of a blood vessel by an embolus.

390

rupture results in brain arterial blockage. A stroke may be preceded by a transient ischaemic attack (TIA), which by definition resolves completely within 24 hours. Approximately 45% of people with a stroke die within a month.

Risk Factors

These include:

- Increasing age
- Hypertension
- Ischaemic heart disease
- Heart disease
- Diabetes
- Smoking
- Alcohol
- Obesity.

Signs and Symptoms

Typical features of stroke are:

- Visual deterioration
- Speech disturbance
- Hemiplegia
- Impaired level of consciousness progressing to coma or death.

Management

- Stroke victims should be admitted to hospital as soon as possible. Treatment lowers the risk of death and disability.
- Protection of the airway including appropriate ventilatory support is crucial.
- Pressure-sensitive nursing is needed to avoid the development of bed sores (pressure ulcers).
- Urinary catheterisation and incontinence pads may be needed.
- Physiotherapy helps reduce muscle wasting.

SYPHILIS

Syphilis is an infection caused by the bacterium *Treponema pallidum*. Over 80% of cases are in homosexual men. Syphilis is rapidly increasing.

- Primary syphilis – syphilis first manifests as a lump, and then an ulcer (primary or Hunterian chancre), usually on the penis or vulva. These are highly infectious.
- Secondary syphilis – follows after six to eight weeks with non-specific features such as fever, headache, malaise, rash and lymph node enlargement. Mouth ulcers (highly infectious mucous patches and snail-track ulcers) may be seen.
- Tertiary syphilis – if untreated, syphilis progresses to a tertiary stage, three to 10 or more years after infection. At this stage it affects the heart and central nervous system. The gumma is the characteristic lesion – deep punched-out ulcers on skin or mucosa.

Management is with antibiotics.

TRANSPLANTATION-RELATED DISORDERS

Transplants are generally needed in patients with severe disease, substantial limitation of daily activities and limited life expectancy. Transplant patients are given immunosuppressive drugs to prevent **transplant or graft rejection**. Therefore they develop low immunity and infections may spread rapidly. Bone marrow transplantation (haematopoietic stem cell transplantation) may additionally cause rashes, mouth ulcers and generalised problems because the graft attacks the recipient. This condition is called graft-versus-host disease (GVHD).

391

**Term to Learn
Transplant or graft rejection:** when the immune system of the person who is receiving a tissue graft or an organ transplant (the recipient) does not accept the new tissue or organ. This means that the immune system of the recipient attacks the transplanted organ or tissue by producing antibodies against it. To prevent this, powerful drugs are given to suppress the immune system, but this makes the recipient vulnerable to a variety of infections.

Dental Implications

- Some immunosuppressive drugs (ciclosporin) can cause gingival swelling. GVHD causes lesions such as lichen planus and Sjögren syndrome.
- Any invasive dental treatment should only be carried out after consultation with the responsible doctor.
- Preventive dentistry is crucial to maintain a healthy mouth and to avoid infections.

In addition, steroid cover may be needed.

TRIGEMINAL NEURALGIA

Trigeminal neuralgia is intermittent, severe pain in the oral and facial regions, which lasts a few seconds only. It affects the areas supplied by the trigeminal nerve. Pain is sometimes triggered by touching areas or by certain daily activities, such as eating, talking, washing the face, shaving or cleaning the teeth.

Management

This includes drugs such as carbamazepine. Surgery is reserved for recalcitrant pain.

TUBERCULOSIS

- Tuberculosis (TB) is an infection caused by the bacterium *Mycobacterium tuberculosis*. It affects about a third of the world population. It is particularly widespread in developing countries, but its incidence is also increasing in Western countries (including the UK).
- Approximately 10% of cases are now antibiotic resistant – they are said to have multi-drug resistant (MDR) TB.
- Some TB is resistant to all drugs – extended resistance TB (XR-TB) – especially in patients with AIDS.
- The infection occurs most often via the respiratory tract so it is primarily a respiratory disease (pulmonary TB). Transmission is by droplet spread.
- Reactivation or progression of primary TB may result in widespread **haematogenous** dissemination of mycobacteria – this is called 'miliary TB'. It affects the CNS and the cardiovascular, gastro-intestinal and genito-urinary systems.

Signs and Symptoms

The initial infection is usually silent (subclinical) causing no symptoms or signs. Active TB typically causes a chronic cough containing blood (haemoptysis), weight loss, night sweats and fever.

Management

- TB is a **notifiable disease** and contact tracing is an important aspect of management.
- Anti-tubercular drug treatment should be instituted as early as possible.
- If patient compliance is considered to be poor, as is often the case since TB is common in the homeless, alcoholics and drug abusers, directly observed therapy (DOT) may be indicated. This means that drugs are dispensed by and taken in the presence of a healthcare professional.

Prevention

- Prevention of TB by BCG vaccination (live attenuated *Mycobacterium bovis* vaccine) is advised for high-risk individuals and healthcare professionals. However, its efficacy is questionable.
- Infection control is important.

392

Term to Learn
Haematogenous: spread of a disease via the blood circulation.

Term to Learn
Notifiable disease: a disease that must be reported to the relevant government authority as per the law.

VON WILLEBRAND DISEASE

von Willebrand disease (vWD) is the most common inherited bleeding disorder. It is characterized by bleeding from mucous membranes – nose bleeds, gingival haemorrhage and gastro-intestinal blood loss. Both males and females can have the disorder. vWD is due to a deficiency of von Willebrand factor (vWF), which takes part in blood clotting (see Subchapter 4.1). There are also reduced levels of factor VIII (the main feature of haemophilia).

Dental Implications

Excessive bleeding may occur after dental treatment and surgery. Thus, before surgery, patients need: factor VIII, or synthetic vasopressin (DDAVP; desmopressin).

FIND OUT MORE

To find out more about human diseases the following websites are good places to visit:
- NHS direct: http://www.nhsdirect.nhs.uk/help/
- Mayo Clinic.com: http://www.mayoclinic.com/
- Medline Plus: http://www.nlm.nih.gov/medlineplus/healthtopics.html
- Healthfinder.gov: http://www.healthfinder.gov/

17.2 GENERAL HEALTH PROMOTION
AVOIDING OR PREVENTING ILL HEALTH

In Subchapter 17.1.1 you saw that diseases arise from interactions of genetic, environmental and lifestyle factors (Figure 17.1.1). Therefore, health may be promoted by avoiding, or minimising, lifestyle or environmental risk factors and, possibly in the future, by **gene manipulation**.

> **Term to Learn**
> **Gene manipulation:**
> the artificial manipulation of genetic material.

393

Genetic Diseases

Already genetic disease effects such as those from haemophilia can be minimised by giving the genetically missing protein (blood clotting factor VIII). Genetic counselling is increasing, especially in relation to disorders such as haemophilia, Down syndrome, Huntington disease, cystic fibrosis and various cancers. In future, genetic manipulation will almost inevitably be more widely possible, but it has raised many ethical questions.

FIND OUT MORE

Can you think of two ethical questions related to gene manipulation?

Environmental and Lifestyle Factors

Environmental and lifestyle factors which when avoided or minimised may prevent many diseases include the following.

ENVIRONMENTAL
- *Trauma* – this can be minimised by avoiding alcohol use, aggression and dangerous environments, activities and sports; and using protective sports and eye wear (e.g. helmets, mouth guards).
- *Infections* – these can be minimised by immunisation, and by using infection control (avoiding needlestick injuries and using barrier protection – gloves, rubber dam, eye protection, condoms). Think about infections when planning overseas visits.

- *Chemicals* – such injuries can be minimised by ensuring containers are safe and labelled appropriately and taking care to avoid exposure to toxic agents.
- *Irradiation* – such injuries can be minimised by reducing exposure to sun, X-rays, lasers, damaging lights etc., and by using safety measures such as protective eyewear and screens.

LIFESTYLE

- Avoid substance dependence. Abstain if possible from the use of:
  - Tobacco
  - Betel
  - Alcohol
  - 'Recreational' drugs.
- Take regular daily exercise for 30 minutes minimum (see p. 400).
- Eat a healthy balanced diet, plenty of fruit and vegetables and avoid food fads.

The most important five lifestyle health measures are 'I HATE':

- **I**njury avoidance
- **H**ave immunisations
- **A**void substance dependence
- **T**ake regular exercise
- **E**at a healthy diet.

KEY POINT *Injuries have causes – they do not usually simply befall us from fate or bad luck – though that can be the case.*

Injury Avoidance

Injuries can of course seem to be the result of simple bad luck but many incidents could have been avoided with more forethought and care. High-risk situations include disasters, conflicts, violence, contact and some other sports and travel.

Groups at particular risk of injury include:

- People who are aggressive, tense, and compulsive
- Young males
- Infants and children
- Certain occupations (e.g. military, police, construction, mining)
- People who are exposed to alcohol, recreational drugs or poisons
- Ethnic minorities
- Sports (e.g. rock climbing, motor sports, water sports, contact sports).

In sports, training can strengthen muscles and make them less susceptible to damage, especially if the training exercises involve movements that mimic those associated with the sport.

Injuries can be fatal or cause significant harm:

- They include soft tissue injuries such as cuts and bruises, and hard tissue injuries such as fractures
- Brain, neck and other neurological damage can be devastating
- Bleeding, burns and poisoning can also be life-threatening.

Have Immunisations

As a member of the dental clinical team you should receive the standard immunisations (Table 17.2.1) (diphtheria, measles, mumps, poliomyelitis, rubella, tetanus, tuberculosis, pertussis, meningitis) and also hepatitis B virus (HBV) and varicella-zoster (chickenpox) before exposure to clinical work.

TABLE 17.2.1 Immunisation Schedules

Age for Immunisation		Vaccines
Months	Years	Routine
2		Diphtheria, tetanus, pertussis (DTP); poliomyelitis (polio); and *Haemophilus influenzae* B (HIB), pneumococcal conjugate vaccine
3		2nd dose: diphtheria, tetanus, pertussis (DTP); poliomyelitis (polio); and *Haemophilus influenzae* B (HIB), group C meningococcus
4		Diphtheria, tetanus, pertussis (DTP), poliomyelitis (polio), *Haemophilus influenzae* B (HIB), and group C meningococcus, pneumococcal conjugate vaccine
12		*Haemophilus influenzae* B (HIB), measles, mumps and rubella (MMR), group C meningococcus and pneumococcal conjugate vaccine
	4–5	'Pre-school' boosters of DTP and MMR
	14–18	Booster DTP
		Certain groups: human papilloma virus (HPV)
	10–14	BCG (against tuberculosis) for at risk groups
	Adults	Tetanus, diphtheria and polio, if not fully immunised as a child
	High-risk groups	Varicella-zoster vaccine
		Hepatitis A vaccine
		Influenza vaccine
		Pneumococcal vaccine
		Rubella vaccine
		Hepatitis B vaccine*

* Contains inactivated hepatitis B virus surface antigen (HBsAg) made biosynthetically using **recombinant DNA technology**. There is as yet no vaccine against hepatitis C virus.

**Term to Learn
Recombinant DNA technology:** these are techniques that allow creation of new DNA by joining segments of DNA taken from one organisation to from a gene that is then placed into another species.

395

FIND OUT MORE

You can find out the government's current advice on immunisations by visiting the Department of Health website (http://www.dh.gov.uk/en/Publichealth/Healthprotection/Immunisation/index.htm)

HEPATITIS B VACCINE

The hepatitis B vaccine produces specific antibodies to the hepatitis B surface antigen (anti-HBs). It takes up to six months to confer adequate protection against HBV. The duration of immunity is not known precisely, but a single booster five years after the primary course may be sufficient to maintain immunity.

As a clinical student or dental clinical staff member, you must have documentary evidence that you have been immunised and your response to the vaccine has been checked. People who fail to respond to the vaccine must undergo further investigation to exclude the possibility of being high-risk carriers of the hepatitis B virus. An employing dentist must hold evidence of their employees' hepatitis B immunisation. They may write a letter similar to the one shown in Box 17.2.1 when requesting this information from the employee's general medical practitioner.

KEY POINT Employers must have the consent of the employee before approaching their doctor and any information provided is confidential and should be used and stored appropriately.

Avoid Substance Dependence

The most common risks from abuse of many recreational drugs are: injury, behavioural disturbances and psychoses, but it may also lead to an

KEY POINT Intravenous use of illegal drugs can also easily lead to life-threatening infections including endocarditis, septicaemias, hepatitis and HIV/AIDS.

BOX 17.2.1 LETTER REQUESTING EVIDENCE OF EMPLOYEE IMMUNE STATUS

Date

Dear Dr Bloggs

You have kindly immunised John Doe against hepatitis B, in line with current recommendations. As employers, we need to know if John has responded to the vaccine (>100 mIU/ml) and is protected against hepatitis B. If he failed to respond, we should know if he is a true non-responder or if he carries the infection (as this may affect day-to-day duties). In work routines, John is exposed to blood and saliva and although we use barrier techniques, it is possible that he could sustain an inoculation injury from an instrument used on an infected patient. Knowing his immune status will allow us to take the most appropriate action. Would it be possible for you to confirm his response to the vaccine or provide us with a copy of his blood test results, please? John has given his consent for you to release this information to us and has countersigned the letter. I look forward to hearing from you in due course.

Yours sincerely,   Countersigned
Dr J M Dentist   John Doe

STI or unwanted pregnancy. High doses can cause mood swings and psychoses – including hallucinations and paranoia – and can also cause respiratory failure and death. Combining use with other drugs or alcohol can result in nausea, difficulty breathing, unconsciousness and death.

TOBACCO

Tobacco is a major hazard to health and promotes many diseases, particularly heart disease, lung disease, and cancers of the lung, oesophagus, mouth and bladder (Table 17.2.2). Tobacco smoke contains nicotine, which is absorbed readily from the lungs on smoking and also when tobacco is chewed. Nicotine is highly addictive and withdrawal results in excessive anger, hostility and aggression.

Term to Learn
Chronic obstructive pulmonary disease: a disease in which the person has long-term obstruction of the airways due to the chronic presence of bronchitis and emphysema. It is most commonly seen in heavy smokers. Symptoms include difficulty breathing, wheezing, and a chronic cough.

TABLE 17.2.2 Possible Systemic Effects of Chronic Tobacco Use

System	Possible Effects
Bladder	Cancer
Cardiovascular system	Ischaemic heart disease (see Chapter 2). If women smokers also take oral contraceptives, they are more prone to cardiovascular and cerebrovascular diseases than are other smokers
Central nervous system	Alzheimer disease, stroke (see Chapter 2)
Mouth	Cancer, candidosis, dry mouth, dry socket, halitosis, implant failure, keratosis, necrotising gingivitis, chronic periodontal disease, teeth staining (see Chapters 5 and 16)
Oesophagus	Cancer
Reproductive system	Women who smoke generally have earlier menopause. Pregnant women who smoke cigarettes run a greater risk of having still-born or premature infants or infants with low birth weight; menopause
Respiratory system	Cancer, **chronic obstructive pulmonary disease**, sinusitis
Growth and development	Children of women who smoked while pregnant have a higher risk for developing behavioural disorders

ORAL HEALTH AND TOBACCO USE

Tobacco use can damage oral health by leading to:

- Oral cancer
- Keratosis
- Periodontal disease, particularly necrotising gingivitis
- Implant failure
- Dry socket
- Candidosis
- Dry mouth
- Halitosis
- Staining of teeth.

Passive smoking can cause lung cancer in adults, greatly increases the risk of respiratory illnesses in children and may cause sudden infant death.

Management

Smoking cessation should be gradual, because withdrawal symptoms are less severe in those who quit gradually than in those who quit quickly. Cessation aids include nicotine chewing gum or patches and various drugs.

ALCOHOL

In many cultures there is nothing wrong with the occasional alcoholic drink, but drinking too much can cause a wide range of serious behavioural and health problems (Table 17.2.3).

Alcohol is also high in calories, so cutting down could help control weight in overweight people.

RECOMMENDED DRINKING AMOUNTS

- Women: up to 2–3 units of alcohol a day.
- Men: up to 3 to 4 units a day.

These amounts appear not to cause significant risk to health.

(A unit is half a pint of standard strength beer, lager or cider, or a measure of spirits. A glass of wine is about 2 units and Alco pops are about 1.5 units.)

TABLE 17.2.3 Possible Systemic Effects of Chronic Alcohol Use

System	Possible Effects
Blood	**Pancytopenia**, folate deficiency, thiamine deficiency, immune defect
Central nervous system	Intoxication, dependency, dementia, **Wernicke–Korsakoff syndrome**
Heart	Arrhythmias, **cardiomyopathy**, hypertension
Intestine	Glucose and vitamin malabsorption
Liver	Hepatitis, fatty liver, cirrhosis, liver cancer
Mouth	Tooth erosion, cancer
Musculoskeletal	Myopathy, gout
Oesophagus	Gastro-oesophageal reflux, **Mallory–Weiss syndrome**, cancer
Pancreas	Pancreatitis
Reproductive system	Impotence, dysmenorrhoea, low birth-weight babies, **fetal alcohol syndrome**
Stomach	Gastritis, ulceration, carcinoma

Term to Learn

Passive smoking: inhaling second-hand smoke, that is, smoke produced from the use of a tobacco product by another person nearby.

Terms to Learn

Mallory–Weiss syndrome: the condition in which tears occur in the mucosal lining of the oesophagus in the area where it joins the stomach, e.g. when a person is coughing severely.

Pancytopenia: a condition in which there are reduced numbers of blood cells and platelets.

Wernicke–Korsakoff syndrome: a disease of the central nervous system, caused by deficiency of vitamin B1, which itself is usually secondary to excessive use of alcohol. Symptoms include vision changes, confusion, impaired memory, impaired co-ordination of muscle movements (ataxia).

Cardiomyopathy: a disease of the muscles of the heart, with impaired pumping action and enlargement of the heart.

Fetal alcohol syndrome: this is a congenital disease which occurs because of the use of alcohol by the pregnant mother. Features include abnormal development of the facial structures and learning disabilities.

397

AMPHETAMINES

Amphetamines are stimulants used for their euphoric effect, and to stave off fatigue. However, they cause dry mouth and caries ('meth mouth'), dilated pupils, increased pulse rate (tachycardia) and breathing rate (tachypnoea), aggression, talkativeness, and hallucinations, leading to seizures, hypertension, dangerously high body temperature (hyperpyrexia), heart arrhythmias and collapse. Mood swings, and psychoses – including hallucinations and paranoia – and respiratory failure can cause death.

Amphetamines have no true withdrawal syndrome and, in this respect, amphetamine addiction is quite different from opioid or barbiturate dependence.

BETEL

Regular chewers of betel leaf and areca (betel) nut as in 'pan' or 'paan' have a higher risk of oral disease and staining of the teeth. Table 17.2.4 lists the various effects of betel chewing on various systems of the body and the oral cavity.

CANNABIS

The main active cannabis (marijuana/'hash' or 'skunk') chemical is THC (delta-9-tetrahydrocannabinol), which binds to the brain. Adverse effects can include depression, anxiety, personality disturbances, impaired memory and learning, distorted perception, difficulty in thinking and problem solving, and impaired co-ordination; it may also trigger psychosis.

Marijuana can also lead to lung infections, affect blood pressure and heart rate and lower the oxygen-carrying capacity of blood. The risk of a heart attack may more than quadruple in the first hour after using it. Marijuana may also cause oral cancer. Babies born to women who use marijuana during pregnancies may be affected.

COCAINE

The major routes of cocaine ('coke' or 'crack') use are snorting, injecting or smoking. Immediate effects include hyperstimulation (euphoria), reduced fatigue and mental clarity, with feelings of well-being and heightened mental activity. Physical effects include constricted peripheral blood vessels, dilated pupils, and raised temperature, pulse rate, and blood pressure. The cocaine addict has aptly been described as a 'sexed-up extrovert with dilated pupils'.

TABLE 17.2.4 Possible Systemic Effects of Chronic Betel Use

System	Possible Effects
Heart	Hypertension, metabolic syndrome, diabetes, coronary heart disease, obesity
Kidneys	Chronic kidney disease, urinary stones
Liver	Cirrhosis, cancer
Mouth	Periodontitis, leukoplakia, **submucous fibrosis**, cancer
Oesophagus	Cancer, submucous fibrosis
Pancreas	Cancer
Reproductive system	Lower birth weight infants

Term to Learn
Submucous fibrosis: a disease in which there is progressive fibrosis of the tissues underlying the mucosa. When it occurs in the mouth, it ultimately leads to severe trismus.

398

Cocaine is powerfully addictive but 'crack' (cocaine that has been processed) is even stronger and can cause paranoia, visual hallucinations ('snow lights') and hallucinations of insects crawling over the skin (formication, 'cocaine bugs'). Adverse reactions of cocaine include angina, arrhythmias, heart attack, stroke, convulsions, depressed breathing and death.

On stopping cocaine, symptoms proceed through a crash phase of depression and craving for sleep, a withdrawal phase of lack of energy and then an extinction phase of recurrence of craving.

ECSTASY (MDMA OR METHYLENE-DIOXYMETHAMPHETAMINE)

Ecstasy is usually taken by mouth, and causes euphoria and appetite suppression, muscle tension, involuntary teeth clenching, nausea, blurred vision, rapid eye movement, faintness, and chills or sweating. Ecstasy is potently hallucinogenic and can cause high body temperature, ataxia and seizures, heart damage, liver or kidney failure or psychological difficulties, including confusion, depression, sleep problems, drug craving, severe anxiety and paranoia – during use and sometimes weeks later.

There is no physical dependence nor withdrawal symptoms.

HEROIN

Heroin is a highly addictive drug, derived from morphine. It can be sniffed, smoked from tin-foil ('chasing the dragon') or injected. The short-term effects are euphoria ('rush') but then an alternately wakeful and drowsy state ('on the nod'). With regular heroin use, physical dependence and addiction develop. Heroin depresses respiration and increases risk of pneumonia, lung abscesses and fibrosis, and infections (abscesses and cellulitis). Infectious diseases, including HIV and hepatitis, are common among users.

Withdrawal causes drug craving, restlessness, muscle and bone pain, insomnia, diarrhoea and vomiting, cold flashes with goose bumps ('cold turkey'), kicking movements ('kicking the habit'), and other symptoms. Sudden withdrawal is occasionally fatal.

Treatment options include behavioural therapies and medications such as methadone.

LSD (LYSERGIC ACID DIETHYLAMIDE)

LSD is taken by mouth and has effects that are unpredictable but prolonged (~12 hrs), producing several different emotions at once or swinging the user rapidly from one emotion to another within 30–90 minutes. Synaesthesia, the overflow from one sense to another when, for example, colours are heard, is common. There is often lability of mood, panic ('bad trip') and delusions of magical powers, such as being able to fly. LSD use also causes dilated pupils, high temperatures, heart rate and blood pressure, sweating, loss of appetite, sleeplessness, dry mouth, and tremors.

Many LSD users later (within a few days or more than a year after use) experience flashbacks, recurrence of certain aspects of a person's experience, without the user having taken the drug again. Severe adverse effects include terrifying thoughts and feelings, and despair, occasionally leading to fatal accidents.

LSD is not considered addictive since it does not produce compulsive drug-seeking behaviour as do cocaine, amphetamine, heroin, alcohol, and nicotine. Most users of LSD voluntarily limit or stop its use over time.

MEPHEDRONE (4-MMC, 'MEOW', 'M-CAT')

Mephedrone has effects similar, but not identical to, Ecstasy, lasting for around two to three hours when taken orally. Effects include a desire to take it again, changes in body temperature (sweating and chills), palpitations, impaired short-term memory, insomnia, tightened jaw muscles, and grinding teeth. After-effects such as insomnia may last for several hours longer.

Take Regular Exercise

Physical inactivity contributes to obesity, diabetes, heart disease, and cancer. In contrast, when exercise is combined with a proper diet, weight can be controlled and obesity prevented. To achieve real health benefit from exercise, at the very least enough regular, moderately intense physical activity to burn an extra 200 calories daily is needed. This means at least 30 minutes of activities such as a brisk walk daily.

> **KEY POINT** Obesity is a major risk factor for many diseases.

Regular exercise has a surprisingly wide range of health benefits, from protecting against heart disease (hypertension, arteriosclerosis, and coronary artery disease) to reducing the chances of cancer and Alzheimer disease. In addition, exercise can:

Term to Learn
Endorphins: chemicals produced in the brain that help reduce the sensation of pain and improve a person's mood.

- Make you feel more energetic
- Increase your stamina
- Improve brain function by releasing **endorphins**
- Reduce stress, depression and anxiety
- Help control weight and build and maintain healthy bones, muscles, and joints
- Reduce the risk of developing diabetes
- Reduce the risk of developing or dying from some of the leading causes of illness and death – such as a heart attack, stroke, or cancer.

TEN GOOD, SCIENTIFICALLY PROVEN, REASONS FOR TAKING REGULAR EXERCISE

- Exercise helps minimise obesity:
  - Obesity is associated with diabetes, heart disease, high blood pressure, stroke and cancer. Obese men are more likely to die from cancer of the colon, rectum, or prostate than are non-obese men
  - Obese women are more likely to die from cancer of the gallbladder, breast, uterus, cervix, or ovaries
  - Other health problems from obesity include gallbladder disease and gallstones; liver disease; osteoarthritis; gout; sleep apnoea; menstrual irregularities and infertility in women; and psycho-social effects
  - Exercise, by burning calories, helps minimise obesity.
- Exercise helps increase levels of HDL or 'good' cholesterol:
  - Blood fat levels seem to predict the risk for coronary heart disease – particularly when levels of high-density lipoproteins (HDL) are low and low-density lipoproteins (LDL) are high
  - Exercise helps increase HDL and lower LDL levels (bad cholesterol) and, by strengthening the heart and lowering blood pressure, protects against arteriosclerosis, heart attacks and stroke (see Chapters 2 and 17.1).
- Exercise helps lower high blood pressure:
  - Blood pressure levels also seem to predict the risk for coronary heart disease and stroke
  - High blood pressure (hypertension) can be reduced by exercise
  - Physical activity also reduces obesity, which is associated with hypertension.
- Exercise helps promote healthy blood sugar levels:
  - Diabetes results in high blood sugar levels – another risk factor for coronary heart disease
  - High blood sugar levels can be lowered by exercise.
- Exercise helps improve the metabolic syndrome:
  - The metabolic syndrome (syndrome X or insulin resistance syndrome) is a cluster of abdominal obesity (excess body fat around the waist), insulin resistance (causing high blood sugar), and increased blood pressure, which increases the risk for diabetes, heart disease and stroke. Having just one of these factors contributes to the risk of serious disease and, in combination, the risk is even greater
  - Exercise reduces these factors.
- Exercise helps build muscle strength:
  - Exercise, by building or preserving muscle mass and strength, and improving the ability to use calories, helps reduce body fat

- By increasing muscle strength and endurance, and improving flexibility and posture, regular exercise also helps prevent back pain
  - Exercise helps build muscle but this benefit fades quickly, if exercise stops for any reason – so *regular* exercise is needed.
- Exercise helps promote bone density:
  - Regular exercise from a young age can increase bone density and help avoid or minimise osteoporosis which is seen mainly in older people, especially in menopausal women.
- Exercise helps improve mobility:
  - People who exercise regularly have been shown to be more mobile and independent, compared with those with a sedentary lifestyle.
- Exercise helps boost the immune system:
  - Exercise helps your immune system fight off simple bacterial and viral infections. The mechanism is unclear but it is known that exercise increases the numbers of leucocytes (white blood cells) circulating in the blood. Leucocytes are part of the body's defence against infections (see Subchapter 4.1)
  - In contrast, when exercise is performed without food intake, and is too continuous, prolonged, or of moderate to high intensity (as in athletes) the immune function can be depressed.
- Exercise helps improve mood:
  - People who exercise regularly have been shown to be generally happier and less liable to depression compared with those having a sedentary lifestyle.

Eat a Healthy Diet

The two keys to a healthy diet are:

- Eating the right amount of food
- Eating a balanced diet that contains a variety of foods:
  - Lots of fruit, vegetables and starchy foods such as wholemeal bread and wholegrain cereals and potatoes
  - Some protein-rich foods such as meat, fish, eggs and lentils
  - Some dairy foods.

BENEFITS OF A HEALTHY DIET

- Generous amounts of vegetables and fruit daily appear to offer some protection against cancers of the stomach, colon and lung, and possibly against cancers of the mouth, larynx, cervix, bladder and breast.
- Carbohydrates as wholegrain unrefined products may offer some protection against colon cancer, diverticulitis and caries.
- A high fibre diet may also offer some protection against hypertension and coronary heart disease.
- A healthy diet is also low in fat (especially saturated fat), salt and sugar.
- Minimising the intake of saturated fats (especially those from dairy sources) and partially hydrogenated vegetable fats may lower the risk of coronary artery disease and some cancers. Consumption of mono-unsaturated fats such as olive oil may be beneficial.

THE CALORIE CONTENT OF FOODS

- The nutritional information provided on food packaging gives the amounts of carbohydrates, fats, proteins, colourings and flavourings, and a figure relating to *energy content*.
- Energy is usually expressed either in *kilocalories* or in *kilojoules*. A calorie is the amount of energy required to heat 1 gram of water by 1 °C, and because this is a small quantity of energy, it is more common to use the kilocalorie or Calorie, which is equivalent to 1000 calories.
- The number of calories multiplied by 4.186 = the number of joules.
- The number of kilocalories multiplied by 4.186 = the number of kilojoules.

Vitamins

Vitamins were discovered when it was noted that some diets – despite having adequate calories, essential fatty acids and minerals – were inadequate to maintain health. Vitamins are **co-factors** essential to a range of biochemical reactions. Vitamins can be classified as:

- *Water-soluble vitamins* (vitamins B and C) – these are readily absorbed from the gastro-intestinal mucosa and needed particularly for healthy nerves and blood.
- *Fat-soluble vitamins* (vitamins A, D, E, and K) – these require the presence of bile for absorption. Vitamin A is needed for healthy eyesight. Vitamin D is needed for healthy bones. Vitamin K is needed for the production of blood clotting factors.

Vitamin deficiency diseases are relatively rare, but may occur due to poor diet patterns in the young, old, people with food fads or alcoholics. Vegans, who eat no animal products, however, can readily become vitamin B12 deficient.

MINERALS AND TRACE ELEMENTS

A number of minerals and trace elements are essential to health. Deficiencies of trace elements can result in serious health problems.

FIND OUT MORE

Visit the HealthCheck Systems website (http://www.healthchecksystems.com/vitamins.htm), where you will find a table listing the vitamins and minerals, their roles and sources.

FAD DIETS

Many commercial diets claim to enhance well-being or reduce weight. But some of these diets have resulted in frank vitamin, mineral, and protein deficiency states. People have developed cardiac, renal, and metabolic disorders and some deaths have resulted too.

VEGETARIANISM

Ovo-lacto vegetarianism is the most common form of vegetarianism. These individuals tend to live longer and to develop fewer chronic disabling conditions than their meat-eating peers. Iron deficiency is the only known risk.

VEGANISM

Complete absence of animal products in the diet can lead to vitamin B12 deficiency. Having said that, the latter is surprisingly uncommon, since yeast extracts and oriental-style fermented foods can provide this vitamin.

FIND OUT MORE

For more about general health promotion, see the Patient UK website (http://www.patient.co.uk/showdoc/16/).

Dietary Recommendations

These recommendations are adapted from the UK Foods Standards Agency '8 tips for eating well' (http://www.eatwell.gov.uk/healthydiet/eighttipssection/8tips/)

1. Base your meals on starchy foods
   - Starchy foods such as bread, cereals, rice, pasta and potatoes are an important part of a healthy diet – a good source of energy and the main source of a range of nutrients. As well as starch, these foods contain fibre, calcium, iron and B vitamins.

- Choose wholegrain varieties of starchy foods whenever you can as they contain more fibre and other nutrients than white or refined starchy foods. We also digest wholegrain foods more slowly so they can help make us feel full for longer.
- Starchy foods should make up about a third of the food we eat.
- Try to include at least one starchy food with each of your main meals. So you could start the day with a wholegrain breakfast cereal, have a sandwich for lunch, and potatoes, pasta or rice with your evening meal.
- Starchy foods, gram for gram, contain less than half the calories of fat. However, you need to watch the fats you add when cooking and serving these foods, because this is what increases the calories.

Wholegrain foods include:

- Wholemeal and wholegrain bread, pitta and chapatti
- Whole-wheat pasta and brown rice
- Wholegrain breakfast cereals.

2. Eat lots of fruit and vegetables
   - Try to eat at least 5 portions of a variety of fruit and vegetables every day. You could try adding up your portions during the day to make it easier. For example, you could have:
     - A glass of juice and a sliced banana with your cereal at breakfast
     - A side salad at lunch
     - A pear as an afternoon snack
     - A portion of peas or other vegetables with your evening meal.

You can choose from fresh, frozen, tinned, dried or juiced, but remember potatoes count as a starchy food, not as portions of fruit and vegetables.

3. Eat more fish
   - Aim for at least two portions of fish a week, including a portion of oily fish (salmon, mackerel, trout, herring, fresh tuna, sardines, pilchards, eel). These are rich in omega 3 fatty acids and can keep the heart healthy. Fish is also an excellent source of protein and contains many vitamins and minerals. You can choose from fresh, frozen or canned – but remember that canned and smoked fish can be high in salt.
   - Do not have more than one portion a week of shark, tuna, swordfish and marlin because of the high levels of mercury in them.

4. Cut down on saturated fat and sugar
   - Having too much saturated fat (meat pies, sausages, meat with visible white fat, hard cheese, butter and lard, pastry, cakes and biscuits, cream, soured cream and crème fraîche, coconut oil, coconut cream or palm oil) can increase the amount of blood cholesterol, which increases the chance of heart disease.
   - Unsaturated fat (vegetable oils (including sunflower, rapeseed and olive oil), oily fish, avocados, nuts and seeds) lowers blood cholesterol.
   - Try eating fewer foods containing added sugar, such as sweets, cakes and biscuits, and drinking fewer sugary soft and fizzy drinks. Having sugary foods and drinks too often can cause dental caries (decay), especially if you have them between meals. Many foods that contain added sugar can also be high in calories, so cutting down could help you control your weight.

5. Try to eat less salt
   - Eating too much salt can raise the blood pressure. And people with high blood pressure are three times more likely to develop heart disease or have a stroke than people with normal blood pressure.
   - Three-quarters (75%) of the salt we eat comes from processed food, such as some breakfast cereals, soups, sauces, bread, biscuits and ready meals.

6. Get active and try to be a healthy weight.

403

Note: Page numbers followed by *f* indicate figures, by *t* indicate tables and by *b* indicate boxes.

412